The Manual of Dermatology

Jennifer A. Cafardi

The Manual of Dermatology

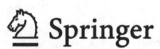
Springer

Jennifer A. Cafardi, MD, FAAD
Assistant Professor of Dermatology
University of Alabama at Birmingham
Birmingham, Alabama, USA
jencafardi@gmail.com

ISBN 978-1-4614-0937-3   e-ISBN 978-1-4614-0938-0
DOI 10.1007/978-1-4614-0938-0
Springer New York Dordrecht Heidelberg London

Library of Congress Control Number: 2011940426

Printed on acid-free paper

Springer is part of Springer Science+Business Media (www.springer.com)

Notice

Dermatology is an evolving field of medicine. Research and clinical experience continue to broaden our approach to illnesses, therapies and our general approach to disease. Readers are advised to check the most current product information available, which is provided by the manufacturer of each medication and device to verify dosages, duration of administration and contraindications. Although every effort has been made to give the most up to date and clinically relevant material, it is the responsibility of the treating physician, relying on experience and knowledge of the patient, to determine the dosages and treatment plans best suited to the individual patient. The author of this book assumes no liability for any injury and/or damage to persons or property arising from this publication.

Contents

List of Abbreviations

5-FU	5-Fluorouracil
5-HIAA	5-Hydroxyindole acetic acid
AA	Alopecia areata
ABX	Antibiotics
ACC	Aplasia cutis congenita
ACTH	Adrenocorticotropic hormone
AD	Autosomal dominant
AE	Adverse events
AFX	Atypical fibroxanthoma
AGEP	Acute generalized exanthematous pustulosis
AK	Actinic keratosis
AKN	Acne keloidalis nuchae
ALA	Aminolevulinic acid
ALT	Alanine transaminase
AN	Acanthosis nigricans
ANA	Antinuclear antigen
AR	Autosomal recessive
ASLO	Antistreptolysin O
AZA	Azathioprine
BCC	Basal cell carcinoma
BP	Bullous pemphigoid
BSLE	Bullous systemic lupus erythematosus
CAH	Congenital adrenal hyperplasia
CARP	Confluent and reticulated papillomatosis
CCB	Calcium channel blockers
CCCA	Central centrifugal cicatricial alopecia
CLL	Chronic lymphocytic leukemia
CMTC	Cutis marmorata telangiectatica congentia
CNH	Chondrodermatitis nodularis helices
CP	Cicatricial pemphigoid
CTCL	Cutaneous T-cell lymphoma
CTD	Connective tissue disease
CVD	Cardiovascular disease
CXR	Chest x-ray

DDx	Differential diagnosis
DFA	Direct fluorescent antibody
DFSP	Dermatofibrosarcoma protuberans
DH	Dermatitis herpetiformis
DHEA-S	Dehydroepiandrosterone sulfate
DHT	Dihydrotestosterone
DIC	Disseminated intravascular coagulation
DIF	Direct immunofluorescence
DIRA	Deficiency of the interleukin-1-receptor
DLE	Discoid lupus erythematosus (also known as chronic cutaneous lupus erythematosus)
DLSO	Distal lateral subungal onychomycosis
DM	Dermatomyositis or diabetes mellitus (depending on context)
DRESS	Drug rash with eosinophilia and systemic symptoms
dz	Disease
E&M	Evaluation and management
EAC	Erythema annulare centrifugum
EB	Epidermolysis bullosa
EBA	Epidermolysis bullosa acquisita
ED&C	Electrodessication and curretage
EDP	Erythema dyschromicum perstans
EDV	Epidermodysplasia verruciformis
EED	Erythema elevatum diutinum
EGFR	Epidermal growth factor receptor
EM	Electron microscopy or Erythema multiforme (depending on context)
EN	Erythema nodosum
EPS	Elastosis perforans serpiginosa
ESR	Erythrocyte sedimentation rate
ESRD	Endstage renal disease
ETOH	Ethanol
FCAS	Familial cold auto-inflammatory syndrome
FFA	Frontal fibrosing alopecia
FH	Family history
FMF	Familial mediterranean fever
G6PD	Glucose-6-phosphate dehydrogenase
GA	Granuloma annulare
GFR	Glomerular filtrate rate
GI	Gastrointestinal
GVHD	Graft versus host disease
HA	Headache
HAIR-AN	Hyperandrogenism (HA), insulin resistance (IR) and acanthosis nigricans (AN)
HCTZ	Hydrochlorothiazide
HIV	Human immunodeficiency virus
HPV	Human papillomavirus

HS	Hidradenitis suppurativa
HSM	Hepatosplenomegaly
HSP	Henoch-schönlein purpura
HSV	Herpes simplex virus
HTN	Hypertension
Hx	History
HZ	Herpes zoster
I&D	Incision and drainage
IFN	Interferon
IIF	Indirect immunofluorescence
IL	Intralesional or interleukin (depending on context)
INH	Isoniazid
IP	Incontinentia pigmenti
IPL	Intense pulsed light
IVIG	Intravenous immunoglobulin
JAAD	Journal of the American academy of dermatology
JXG	Juvenile xanthogranuloma
KD	Kawasaki disease
KOH	Potassium hydroxide
KS	Kaposi's sarcoma
LABD	Linear IgA bullous dermatosis
LCH	Langerhans cell histiocytosis
LCV	Leukocytoclastic vasculitis
LFT	Liver function tests
LN	Lymphadenopathy
LP	Lichen planus
LPP	Lichen planopilaris
LR	Livedo reticularis
LsA	Lichen sclerosus et atrophicus
MAL	Methyl aminolevulinate
MCC	Merkel cell carcinoma
MF	Mycosis fungoides
MMF	Mycophenolate mofetil
MPS	Mucopolysaccharidoses
MR	Mental retardation
MSM	Men who have sex with men
MTX	Methotrexate
NASH	Nonalcoholic steatohepatitis
NbUVB	Narrowband UVB
NF	Neurofibromatosis
NICH	Noninvoluting congenital hemangioma
NI	Normal
NL	Necrobiosis lipoidica (previously called Necrobiosis lipoidica diabeticorum)
NSF	Nephrogenic systemic fibrosis

OCPs	Oral contraceptives
PAPA	Pyogenic arthritis, pyoderma gangrenosum and acne syndrome
PASI	Psoriasis area and severity index
PCN	Penicillin
PCOS	Polycystic ovarian syndrome
PCP	Pneumocystis pneumonia
PCR	Polymerase chain reaction
PCT	Porphyria cutanea tarda
PDL	Pulsed dye laser
PDT	Photodynamic therapy
PF	Pemphigus foliaceous
PFB	Pseudofolliculitis barbae
PG	Pyoderma gangrenosum or pyogenic granuloma (depends on context)
PHACES	Posterior fossa, hemangioma, arterial lesions, coarctation of aorta & cardiac anomalies, eye abnormalities and sternal clefting/ supraumbilical abdominal raphe
PLC	Pityriasis lichenoides chronica
PLEVA	Pityriasis lichenoides et varioliformis acuta
PMH	Past medical history
PMLE	Polymorphous light eruption
PNP	Paraneoplastic pemphigus
PO	By mouth
POD	Perioral dermatitis
POEMS	Polyneuropathy, organomegaly, endocrinopathy, monoclonal gammopathy, and skin changes
PPK	Palmar plantar keratoderma
PPV	Phakomatosis pigmentovascularis
PR	Pityriasis rosea
PRP	Pityriasis rubra pilaris
PSA	Prostate-specifica antigen
PSO	Proximal subungal onychomycosis
Pt	Patient
PT	Pili torti
PUD	Peptic ulcer disease
PUPPP	Pruritic urticarial papules and plaques of pregnancy
PUVA	Psoralen + UVA
PV	Pemphigus vulgaris
RA	Rheumatoid arthritis
RAS	Recurrent aphthous stomatitis
RAST	Radioallergosorbent test
RICH	Rapidly involuting congenital hemangioma
ROM	Range of motion
ROS	Review of systems
RPC	Reactive perforating collagenosis
RPR	Rapid plasma reagin

Rx	Prescription
SAHA	Seborrhoea, acne, hirsutism and alopecia
SCC	Squamous cell carcinoma
SCLE	Subacute cutaneous lupus erythematosus
SH	Social history
SHBG	Sex hormone binding globulin
SJS	Stevens Johnson syndrome
SK	Seborrheic keratosis
SLE	Systemic lupus erythematosus
soln	Solution
SSRI	Selective serotonin reuptake inhibitor
SSSS	Staphylococcal scalded skin syndrome
TCA	Trichloroacetic acid
TCN	Tetracycline
TEN	Toxic epidermal necrolysis
TLR	Toll-like receptor
TMEP	Telangiectasia macularis eruptiva perstans
TMP-SMX	Trimethoprim-sulfamethoxazole
TN	Trichorrhexis nodosa
TNF	Tumor necrosis factor
tPA	Tissue plasminogen activator
TPMT	Thiopurine methyltransferase
TRAPS	Tumor necrosis factor associated receptor syndromes
TSH	Thyroid stimulating hormone
TSS	Toxic shock syndrome
TTD	Trichothiodystrophy
Tx	Treatment
UA	Urinalysis
UP	Urticaria pigmentosa
WSO	White superficial onychomycosis
XLD	X-linked dominant
XLR	X-linked recessive

Coding

Outpatient Coding

New patients you need to meet the level in each of the three areas (HPI, PE, Plan)

HPI: always include four points of history (location, duration, symptoms, severity, alleviating, or aggravating factors

PE: for a new level 3, need to discuss five body parts. (so ... new alopecia patients. are level 2 since only scalp examined but acne patients. should still be level 3 as you need to check upper back, chest, neck, and upper arms for pustules) Remember to dictate every body part you examine even if findings are negative – Ex: no other worrisome lesions noted on exam of the face, neck, scalp, arms, legs, back, chest, etc.

Impression: number each complaint separately

Plan: corresponds to the numbers in plan to match the numbered diagnoses in impression. BE SURE to mention any Rx. written as this supports higher coding. Mention any notes, biopsies, labs reviewed, and any follow-up and any thoughts or considerations on diagnosis or future options as this is "medical decision making."

For return patients, you only need two of three areas to reach your code

–Ex: level 3 return–> you can have a one word HPI as long as you discuss level 3 PE (five body parts) and level 3 medical decision making (Rx. given)

–or the 2 out of 3 can be a good HPI covering four points as above with a brief one area PE then a level 3 plan

J.A. Cafardi, *The Manual of Dermatology*,
DOI 10.1007/978-1-4614-0938-0_1, © Springer Science+Business Media, LLC 2012

Table 1   Outpatient medical decision-making grid – history

History of present illness (Chief complaint) Location Timing Quality Modifying factors Duration Assoc signs/symptoms Context severity		Brief (1–3)	4+	Extended (four or more) OR >three chronic or inactive conditions
Review of systems All/immunology, GI Psych, CV, GU, Resp, Endo, Constit, skin, ENT Heme/ Lymph, neuro, Eyes, MSK	None	Pertinent to Problem (one system)	Extended (two to nine systems)	Complete (10+ systems) OR > one system and All others negative
PMH, FH, SH Established patients: two areas New patient/consult: three areas		None	Pertinent to (one history area)	Complete – Est: two areas New patient or consult: three areas
History level	**Problem focused**	**Expanded problem focused**	**Detailed**	**Comprehensive**

Physical exam	
System/body area	**Elements of examination**
Constitutional	• Measurement of any three of the following seven signs: 　1. Sitting or standing blood pressure 　2. Supine blood pressure 　3. Pulse rate and regularity 　4. Respiration 　5. Temperature 　6. Height 　7. Weight (may be measured and recorded by ancillary staff) • General appearance of patient (e.g., development, nutrition, body habitus, deformities, attention to grooming)
Eyes	• Inspection of conjunctivae and lids
Ears, Nose, Mouth, and Throat	• Inspection of lips, teeth, and gums • Examination of oropharynx (e.g., oral mucosa, hard and soft palates, tongue, tonsils, posterior pharynx)
Neck	• Examination of thyroid (e.g., enlargement, tenderness, mass)
Cardiovascular	• Examination of peripheral vascular system by observation (e.g., swelling, varicosities) and palpation (e.g., pulses, temperature, edema, tenderness)
Gastrointestinal (abdomen)	• Examination of liver and spleen • Examination of anus for condyloma and other lesions
Lymphatic	• Palpation of lymph nodes in neck, axillae, groin, and/or other location

(continued)

Table 1 (continued)

Physical exam	
System/body area	**Elements of examination**
Extremities	• Inspection and palpation of digits and nails (e.g., clubbing, cyanosis, inflammation, petechiae, ischemia, infections, nodes)

Skin	• Palpation of scalp and inspection of hair of scalp, eyebrows, face, chest, pubic area (when indicated), and extremities
	• Inspection and/or palpation of skin and subcutaneous tissue (e.g., rashes, lesions, ulcers, susceptibility to and presence of photo damage) in eight of the following ten areas:
	   ○ Head, including the face
	   ○ Neck
	   ○ Chest, including breasts and axillae
	   ○ Abdomen
	   ○ Genitalia, groin, buttocks
	   ○ Back
	   ○ Right upper extremity
	   ○ Left upper extremity
	   ○ Right lower extremity
	   ○ Left lower extremity
	• **Note:** For the comprehensive level, the examination of at least eight anatomic areas must be performed and documented. For the three lower levels of examination, each body area is counted separately. For example, inspection and/or palpation of the skin and subcutaneous tissue of the right upper extremity and the left upper extremity constitute two elements
	• Inspection of eccrine and apocrine glands of skin and subcutaneous tissue with identification and location of any hyperhidrosis, chromhidrosis, or bromhidrosis

Neurological/Psychiatric	Brief assessment of mental status including: • Orientation to time, place, and person • Mood and affect (e.g., depression, anxiety, agitation)
Content and Documentation Requirement for Skin Examination	
Problem Focused ————————————▶	**One to five elements identified by a bullet**
Expanded Problem Focused ————————▶	**At least six elements identified by a bullet**
Detailed ————————————————▶	**At least 12 elements identified by a bullet**
Comprehensive ——————————————▶	**Perform all elements identified by a bullet; document every element in each shaded box and at least one element in each unshaded box**

Outpatient Medical Decision-Making Grid

Table 2   Number of diagnosis or treatment options

Problem(s) Status	No.	Point	Result	Amount/complexity of data	
Self-limited or minor (max = 2)		1		Review/order lab test	1
				Review/order radiology tests	1
Established problem: stable		1		Review/order service in medicine section	1
Established problem: worsening		2		Discussion of test with performing MD	1
New problem: no additional workup (max = 1)		3		Obtain old records / Hx from other provider	1
				Review/summarize old records / Hx from and discuss with other provider	2
New problem: additional workup		4		Independent visualization of image, tracing, specimen itself (not review of report)	2
Total				Total	

Table 3 Table of risk: only one required

Risk	Presenting problem(s)	Diagnostic procedure(s) ordered	Management options selected
Minimal	One self-limited problem, e.g., cold, etc.	Lab tests; x-rays; ultrasound; EKG/EEG	Rest; gargles; superficial dressings
Low	– Two or more self-limited/minor problems – One stable chronic illness, e.g., well-controlled HTN, non-insulin-dependent diabetes, BPH – acute uncomplicated illness/injury	– Physiologic tests not under stress, e.g., PFT – Skin biopsy; superficial needle biopsy – Non-cardiovascular imaging studies with contrast, e.g., barium enema – Clinical lab tests requiring arterial puncture	– OTC drugs; physical therapy; IV fluids w/o additives – Minor surgery w/no identified risk factors – Physical and/or occupational therapy
Moderate	– One or more chronic illnesses w/mild exacerbation, progression of SE of treatment – Two or more stable chronic illnesses – Undiagnosed new problem w/uncertain prognosis – Acute illness with systemic sx – Acute complicated injury, e.g., head injury	– Physiologic tests under stress, e.g., Cardiac stress test, fetal stress test – Diagnostic endoscopies w/no identified risk factors – Deep needle or incisional bx – Obtain fluid from body cavity	– Minor surg w/identified risk factors – **Prescription drug management** – Therapeutic nuclear med – IV fluids with additives – Elective major surg (open, percutaneous or endoscopic) w/no identified risk factors
High	– One or more chronic illnesses w/severe exacerbation or SE of tx Acute or chronic illness/injury that poses a threat to life or bodily fxn, e.g., acute MI, multiple trauma, PE – Psychiatric illness w/ potential threat to self/others; peritonitis; acute renal failure – Abrupt change in neurologic status, e.g., seizure, TIA, weakness, sensory loss	– Cardiovascular imaging studies w/ contrast w/identified risk factors – Diagnostic endoscopies w/ identified risk factors – Discography – Cardiac electrophysiology tests	– Elective major surg (open, percutaneous, or endoscopic) w/identified risk factors – Emergency major surgery – Drug therapy requiring intensive monitoring for toxicity – Parenteral controlled substances

Table 4   Final results for complexity: two of three required

Number of diagnosis or management options	Minimal: 1	Limited: 2	Multiple: 3	Extensive: 4
Amount and complexity of data reviewed	Minimal: 1	Limited: 2	Multiple: 3	Extensive: 4
Risk	Minimal	Low	Moderate	High
Level of decision making	**Straight forward**	**Low complexity**	**Moderate complexity**	**High complexity**

New patient (three of three)				
History		Exam	MDM	Time
99201	PF	PF	StFwd	10
99202	Ex PF	Ex PF	StFwd	20
99203	Detailed	Detailed	Low	30
99204	Comp	Comp	Mod	45
99205	Comp	Comp	High	60

Established patient (two of three)				
History		Exam	MDM	Time
99211	MD presence not required			5
99212	PF		PF	StFwd	10
99213	ExPF		ExPF	Low	15
99214	Detailed		Detailed	Mod	25
99215	Comp		Comp	High	40

Consult (three of three)				
History		Exam	MDM	Time
99241	PF	PF	StFwd	15
99242	Ex PF	Ex PF	StFwd	30
99243	Detailed	Detailed	Low	40
99244	Comp	Comp	Mod	60
99245	Comp	Comp	High	80

*Consults – must name the requesting physician, identify the reason for the consult, and a report should be sent to the requesting physician. (The requesting physician also needs a note in *their chart* that they're requesting this consult.)

Commonly Used Modifiers in Dermatology

From AMA CPT® 2011 codes

Global Period Modifiers

24 – Unrelated Evaluation and Management Service by the Same Physician During a Postoperative Period: The physician may need to indicate that an evaluation and management service was performed during a postoperative period for a reason(s) unrelated to the original procedure. The circumstance may be reported by adding modifier -24 to the appropriate level of E/M service.

- Postop Periods
  - Minor surgery
    - Acne Surgery (10040) – 10 days
    - I&D, simple or single (10060) – 10 days
    - I&D, complex or multiple (10061) – 10 days
    - Skin tags (11200) – 10 days
    - Inflamed SK, HPV, molluscum, milia, 1–14 (17110) – 10 days
    - Inflamed SK, HPV, molluscum, milia, 15+ (17111) – 10 days
  - Biopsy
    - Skin (11100, 11101) – 0 days
    - Special sites
      - External ear (69100) – 0 days
      - External auditory canal (69105) – 0 days
      - Eyelid (67810) – 0 days
      - Intranasal (30100) – 0 days
      - Lip (40490) – 0 days
      - Penis (54100) – 0 days
      - Vulva/perineum (56605) – 0 days
      - Nail (11755) – 0 days
  - Destruction premalignant/benign lesions
    - Actinic keratoses, (17000, 17003, 17004) – 10 days
  - Surgical excisions – 10 days
  - Injection of intralesional Kenalog – 0 days

25 – Significant, Separately Identifiable Evaluation and Management Service by the Same Physician on the Same Day of the Procedure or Other Service: It may be necessary to indicate that on the day a procedure or service identified by a CPT® code was performed, the patient's condition required a significant, separately identifiable E/M service above and beyond the other service provided or beyond the usual preoperative and postoperative care associated with the procedure that was performed. A significant, separately identifiable E/M service is defined or substantiated by documentation that satisfies the relevant criteria for the respective E/M service to be reported. The E/M service may be prompted by the symptom or condition for which the procedure and/or service was provided. As such, different diagnoses are not required for reporting of the E/M services on the same date. This circumstance may be reported by adding modifier -25 to the appropriate level of E/M service.

- Notes – This modifier is not used to report an E/M service that resulted in a decision to perform surgery. See modifier -57. For significant, separately identifiable non-E/M services, see modifier -59.

57 – Decision for Surgery: An evaluation and management service that resulted in the initial decision to perform the surgery may be identified by adding modifier -57 to the appropriate level of E/M service.

58 – Stage or Related Procedure or Service by the Same Physician During the Postoperative Period: It may be necessary to indicate that the performance of a procedure or service during the postoperative period was: (a) planned or anticipated (staged); (b) more extensive than the original procedure; or (c) for therapy following a surgical procedure. The circumstance may be reported by adding modifier -58 to the staged or related procedure.

- Notes – For treatment of a problem that requires a return to the operating/ procedure room (e.g., unanticipated clinical condition), see modifier 78.

59 – Distinct Procedural Service: Under certain circumstances, it may be necessary to indicate that a procedure or service was distinct or independent from other non-E/M services performed on the same day. Modifier -59 is used to identify procedures/services, other than E/M services, that are not normally reported together, but are appropriate under the circumstances. Documentation must support a different session, different procedure or surgery, different site or organ system, separate incision/excision, separate lesion, or separate injury (or area of injury in extensive injuries) not ordinarily encountered or performed on the same day by the same individual. However, when another already established modifier is appropriate, it should be used rather than modifier -59. Only if no more descriptive modifier is available, and the use of modifier -59 best explains the circumstances, should modifier -59 be used.

- Notes – Modifier -59 should not be appended to an E/M service. To report a separate and distinct E/M service with a non-E/M service performed on the same date, see modifier 25.

79 – Unrelated Procedure or Service by the Same Physician During the Postoperative Period: The physician may need to indicate that the performance of a procedure or service during the postoperative period was unrelated to the original procedure. This circumstance may be reported by using modifier -79.

Modifiers for Special Surgical Situations

50 – Bilateral Procedure: Unless otherwise identified in the listings, bilateral procedures that are performed at the same session should be identified by adding modifier -50 to the appropriate 5-digit code. Report such procedures as a single line item with a unit of 1.
- Example – When procedure code 29580 unna boot is performed bilaterally, report 29580-50.

51 – Multiple Procedures: When multiple procedures, other than E/M services, Physical Medicine, and Rehabilitation services or provision of supplies (e.g., vaccines), are performed at the same session by the same provider, the primary procedure or service may be reported as listed. The additional procedure(s) or service(s) may be identified by appending modifier -51 to the additional procedure or service code(s).
- Note – This modifier should not be appended to designated "add-on" codes.

53 – Discontinued Procedure: Under certain circumstances, the physician may elect to terminate a surgical or diagnostic procedure. Due to extenuating circumstances or those that threaten the well-being of the patient, it may be necessary to indicate that a surgical or diagnostic procedure was started but discontinued. This circumstance may be reported by adding modifier -53 to the code reported by the physician for the discontinued procedure.
- Notes – This modifier is not used to report the elective cancelation of a procedure prior to the patient's anesthesia induction and/or surgical preparation in the operating suite. Include documentation describing the circumstance in your claim or it may be denied.

54 – Surgical Care Only: When one physician performs a surgical procedure and another provides preoperative and/or postoperative management, surgical services may be identified by adding modifier -54 to the usual procedure number.

55 – Postoperative Management Only: When one physician performed the postoperative management and another physician performed the surgical procedure, the postoperative component may be identified by adding modifier -55 to the usual procedure number.

62 – Two Surgeons: When two surgeons work together as primary surgeons performing distinct part(s) of a procedure, each surgeon should report his/her distinct operative work by adding modifier -62 to the procedure code and any associated add-on code(s) for that procedure as long as both surgeons continue to work together as primary surgeons. Each surgeon should report the co-surgery once using the same procedure code. If additional procedure(s) (including add-on procedure(s) are performed during the same surgical session, separate code(s) may also be reported with modifier -62 added.

■ Note – If a co-surgeon acts as an assistant in the performance of additional procedure(s) during the same surgical session, those services may be reported using separate procedure codes(s) with modifier -80 or modifier -82 added, as appropriate.

80 – Assistant Surgeon: Surgical assistant services may be identified by adding modifier -80 to the usual procedure number(s).
■ Note – this modifier is for assistance in a nonteaching setting.

82 – Assistant Surgeon (when qualified resident surgeon not available): The unavailability of a qualified resident surgeon is a prerequisite for use of modifier -82 appended to the usual procedure code number(s).
■ Note – used in teaching hospitals if there is no approved training program related to the medical specialty required for the surgical procedure or no qualified resident was available.

Other Modifiers

22 – Increased Procedural Services: When the work required to provide a service is substantially greater than typically required, it may be identified by adding modifier -22 to the usual procedure code. Documentation must support the substantial additional work and the reason for the additional work (i.e., increased intensity, time, technical difficulty or procedure, severity of patient's condition, physical and mental effort required).
■ Notes – Supportive documentation must be submitted with the claim (progress notes, orders, pathology sheets, etc). This modifier only applicable to those procedure codes which have a global period of 0, 10, or 90 days whether the procedure code is surgical in nature or not.

63 – Procedure Performed on Infants less than 4 kg: Procedures performed on neonates and infants up to a present body weight of 4 kg may involve significantly increased complexity and physician work commonly associated with these patients. This circumstance may be reported by adding modifier -63 to the procedure number.
■ Notes – Unless otherwise designated, this modifier may only be appended to procedures/services listed in the 20000-69990 code series. Modifier -63 should not be appended to any CPT® codes listed in the E/M services, anesthesia, radiology, pathology/laboratory, or medicine sections.

76 – Repeat Procedure by Same Physician: It may be necessary to indicate that a procedure or service was repeated by the same physician or other qualified health care professional subsequent to the original procedure or service. This circumstance may be reported by adding modifier -76 to the repeated procedure or service.

■ Notes – When medically necessary to repeat the service, the first service should be reported as usual. The repeat service should be reported on the next line with modifier -76. Always document medical necessity in the patient's record.

Additional Anatomic Modifiers

E1 – Upper left, eyelid
E2 – Lower left, eyelid
E3 – Upper right, eyelid
E4 – Lower right, eyelid

FA – Left hand, thumb
F1 – Left hand, 2nd digit
F2 – Left hand, 3rd digit
F3 – Left hand, 4th digit
F4 – Left hand, 5th digit
F5 – Right hand, thumb
F6 – Right hand, 2nd digit
F7 – Right hand, 3rd digit
F8 – Right hand, 4th digit
F9 – Right hand, 5th digit

LT – Left side of body
RT – Right side of body

TA – Left foot, great toe
T1 – Left foot, 2nd digit
T2 – Left foot, 3rd digit
T3 – Left foot, 4th digit
T4 – Left foot, 5th digit
T5 – Right foot, great toe
T6 – Right foot, 2nd digit
T7 – Right foot, 3rd digit
T8 – Right foot, 4th digit
T9 – Right foot, 5th digit

Inpatient Consults– Coding

Courtesy of Dr. Lauren Hughey

Initial

99253   History: Detailed (four elements)
PE: Detailed (12 bullets)
Decision: low (**old problem or new low-level problem**)

99254   History: Comprehensive (**four elements**)
PE: Comprehensive (**every bullet**)
Decision: Moderate: two of the three bullets below:

    * **New problem**
    * Need three points: Reviewed labs (1)
                                 Radiology (1)
                                 Medicine note (1)
                                 Old records (1)
                                 Discussed with other physician (2)
                                 Any test done by dermatology: Tzank, KOH (2)

    * Need one of the following:
                                 Chronic illness w/exacerbation
                                 Two stable chronic illnesses
                                 Undiagnosed problem w/uncertain prognosis
                                 Acute illness with systemic symptoms
                                 Complicated injury
                                 Incisional biopsy
                                 Rx drug management

99255   History: Comprehensive (**four elements**)
PE: Comprehensive (**every bullet**)
Decision: High: two of the three bullets below:

    * **New problem requiring workup**
    * Need four points: Reviewed labs (1)
                                 Radiology (1)
                                 Medicine note (1)
                                 Any old records (1)
                                 Discussed with other physician (2)
                                 Any test done by dermatology: Tzank, KOH (2)

    * Need one of the following:
                                 Life-threatening illness
                                 Severe exacerbation of chronic illness or severe
                               Side effects from treatment
                               Abrupt changes in neuro status
                               Drug therapy requiring monitoring
                               "Do Not Resuscitate status" (DNR) b/c poor prognosis

Inpatient Consults– Coding for Subsequent Visits

Subsequent	
99231	STABLE, RECOVERING, IMPROVING **History:** brief **ROS:** pertinent to problem (one system only needed – skin is a system) **PE:** only need comment on one skin area **Plan:** brief plan
99232	NOT RESPONDING, MINOR COMPLICATION **History:** 1–3 components of history (interval change, location, severity, quality, etc.) **ROS:** pertinent to problem (one system only needed – skin is a system) **PE:** six bullets from the template, ALWAYS include constitutional! **Plan:** (Moderate) discuss if any **notes or results of tests or biopsies reviewed** Review plan. Include any **Rx meds** recommending. Report on what **follow-up** patient will have with derm (i.e., will follow or patient can follow-up with derm as outpatient)
99233	VERY UNSTABLE, CRITICALLY ILL, SIGNIFICANT COMPLICATIONS **History:** four components of history (interval change, location, severity, quality, duration, context, timing, modifying factors, associated symptoms) **ROS:** at least two body SYSTEMS must be mentioned (skin is only one system – can use constitutional or Eyes to get second) **PMH (or FH):** need to mention at least one history hopefully pertinent to problem **PE:** 12 bullets from the template **Plan:** (High life-threatening or severe organ impact) discuss if ANY **notes or labs, test, or biopsy results reviewed** – i.e., CBC, blood cultures, febrile? Include any **Rx meds requiring monitoring**. Review plan and report on what **follow-up** patient will have with derm (i.e., will follow vs. patient can follow-up with derm as outpatient)

Hair Disorders

Alopecia Classification

Non-Cicatricial (non-scarring) Alopecias

1. Androgenetic alopecia
2. Telogen effluvium
3. Trichotillomania
4. Alopecia areata
5. Postoperative (Pressure-Induced) alopecia
6. Temporal triangular alopecia
   ○ Patch of alopecia with normal follicles, but almost all are vellus hairs
   ○ Present at birth or acquired in first decade
7. Lipedematous alopecia (lipedematous scalp)
   ○ Doubling in scalp thickness
8. Congenital atrichia with papules
   ○ Very rare condition, previously known as congenital alopecia universalis
   ○ Fail to regrow hair after shedding their initial growth of hair shortly after birth

Cicatricial (scarring) Alopecia

1. **Group 1: Lymphocytic**
   ○ Chronic cutaneous lupus erythematosus (DLE)
   ○ Lichen planopilaris (LPP)
     ■ Classic LPP
     ■ Frontal fibrosing alopecia
     ■ Graham-Little syndrome
   ○ Brocq's alopecia
   ○ Central centrifugal cicatricial alopecia (CCCA)

- ○ Alopecia mucinosa
- ○ Keratosis follicularis spinulosa decalvans
  - ■ Corneal dystrophy with cutaneous findings including cicatricial alopecia of the scalp, eyebrows, and eyelashes in association with perifollicular erythema and follicular hyperkeratosis

2. **Group 2: Neutrophilic**
   - ○ Folliculitis Decalvans – used by different authors to mean different things; usually means the inflammatory phase of CCCA
   - ○ Dissecting cellulitis
3. **Group 3: Mixed**
   - ○ Acne keloidalis
   - ○ Acne necrotica
   - ○ Erosive pustular dermatosis
4. **Group 4: Nonspecific**

Reference:

Olsen EA, Bergfield WF, Cotsarelis G, et al. *Summary of North American Hair Research Society (NAHRS)-sponsored workshop on Cicatricial Alopecia. Duke University Medical Center, February 10 and 11, 2001.* J Am Acad Dermatol 2003; 137: 1465–71.

Alopecia Areata

Etiology and Pathogenesis

- Most widely accepted hypothesis is that alopecia areata is a T-cell mediated auto-immune condition that is most likely to occur in genetically predisposed individuals

Clinical Presentation and Types

- Recurrent non-scarring type of hair loss that can affect any hair-bearing area
- Usually asymptomatic, but some experience a burning sensation or pruritus in the affected area
- May have few or many patches. No correlation exists between the number of patches at onset and subsequent severity
- Dermoscopy – yellow "dots" around hair follicles (not seen in other alopecias)
- **Pattern Types**
  - Alopecia **areata, localized** – usually localized and patchy
    - **Circumscribed** – isolated oval patches
    - **Ophiasis** – hair loss localized to the sides and lower back of head
    - **Sisaipho** (ophiasis spelled backward) – hair loss spares sides of back of head
  - **Reticular pattern** – innumerable small patches that coalesce
  - **Alopecia areata, diffuse** – usually see circumscribed patches with alopecia areata, but can sometimes see a diffuse pattern which mimics telogen effluvium
  - **Alopecia totalis** – complete loss of all scalp hair
  - **Alopecia universalis** – complete loss of all body hair
- **Associated Conditions**
  - Thyroid disease
    - **Presence of microsomal antibodies is found in 3.3–16% of patients. Antibodies** can be found +/– symptoms of thyroid disease, but patients with positive autoantibodies have higher incidence of functional abnormalities found on thyroid-releasing hormone tests (26% vs. 2.8%)
  - Vitiligo
  - Atopic dermatitis
  - Collagen vascular diseases have been found in 0.6–2% of patients with AA
  - Emotional stress and psychiatric disease
  - Pernicious anemia, myasthenia gravis, ulcerative colitis, lichen planus, and *Candida* endocrinopathy syndrome also have been associated with AA in some studies
  - Down syndrome

Differential Diagnosis (DDx) – androgenetic alopecia, pseudopelade, syphilis, telogen effluvium, tinea capitis, trichotillomania

Treatment

- Rule out tinea if scale is present. Rule out syphilis if presentation or history suggests
- **Corticosteroids**
  - ○ Topicals – such as Olux foam, Luxiq foam, Temovate scalp soln, clobetasol ointment, Diprolene lotion, Lidex solution, etc.
    - ■ Itching + Alopecia → 2% sulfur ppt + 0.25% menthol in Lidex oint (or aquaphor or 2.5% hydrocortisone). Disp: 60 g tube
  - ○ Intralesionals – first-line in adult patients for localized patches
    - ■ Kenalog concentrations vary from 5–20 mg/mL; q 4–6 weeks
      - □ Hair growth may be seen for 6–9 months after injection
      - □ Less than 0.1 mL is injected per site; injections spread out to cover affected areas (approximately 1 cm between injection sites)
      - □ Avoid reinjecting areas of denting, which usually is sufficient to allow atrophy to revert
      - □ If you see bleb form while injecting = too superficial; may cause atrophy
- **Topical immunotherapy** – the induction and periodic elicitation of an allergic contact dermatitis by topical application of potent contact allergens
  - ○ Commonly used agents for immunotherapy include **squaric acid dibutylester** (SADBE) and diphencyprone (DPCP)
    - ■ Dinitrochlorobenzene (DNCB) has become less popular as a result of reports that it is mutagenic in the Ames assay (a bacterial assay)
    - ■ A lag period of 3 months usually present between onset of tx and presence of regrowth. The median time to achieve significant regrowth was 12.2 months
    - ■ If no benefit in 12–24 months, discontinue therapy
    - ■ The most common side effect, which is desired, is a mild contact dermatitis (redness, scaling, itching); pigment changes can occur
  - ○ Squaric acid treatment
    - ■ Patient is sensitized directly with 2% concentration on a 2 cm area (scalp or buttock)
    - ■ The following week, a low concentration (0.05%) is applied 3x/week to start
    - ■ The frequency and concentration may be slowly titrated as tolerated
    - ■ Patients advised to avoid light exposure on scalp for 48 h, since light degrades chemical. Patients also advised not to wash the scalp for 48 h

- ○ Anthralin
  - ▪ Both short-contact and overnight treatments have been used
  - ▪ Anthralin concentrations varied from 0.2–1%; Most → irritant contact dermatitis
  - ▪ AE – pruritus, burning, staining of clothes, folliculitis, localized pyoderma, LN
- • PUVA – topical and oral
- • Tacrolimus – May or may not help
- • Cyclosporine – patients relapse within 3 months of discontinuing med; limited use
- • Interferon alfa-2 – (1.5 million IU, 3 times per week for 3 week); no benefit in small study
- • Dapsone – 50 mg BID was used in a 6-month, double-blind, placebo-controlled study
  - ○ Did show efficacy but many dropped out due to side effects (malaise)
- • Minoxidil (Rogaine)
  - ○ Foam less likely to cause irritation than soln b/c no propylene glycol
  - ○ Can be added to other regimens to help facilitate hair growth

Pearls and Pitfalls

- – Patients and their families often need extensive counseling about this disorder, especially in pediatric setting
- – Worse prognosis = ophiasis, age of onset < 5 years with alopecia totalis or alopecia universalis, association with atopy
- – Recommend the National Alopecia Areata Foundation (www.naaf.org)

Alopecia – Androgenetic Type

Etiology and Pathogenesis

- Androgenetic alopecia is postulated to be a dominantly inherited disorder with variable penetrance and expression. However, it may be of polygenic inheritance
- Women who develop balding shortly after puberty are more likely to have a family history for pattern baldness. Women who develop this in the perimenopausal and menopausal phases have contributing genetic and hormonal factors
- Male androgenetic alopecia partially related to dihydrotestosterone (DHT). Testosterone converted to DHT by 5α-reductase. Type II 5α-reductase dominates in scalp, beard and chest hair, as well as in liver and prostate. Genetic absence of Type II 5α-reductase prevents male androgenetic alopecia

Clinical Presentation

- Affects roughly 50% of men and perhaps as many women older than 40 years. As many as 13% of premenopausal women reportedly have some evidence of androgenetic alopecia.
- **Ludwig Pattern**
  - Grade I – minimal widening of part width
  - Grade II – moderate thinning
  - Grade III – significant thinning and widening of part width
- **Hamilton/Norwood Classification** – pattern of balding seen in men, rarely in women
- Men
  - Gradual thinning in the temporal areas, producing a reshaping of the anterior part of the hairline. Evolution of baldness progresses according to Norwood/Hamilton classification
  - Associations:
    - Males with androgenetic alopecia *may* have an increased incidence of myocardial infarction
    - Increased incidence of benign prostatic hypertrophy has also been associated
- Women
  - Usually present with diffuse thinning on the crown. Bitemporal recession does occur in women but usually to a lesser degree than in men. Women generally maintain a frontal hairline

Labs

- Females with early onset or severe patterned hair loss could have pathologic hyperandrogenism
  - Check – total and free testosterone, DHEAS, 17-hydroxyprogesterone
- Evaluate for thyroid disease – TSH, free T4
- Evaluate for anemia – CBC + diff, ferritin, TIBC, transferring sat, total iron
  - A normal CBC does not exclude iron deficiency as a cause of hair loss
  - Check ESR in addition to ferritin. If both elevated, then ferritin may be inappropriately normal as a result of acute inflammation (both are acute phase reactants)

Histology

- Normal *total* number of follicles (about 35 in Caucasians or 20 in AA per 4-mm plug)
- Reduced number of hairs (mixture of terminal and indeterminate) when counted at the dermal/fat junction
- Increased numbers and percentage of vellus and indeterminate hairs when counted at the level of the upper dermis
- Presence of fibrous "streamers" below miniaturized hairs
- Slightly increased telogen count compared with "unaffected" scalp
- Uninvolved scalp (e.g., occiput) appears normal or relatively normal
- No significant inflammation

Treatment

- Minoxidil BID, (2% or 5% soln, 5% foam)
  - Appears to lengthen anagen phase, and may increase blood supply to follicle. Regrowth at vertex > frontal areas; is not noted for at least 4 months. Continue
  - Topical treatment with drug indefinitely; discontinuation of treatment produces rapid reversion to pretreatment balding pattern
  - Women respond better → recommend men's formulation
- Finasteride (Propecia) 1 mg PO qd
  - 5-α-reductase inhibitor which inhibits type 2
  - Can produce ambiguous genitalia in developing male fetus. Don't use in young women who may get pregnant
  - Affects vertex balding > frontal hair loss. Must be continued indefinitely because discontinuation results in gradual progression of the disorder

- Dutasteride (Avodart) 2.5 mg PO QD – may work better than finasteride
  - [Olsen EA, et al. The importance of dual 5-alpha-reductase inhibition in the treatment of male pattern hair loss: results of a randomized placebo-controlled study of dutasteride versus finasteride. JAAD 2006; 55(6): 1014–23.
  - 5a-reductase inhibitor – inhibits type 1 and type 2
- Females – can try spironolactone, oral contraceptives
  - Evidence exists of an association between androgenetic alopecia, hypertension, and hyperaldosteronism. Spironolactone could play a dual role in treatment
    - Spironolactone = Preg Category X. Need concomitant birth control
  - Oral contraceptives helpful if hyperandrogenism present (to suppress ovarian androgen production)
- Hair transplantation and scalp reduction

Pearls and Pitfalls

– Finasteride will decrease PSA levels by 40% (men ages 40–49) and 50% (men ages 50–60)
– Finasteride will stop hair loss in 90% of men and cause regrowth in 65%. Continued therapy need to see benefits

Alopecia – Brocq's Alopeica

Etiology and Pathogenesis

- Brocq's Alopecia (or Pseudopelade of Brocq) is felt to be the end stage of several different forms of scarring alopecia, especially lichen planopilaris and chronic cutaneous lupus erythematosus. Therefore, the cause of pseudopelade of Brocq is linked to the etiology of the underlying skin disease
  - If a definitive diagnosis of DLE, LPP, or another condition can be made based on clinical, histologic, or immunofluorescent features, then the term pseudopelade of Brocq cannot be used

Clinical

- Lesions are discrete, randomly distributed, irregularly shaped, and often clustered in patches on the scalp; asymptomatic
- The individual lesion is hypopigmented (porcelain white is the classic description) and slightly depressed (atrophic)
  - "footprints in the snow" refers to dermal atrophy causing a slight depression below the surrounding normal scalp
- Condition may worsen in "spurts" with periods of activity, followed "dormant" phase
- Unlike the steady disease progression seen in CCCA

Histology – shows a "burnt-out" alopecia. If typical findings of LPP, CCCA or other types of scarring alopecia are found, the diagnosis of Brocq's alopecia can be excluded

- Decreased number of hairs, especially terminal hairs
- Loss of sebaceous glands
- Residual, "naked" hair shafts surrounded by mild, granulomatous inflammation
- Follicular stelae without overlying follicles
- Cylindrical columns of connective tissue at the sites of former follicles

Labs to Consider → ANA if suspect lupus. Rule out systemic causes – anemia, thyroid, etc.

Treatment

- When lesions of pseudopelade of Brocq are burnt out, treatment is neither necessary nor possible. Unfortunately, the condition can reactivate episodically and unpredictably. If active inflammation is present, consider an alternative diagnosis, and potent topical corticosteroids, such as fluocinonide or clobetasol, can be tried

References:

(1) Sperling LC. An Atlas of Hair Pathology with Clinical Correlations. New York: Parthenon, 2003.
(2) Sperling LC. Alopecias. In: Bolognia, Jorizzo, Rapini (eds). Dermatology, 2nd edition. Spain: Mosby Elsevier, 2008: 997–8.

Alopecia – Central Centrifugal Cicatricial Alopecia (CCCA)

Etiology and Pathogenesis

- The most common form of scarring alopecia in African-Americans; Females: Males is 3:1
  - ○ Average age of presentation – 36 for women, 31 for men
  - ○ Virtually all women with CCCA are using or have used chemical hair relaxers, but few men have used anything except pomades
  - ○ Progression of the disease even after all chemical tx (if any) are discontinued
  - ○ Patients may be predisposed to follicular damage b/c of premature desquamation of the inner root sheath
- CCCA = Recently coined term used to incorporate several variants of inflammatory, scarring alopecia. The entities grouped under CCCA include *pseudopalade* (*not* Brocq's pseudopelade), the *follicular degeneration syndrome*, and *folliculitis decalvans*. As variants of CCCA, they have the following features in common:
  - ○ Chronic, progressive, with eventual spontaneous "burn out" after years
  - ○ Predominantly centered on the crown or vertex
  - ○ Progress in a symmetrical fashion, with the most active disease activity occurring in a peripheral zone of variable width, surrounding a central zone of alopecia
  - ○ They show both clinical and histological evidence of inflammation in the active, peripheral zone

Clinical Presentation

- Symptoms may be mild or absent; most note only mild, episodic pruritus or tenderness of involved areas
- Scarring alopecia
  - ○ The follicular ostia between remaining hairs are obliterated and the scalp is smooth and shiny (evidence of scarring)
  - ○ A few isolated hairs may have tufting; "Baby doll hair"
- Early or mild disease → partially bald patch only a few cm in diameter
- Long-standing or severe disease → can result in hair loss covering entire crown of scalp
- "Transitional zone" – few inflammatory, follicular papules
- Even "normal" scalp skin can have foci of alopecia and an occasional follicular papule or perifollicular scaling
- Pustules come and go – likely related to bacterial superinfection and/or immune response to degenerating follicular components

DDx – folliculitis decalvans (for those who feel this is a separate entity), tinea capitis/kerion, true bacterial infection of scalp

Histology

- Biopsy the peripheral, partially alopecic fringe; note – *involved* follicles are selectively *destroyed*, with sparing of the relatively normal follicles
- **Premature desquamation of the inner root sheath** – most distinctive and earliest finding; can be found even in normal-appearing scalp skin
- As disease progresses …
  - Eccentric epithelial atrophy (thinning) with hair shafts in close proximity to the dermis
  - Concentric lamellar fibroplasias (onion skin-like fibrosis) of affected follicle
  - Variably dense lymphocytic perifollicular inflammation primarily at upper isthmus and lower infundibulum
  - Occasional fusion of infundibula (polytrichia)
  - Later, total destruction of hair shaft

Treatment

- Short course of corticosteroids can temporarily eliminate purulent component of CCCA
- Relatively noninflammatory disease
  - Combination of long-acting oral TCN (doxycycline, TCN, minocycline) plus potent topical steroid (e.g., clobetasol or fluocinonide) – can be safely maintained for years
- Highly inflammatory disease ("folliculitis decalvans")
  - PO rifampin + PO clindamycin (both at 300 mg BID) × 10–12 weeks
  - Maintenance therapy such as oral doxycycline plus topical clobetasol should follow
- Some physicians use methotrexate to decrease inflammation

References:

(1) Sperling LC. An Atlas of Hair Pathology with Clinical Correlations. New York: Parthenon, 2003.
(2) Sperling LC. Alopecias. In: Bolognia, Jorizzo, Rapini (eds). Dermatology, 2nd edition. Spain: Mosby Elsevier, 2008: 997–8.

Alopecia – Discoid Lupus (DLE)

Etiology and Pathogenesis

- AKA – Chronic cutaneous lupus erythematosus
- One form of cutaneous lupus that often involves the scalp and can commonly cause scarring
- Autoimmune

Clinical Presentation

- Majority of patients with DLE do not have systemic lupus
- Alopecia, erythema, epidermal atrophy and dilated, plugged follicular ostia
  ○ Scales difficult to remove and show spines on undersurface (resembling carpet tacks)
- Central hypopigmentation and peripheral hyperpigmentation are characteristic of lesions in dark-skinned individuals
- Plaques may coalesce to form large, irregular-shaped zones of scarring alopecia
- Lesions commonly involve scalp, ears, face
- < 5% have mucosal involvement

DDx – alopecia areata (initially), lichen planopilaris, central centrifugal cicatricial alopecia, linear morphea, tinea capitis

Labs and Workup – ANA with quantitation, general alopecia labs, biopsy. Occasionally, leukopenia is present

Histology

- Superficial and deep inflammation
- Vacuolar interface alteration of dermal–epidermal junction and at the follicular epithelium
- Increased dermal mucin
- Chronic inflammation (often including plasma cells) of the eccrine sweat glands and erector pili is sometimes present
- Typically, see granular deposits of IgG and C3 (less commonly IgM or IgA) at the dermal–epidermal junction and/or the junction of the follicular epithelium and dermis

Treatment

- Sunscreens with physical blockers (zinc oxide, titanium dioxide)
- Topical and intralesional corticosteroids
- Topical tacrolimus or pimecrolimus may be helpful
- Hydroxychloroquine 200 mg PO BID
- Quinacrine 100 mg PO TID added to hydroxychloroquine regimen (OK to use these together)
- Hyperkeratotic lesions respond well to acitretin
  ○ Not for use in females of child-bearing potential

Pearls and Pitfalls

- Risk of SCC in long-standing DLE lesions. Consider adding acitretin if this is a recurrent issue
- Be aggressive in treating this condition since scarring is often disfiguring
- Quinacrine may lead to yellowing of the skin

Alopecia – Dissecting Cellulitis of the Scalp

Etiology and Pathogenesis

- AKA – perifolliculitis capitis abscedens et suffodiens
- Part of the "follicular occlusion tetrad" which includes hidradenitis suppurativa, acne conglobata, and pilonidal sinus. Scalp disease often stands alone

Clinical Presentation

- Tends to affect young adult men, especially African-Americans
- Lesions begin as multiple, firm scalp nodules, typically on the crown, vertex and upper occiput. Nodules rapidly enlarge into boggy, fluctuant, oval and linear ridges that discharge purulent material
- Lesions often interconnect, so that pressure on one fluctuant area may result in purulent discharge from perforations several centimeters away
- Despite massive inflammation, there can be surprisingly little pain
- Patients seek help because of hair loss and foul-smelling discharge
- Disease waxes and wanes for years, but eventually leads to dense dermal fibrosis, sinus tract formation, permanent alopecia, and hypertrophic scarring

DDx – tinea capitis (on occasion), highly inflammatory forms of cicatricial alopecia ("folliculitis decalvans")

Histology

- Very early lesions are seldom evaluated, but may show moderately dense, lymphocytic, perifollicular inflammation surrounding the lower half of the follicle
- Increase in catagen and telogen hairs
- Sebaceous glands may persist well into the course of the disease
- Fully developed fluctuant lesions show perifollicular and mid-to-deep dermal abscesses composed of neutrophils, lymphocytes, and often copious plasma cells
- Eventually – granulation tissue, epithelium-lined sinus tracts, and fibrosis are seen

Treatment

- Rule out tinea capitis
- Culture purulent material, although usually no growth

- Isotretinoin – 0.5–1.5 mg/kg/day until 4 months after achieving a clinical remission
  - Relapses are common
- Intralesional corticosteroids
- Oral antibiotics – such as long-acting TCNs (doxycycline, tetracycline, minocycline)
  - Oral quinolones (such as ciprofloxacin) – successful case reports
- Clindamycin + rifampin, 300 mg PO BID (for each)
- Surgical approaches – ranging from incision and drainage to grafting
- Adalimumab has been successful in some case reports
- Radiation therapy – may be successful in severe, refractory cases
- Oral zinc may be helpful in some cases

Pearls and Pitfalls

- Rare reports of dissecting cellulitis being associated with spondylarthropathy
- SCC can rarely occur in the setting of long-standing disease
- Rare reports of Keratitis–Ichthyosis–Deafness (KID) syndrome being associated with follicular occlusion tetrad

References:

(1) Sperling LC. An Atlas of Hair Pathology with Clinical Correlations. New York: Parthenon, 2003.
(2) Sperling LC. Alopecias. In: Bolognia, Jorizzo, Rapini (eds). Dermatology, 2nd edition. Spain: Mosby Elsevier, 2008: 997–8.

Alopecia – Folliculitis Decalvans

Etiology and Pathogenesis

- *Staph. aureus* seems to play important role in pathogenesis; can be isolated in almost every case
  - Has been suggested that "superantigens" or cytotoxins that bind to MHC class II molecules may stimulate T cells, but "escape" detection by the host immune system, and play a role in pathogenesis

Clinical Presentation

- Predominantly involves the vertex and occipital area of the scalp
- Initial lesion is an erythematous follicular papule
- Hallmark – development of scarred areas and pustules
- Livid to bright erythema together with yellow-gray scales can be present, especially around follicles; also follicular hyperkeratosis, erosions and hemorrhagic crusts
- Pain, itching, and/or burning sensations
- With progressive disease, develop ivory-white patches of cicatricial alopecia
- Tufting (polytrichia) is a common feature
  - Also seen in several forms of cicatricial alopecia (DLE, LPP, CCCA, acne keloidalis, dissecting cellulitis, pemphigus of the scalp and tinea capitis)

Diagnosis

- Bacterial cultures should be taken from intact pustule or from scalp swab
- A nasal swab should be performed to identify an occult *S. aureus* reservoir
- Skin biopsy of an active lesion
  - One 4-mm punch biopsy which includes subcutaneous tissue – from clinically active area, processed for horizontal sections, and stained with H&E
  - Biopsy should be taken from an active hair-bearing margin of the lesion and has to follow the direction of the hair growth
  - PAS – to rule out fungal organisms
  - Elastin – helpful to identify classic pseudopelade of Brocq
  - Can do DIF if suspicious for DLE

Histology

- Characterized as a neutrophilic primary cicatricial alopecia
- Early lesions
  - ○ Keratin aggregation and a dilatation of the infundibulum in combination with numerous intraluminal neutrophils
  - ○ Sebaceous glands are destroyed early in the process
  - ○ Intrafollicular and perifollicular predominantly neutrophilic infiltrate found
- Advanced lesions

  - ○ Infiltrate may consist of neutrophils, lymphocytes, and numerous plasma cells – extend into dermis and around blood vessels
  - ○ Granulomatous inflammation with foreign-body giant cells are a common finding – believed to result from ectopic pieces of hair shafts
  - ○ Follicular tufts can frequently be found
  - ○ Sinus tracts are NOT found in folliculitis decalvans (in contrast to dissecting cellulitis)

DDx – dissecting cellulitis, acne keloidalis nuchae, erosive pustular dermatosis, acne necrotica varioliformis, deep fungal infection of scalp, DLE, CCCA, lichen planopilaris, pseudopelade of Brocq

Treatment of Folliculitis Decalvans

- Educate patient about hygiene – ok to wear bandanas, caps, hats, hair pieces and wigs – BUT these can be a reservoir for *S. aureus*. All headdresses have to be cleaned with antiseptic diligently and the patient should switch between hairpieces
- Oral antibiotics
  - ○ Relapse is common after stopping ABX; patients often on low-dose ABX for years
  - ○ **Rifampin 300 mg BID over 10–12 weeks** is believed to be the best anti-staphylococcal agent. May also be effective in eliminating carrier state
    - ▪ Strongly recommended to **use rifampin in combination with Clindamycin 300 mg BID** to avoid rapid emergence of resistance
    - ▪ SE Rifampin – hepatitis, induction of hepatic microsomal enzymes, OCP failure, influenza-like syndrome, hemolytic anemia, thrombocytopenia, interaction with warfarin
    - ▪ **Ciprofloxacin** or **Clarithromycin** can alternatively be used in combination with Rifampin
- Topical antibiotics and antiseptics → Combine with oral therapy
  - ○ 2% mupirocin
  - ○ 1% clindamycin
  - ○ 2% erythromycin

- Shampoos
  - Use shampoo with antiseptic cleanser → Teraseptic® cleanser – contains 0.5% triclosan cleanser; can be drying, so use in conjunction with antibiotic ointment
- Topical and Intralesional corticosteroids
  - Can help with the itching, burning, and pain
  - IL Kenalog 10 m/mL q4–6 weeks
  - Topical class I or II corticosteroids can be used BID
  - Oral corticosteroids
  - Consider PO prednisone only for highly active and rapidly progressing cases
  - *Aggressive regimen* – Prednisolone 20 mg QD tapered over 3 weeks + isotretinoin 40 mg QD, which is reduced to maintenance of 30 mg QD + PO clindamycin 300 mg QD × 6 weeks
- Isotretinoin
  - Limited used in folliculitis decalvans (but works well in dissecting cellulitis)
- Dapsone
  - 50–100 mg PO daily alone or in combination with an antibiotic
  - Long-term tx with 25 mg daily may stabilize the disease
- Isolated reports – Oral zinc sulfate, oral L-tyrosine, laser epilation with Nd:YAG. Careful with scalp surgery → can flare the disease. Proceed with caution

Pearls and Pitfalls

– Websites: www.nahrs.org and www.carfintl.org

Reference:

Otberg N, Kang H, Alzolibani AA and Shapiro J. Folliculitis Decalvans. Dermatologic Therapy; 21(4): 238–44.

Alopecia – Lichen Planopilaris (LPP)

Etiology and Pathogenesis

- Etiology not known, but is presumably related to the cause(s) of lichen planus
- Type of alopecia whose clinical course may be insidious or fulminant; pattern of scalp hair loss is highly variable

Clinical Presentation

- Caucasians more often affected than dark-skinned individuals; middle-aged women
- Up to 50% have other findings of lichen planus – nails, skin, oral mucosa
- Most common – several scattered foci of partial hair loss; irregularly shaped and widely scattered over the scalp
- Perifollicular erythema and scaling almost always present
- Pattern of hair loss suggestive of CCCA or pseudopelade of Brocq can also occur
- Can heal with the formation of polytrichia (tufting) – seen with any inflammatory scarring alopecia
- Indolent dz – may be asymptomatic, but itching and tenderness often present
- "Confetti-like" pattern of numerous small and widely distributed lesions is a relatively common clinical variant of LPP
- *Cannot* make diagnosis of LPP based on clinical features alone
- Clinical Variants of LPP
  - **Graham-Little Syndrome** – scarring alopecia of the scalp, loss of pubic and axillary hair, and the rapid development of keratosis pilaris. Rare
    - Considered by some to be a variant of LPP; however … typical lichen planus lesions are not found and the histological findings are usually not lichenoid
  - **Frontal Fibrosing Alopecia** – Elderly women with progressive hair loss along the anterior hairline and the eyebrows. Histopathology similar to those in LPP
    - Lesions of lichen planus are usually <u>not</u> seen and the lichenoid inflammation does not affect the interfollicular epidermis

Histology

- Band-like infiltrate obscures interface between epidermis and dermis. Vacuolar changes at the interface and wedge-shaped hypergranulosis within affected infundibula is typical
- Often see prominent dyskeratosis with individually necrotic basal keratinocytes

- Colloid or Civatte bodies occasionally found as part of the interface alteration, but less common than in LP of the epidermis
- Inflammation most severe at upper portion of follicle – infundibulum and isthmus – but can extend down follicle
- Perivascular and perieccrine lymphocytic infiltrates (as seen in lupus) are absent in LPP
- Occasionally, interfollicular changes of LP are found – strongly supports a dx of LPP
- Eventually, the infundibulum and isthmus become distended and plugged with keratinous
- Basilar keratinocytes often become pink, flattened, and an artifactual cleft can form b/n epithelium and stroma – late stage of LPP; can be seen in other forms of scarring alopecia
- Follicles eventually replaced by columns of connective tissue
- **Grouped, globular immunofluorescence (especially IgM), especially when found adjacent to the follicular epithelium, is the characteristic pattern in LPP**
  - Note – Lupus has linear deposits of immunoreactants

Treatment

- Difficult condition to treat
- Corticosteroids (topical, intralesional, oral)
- Oral antibiotics with anti-inflammatory properties – doxycycline
- **Hydroxychloroquine**
  - Effective at decreasing signs and symptoms of LPP and FFA even at 6 and 12 months
  - Dose = 200 mg BID
- Mycophenolate mofetil
  - Very effective in small studies, even in patients who have failed many other treatments
  - Improvement typically seen within 6 months
  - Dose = 500 mg BID × 4 weeks, then 1 g BID
- Anecdotal reports of success with …
  - Cyclosporine, PO
  - Systemic retinoids
  - Low-dose weekly oral methotrexate
  - (Note – the above tx should be used with caution as they themselves may cause some degree of alopecia)
- Some cases can resolve spontaneously, but others often go on for years

Pearls and Pitfalls

– Keep flowchart of patient's signs and symptoms – will help you see if progress
  is occurring and will help facilitate treatment decisions
  ○ See JAAD article for example and LPP Activity Index
  ○ Things to include:
    ▪ Pruritus, pain, burning, erythema, perifollicular erythema, perifollicular
      scale
    ▪ Pull test – anagen hair? Telogen hair?
    ▪ Spreading?
    ▪ Dimensions/extent?
    ▪ Tufting
    ▪ Atrophy and telangiectasis
    ▪ Pigment changes
    ▪ Other skin changes – skin, nails, mucosa
    ▪ Labs – CBC, AST/ALT/Alk phos, G6PD, Eye exam, BUN/Cr, Blood
      pressure
    ▪ Cultures and sensitivities
    ▪ Treatments/comments
    ▪ Biopsy
    ▪ Photographs

References:

(1) Sperling LC. An Atlas of Hair Pathology with Clinical Correlations. New York: Parthenon,
    2003.
(2) Sperling LC. Alopecias. In: Bolognia, Jorizzo, Rapini (eds). Dermatology, 2nd edition. Spain:
    Mosby Elsevier, 2008: 997–8.
(3) Chiang C, Sah D, Cho BK, et al. Hydroxychloroquine and lichen planopilaris: efficacy and
    introduction of Lichen planopilaris Activity Index scoring system. J Amer Acad Dermatol
    2010; 62(3): 387–92.

Alopecia Mucinosa

Etiology and Pathogenesis

- AKA – Follicular mucinosis. Etiology unknown
- Occurs in three settings:
  - Idiopathic – Usually a benign idiopathic condition in majority of cases involving those younger than age 40; CTCL rarely associated in children but must be followed closely
  - In association with MF/CTCL – In patients older than age 40, alopecia mucinosa may be first sign of CTCL
  - In association with other neoplastic and inflammatory conditions – such as atopic dermatitis or in association with known CTCL

Clinical Presentation

- Inflammatory disorder characterized by follicular papules or infiltrated plaques with scaling, alopecia, and accumulation of mucin in sebaceous glands and the outer root sheaths of hair follicles
- Three morphologic forms:
  - Grouped follicular papules coalescing into rough patches
  - Grouped follicular papules coalescing into scaly plaques
  - Nodular, boggy plaque with overlying erythema and scaling
- Lesions usually measure 2–5 cm in diameter and are typically devoid of hair
- Distribution – face, scalp, neck, shoulders (occasionally on trunk and extremities)

DDx – lichen spinulosus, pityriasis rubra pilaris, tinea, pityriasis alba, granulomatous diseases, and papulosquamous disorders, urticarial-like follicular mucinosis (head/neck on seborrheic background but neither follicular plugging nor alopecia present)

Histology

- Accumulation of mucin within follicular epithelium and sebaceous glands, causing keratinocytes to disconnect
- More advanced lesions → follicles converted into cystic spaces containing mucin, inflammatory cells, and altered keratinocytes. A perifollicular infiltrate of lymphocytes, histiocytes, and eosinophils are seen

Treatment

- Spontaneous healing may occur in idiopathic forms
- Topical and intralesional corticosteroids
- Antimalarials – hydroxychloroquine
- Minocycline
- Indomethacin
- Dapsone
- PUVA or UVA-1 phototherapy
- Oral isotretinoin

Pearls and Pitfalls

- Follow patients closely . Detection of clonal T-cell gene rearrangements does not seem to help differentiate between primary and secondary forms

Alopecia – Telogen Effluvium

Etiology and Pathogenesis

- Interval between precipitating event and the onset of shedding corresponds to the length of the telogen phase, usually 3 months (can be 1–6 months)
- Acute illness – febrile illness, severe infection, major surgery, severe trauma, etc.
- Chronic illness – malignancy (especially lymphoproliferative disorders), systemic lupus erythematosus, end-stage renal disease, liver disease, HIV
- Hormonal changes – pregnancy and delivery (can affect both mother and child), hypothyroidism, and discontinuation of estrogen-containing medications
- Changes in diet like crash dieting, anorexia, low protein intake, and chronic iron deficiency
- Sudden weight loss
- Heavy metals such as selenium, arsenic, and thallium
- Medications –
  - ACE-inhibitors, allopurinol, amphetamines, **anticoagulants,** azathioprine, **beta-blockers (especially propranolol),** boric acid, chloroquine, iodides, lithium, methysergide, contraceptives, **retinoids (including excess vitamin A), propylthiouracil (induces hypothyroidism), carbamazepine, and immunizations**
- Allergic contact dermatitis of the scalp

Clinical

- Thinning of hair which involves the entire scalp; sometimes in pubic and axillary regions
- Gentle hair pull may be positive for two or more hair shafts per pull → telogen hairs
- Forcible hair pluck (trichogram) → mix of normal anagen and telogen hairs; 20% or more telogen

Labs to Consider (based on history and physical) – CBC+diff, Ferritin, ESR, TIBC, TSH, free T4, RPR, 17-OH-testosterone, DHEA-S, Free and total testosterone, vitamin D

Other Tests

- The patient should be instructed to collect all hairs shed in a 24-h period on a non-shampoo day. Process should be repeated every other week, for a total of three or four collections

- Collections totaling 100 hairs or more in a given 24-h period are indicative of ongoing telogen effluvium. If the collections are performed over several weeks while the telogen effluvium is resolving, the number of hairs collected each time should decrease
- Scalp biopsy (**histology**):
  - ○ Normal total number of hairs and normal number of terminal hairs
  - ○ Increase in telogen count to greater than 20%
  - ○ Absence of inflammation and scarring
  - ○ Telogen count rarely exceeds 50%; greater than 80% inconsistent with telogen effluvium

Treatment

- Assess for etiology: Evaluate medication list, history, precipitating events, thyroid, anemia, etc.
- Minoxidil foam BID (men's)
- Biotin forte (3 mg) or Appearex (2.5 mg biotin)

Pearls and Pitfalls

- A chronic form of telogen effluvium can rarely occur and is a diagnosis of exclusion
- Regrowth takes months to years (in some cases)

Alopecia – Traction Alopecia

Etiology and Pathogenesis

- A form of mechanical, traumatic alopecia. Trauma is usually mild and chronic
- Most cases are caused by hairstyles involving tight braiding or banding of the hair, especially in AAF
- Biphasic form of hair loss
  - Initially the hair loss is temporary, hair regrowth occurs, and the condition behaves like a non-scarring form of alopecia. If excessive traction is maintained for years, the hair loss may eventually become permanent
  - There may be a lag period of a decade or more between the period of traction and the onset of permanent hair loss
    - Many AAF present in their 30s and 40s with a several-year history of persistent, bitemporal, or frontal hair loss
    - These women may deny having worn tight braids since childhood, although often other forms of traumatic styling (e.g., "curlers") have been employed

Clinical Presentation

- Peripheral or marginal form of alopecia involving the frontal, temporal, and parietal margins of the scalp; pruritus often present
- In girls who wear tight braids, perifollicular erythema and pustule formation may be seen

DDx – Alopeica areata, temporal triangular alopecia, trichotillomania, tinea capitis

Histology

- Early or acute disease
  - Normal size of follicles
  - Total number of hairs (both terminal and vellus) is normal
  - Most prominent finding is ↑ number of catagen and/or telogen hairs
  - Trichomalacia and pigment casts occasionally found
  - Incomplete, disrupted follicular anatomy rarely found
  - No significant inflammation (peribulbar inflammation absent)

- End-stage or "burnt out" disease
  - Marked ↓ in total # of follicles, terminal follicles, with retention of vellus hairs
  - Dermal collagen relatively normal; occ fibrous tracts at sites of former follicles
  - Many or most follicular units still have associated sebaceous glands
  - No significant inflammation (peribulbar inflammation absent)

Treatment and Prevention

- Immediately after traction alopecia is diagnosed, any practices that exert traction on the hair must be discontinued
- Topical steroids can decrease inflammation
- Oral antibiotics that decrease inflammation – TCN, doxycycline, minocycline
- No treatment to reverse late-stage disease

Pearls and Pitfalls

- Patients often present to dermatology with other concerns, but traction alopecia is noted. Take advantage of the teachable moment and gently counsel the patient/ parents about this condition
- Parents often deny that hairstyles are "too tight", so a trial of wearing the hair down until the condition resolves may be helpful
- "Eyebrow test" – if the hairstyle literally raises the child's eyebrows, it is too tight

References:

(1) Sperling LC. An Atlas of Hair Pathology with Clinical Correlations. New York: Parthenon, 2003.
(2) Sperling LC. Alopecias. In: Bolognia, Jorizzo, Rapini (eds). Dermatology, 2nd edition. Spain: Mosby Elsevier, 2008: 997–8.

Alopecia – Trichotillomania

Etiology and Pathogenesis

- Impulse control disorder in DSM-IV
  1. Recurrent pulling out of one's hair resulting in noticeable hair loss
  2. An increasing sense of tension immediately before pulling out the hair or when attempting to resist the behavior
  3. Pleasure, gratification, or relief when pulling out the hair
  4. The disturbance is not better accounted for by another mental disorder and is not due to a general medical condition (e.g., dermatologic condition)
  5. The disturbance provokes clinically marked distress and/or impairment in occupational, social, or other areas of functioning
- May encompass a spectrum of patients who pull hair as a habit to those with impulse-control and personality disorder, body dysmorphic disorder, mental retardation or psychosis
  - Contrast to hair pulling which occurs in infancy and early childhood, where the behavior disappears with or without minimal treatment

Clinical Presentation

- Patchy or full alopecia of the scalp (and sometimes eyebrows, eyelashes)
- Areas of alopecia often have bizarre shapes, irregular borders, and contain hairs of varying lengths
- Plucking associated with hair shaft fractures making hair ends feel rough
- Can weekly shave a small area of involved scalp to demonstrate normal, dense regrowth

DDx – alopecia areata, tinea capitis

Histology

- Follicles are normal size and total number of hairs is normal
- Incomplete, disrupted follicular anatomy
- Trichomalacia and pigment casts
- Minimal inflammation
- Increased number of catagen and/or telogen hairs

Treatment

- Behavioral modification therapy
- Selective serotonin reuptake inhibitor (SSRI) such as fluvoxamine, fluoxetine, paroxetine, sertraline, citalopram, etc.
- Topical minoxidil to help regrow hair

Pearls and Pitfalls

- It is difficult to convince parents that the child is pulling out hair, as it is commonly not seen directly by them. A biopsy can be very helpful in convincing them if there is any question about the diagnosis

Alopecia – Other Types

Pressure-Induced Alopecia

- Occurs with prolonged contact in one position (usually the occipital scalp)
- Initially, see erythema and some induration → almost complete hair loss in demarcation area of pressure
- Usually see complete hair regrowth

Temporal Triangular Alopecia

- AKA – congenital triangular alopecia
- May present at birth or acquired during first decade of life
- Rarely occurs outside of the temporal area or presents during adulthood
- See "lancet-shaped" lesions which point superiorly and posteriorly
- Area appears hairless but actually has fine, vellus hairs
- The patches of alopecia persist for life
- Histology
  - Normal number of follicles, but almost all are vellus hairs
  - Inflammation absent
  - Epidermis, dermis, adnexae – normal

Congenital Atrichia with Papules

- Individuals shed all their hair shortly after birth and fail to regrow it
- Follicular cysts and milia-like lesions appear on skin later in life
- Associated with mutations in two different genes:
  - The *hairless gene*
  - The vitamin D receptor gene

Lipedematous Alopecia

- Thick boggy scalp associated with hair loss
- Usually seen in darker-skinned females
- See doubling of scalp thickness as a result of edema and expansion of the subcutaneous fat layer
  - Unclear how this leads to hair loss as follicular structures appear relatively normal but ectatic lymphatic vessels sometimes seen

Hair Shaft Abnormalities

Table 5   Hair shaft disorders characterized by hair fragility

Increased fragility
Trichorrhexis nodosa
Trichoschisis
Trichorrhexis invaginata
Pili torti
Monilethrix
Without increased fragility
Pili annulati
Loose anagen hair syndrome
Uncombable hair syndrome

Trichorrhexis Nodosa (TN)

- Beaded swellings with loss of cuticle and frayed "paintbrushes" against each other
- Seen in → excessive perming and chemical treatments, mechanical trauma
- Genetic disorders
    1. **Argininosuccinic aciduria** – 50% have TN. Defect in urea synthesis (argininosuccinate lyase deficiency)
        - Seizures, neurologic damage, growth retardation, coma from ↑ ammonia
        - Hair usually normal at birth with development of dull, dry hair and TN in infancy and early childhood
        - Labs – ↓ serum arginine and ↑ citrulline (serum and urine)
        - Mutations in ASL gene, autosomal recessive
    2. **Citrullinemia** – defect in urea synthesis (argininosuccinic acid synthetase)
        - Infantile onset – TN, atrophic hair bulbs, and/or pili torti. Some get rash similar to acrodermatitis enteropathica. Clinical similar to argininosuccinic aciduria.
        - Adult onset – argininosuccinic acid synthetase is liver-specific with an abnormal transporter protein citrin

Trichoschisis

- Clean, transverse fracture of the hair shaft
- Low cysteine (sulfur) content of hair is postulated to account for cuticular and cortical weakness
- Usually seen on light microscopy
- Polarized light – "tiger tail" of alternating bright and dark diagonal bands; its absence does not exclude diagnosis

- Genetic disorders
  1. **Trichothiodystrophy** (TTD) – AR
     - Brittle hair and low sulfur content of hair
     - Trichoschisis is common finding
     - Involvement of all body hair reported
     - Eight subgroups:
       □ BIDS – brittle hair, intellectual impairment, decreased fertility, short stature
       □ IBIDS – BIDS + ichthyosis
       □ PIBIDS – IBIDS + photosensitivity
       □ SIBIDS – IBIDS + osteosclerosis
       □ ONMR – onychotrichodysplasia, chronic neutropenia, mental retardation
       □ Tay, sabinas, and pollitt syndromes
  2. **TTD, Photosensitivity, and Impaired DNA**
     - DNA repair defects linked to defects in nucleotide excision repair (NER)
     - 95% of patients with TTD and photosensitivity and NER have xeroderma pigmentosum complement group D
       □ Some have xeroderma pigmentosum type B and defects in TTD-A gene
- NOT at increased risk for developing skin cancer
  3. **Non-photosensitive TTD** → Amish brittle-hair syndrome and non-photosensitive TTD with mental retardation and/or decreased fertility

Trichorrhexis Invaginata

- Bamboo hair or "golf-tee" hair (distal hair shaft invaginates into proximal hair shaft)
- Genetic disorders:
  1. **Netherton syndrome** – SPINK5 – encodes serine protease inhibitor LEKTI
     - Triad – ichthyosis linearis circumflexa, trichorrhexis invaginata, atopic diathesis
     - Usually appears in infancy, may be born with collodion membrane, generalized scaling or erythema
     - Scalp hair short and brittle. Eyebrows may be affected. Hair breakage may improve with age
     - Many patients – atopic derm, hay fever, food allergies, angioedema, urticarial, allergic rhinitis, hypereosinophilia, recurrent skin infections, ↑ IgE
     - Failure to thrive, recurrent infections, and dehydration (may be due to impaired epidermal barrier)
     - EM – premature lamellar body secretion in stratum corneum

- Treatment
  - □ Use topical medications with *extreme caution* – meds absorbed very easily and can cause systemic toxicity
  - □ Use of oral retinoids has yielded mixed results

Pili Torti

- Characterized by hair shafts which are flattened and twist with an angle of 180°
- Fractures occur within the twists, which is weakest point
- Early auditory testing important in all kids with pili torti
  1. **Classic PT** – presents in first 2 years of life. Inheritance – AD, AR, or sporadic
  2. **Late-onset PT** – AD, onset in childhood, or after puberty. Caucasian patient with black unruly hair. Mental deficiency. Typically presents with breakage of eyebrows and eyelashes
  3. **PT and hearing loss → Björnstad syndrome and Crandall syndrome**
     - **Björnstad syndrome** – congenital sensorineural hearing loss and PT; BCS1L mutation
     - **Crandall syndrome** – hearing loss, PT, hypogonadism. MR rare. Typically develop symptoms in first 2 years of life and hearing loss by age 4. Severity of hair shaft abnormalities correlates with severity of deafness
  4. **PT and ectodermal dysplasias** – widely spaced teeth and enamel hypoplasia, acrofacial dysostosis, tooth agenesis, arthrogryposis, nail dystrophy, clefting, corneal opacities, ichthyosis, hypohidrotic ectodermal dysplasia
  5. **Menkes syndrome** – XLR; gene ATP7A
     - Defective copper export from cells with normal copper absorption into cells
     - Primary finding is pili torti, but can get trichorrhexis nodosa
     - Skin and hair hypopigmentation, progressive neurodegeneration, MR, soft doughy skin, joint laxity, vascular abnormalities (aneurysms), and bladder diverticula
     - Hair – short, sparse, brittle, depigmented. Looks like steel wool
     - Labs – ↓ serum copper and ↓ ceruloplasmin
     - Tx – infusions with copper-histidine. Increases serum copper levels and can permit survival into adolescence. Many die secondary to neurodegeneration and oral failure

Monilethrix

- Beaded hair – elliptical nodes at regular intervals with intervening, nonmedullated tapered fragile constrictions
- Usually AD and presents in early childhood

- Hairs rarely grow beyond 1–2 cm in length because of breakage → gives stubbly appearance
- Common – keratotic follicular papules at base of nape of neck, keratosis pilaris and TN
- Light microscopy – nodes and internodes
- EM – at internodes, see increased longitudinal ridging with fluting
- Treatment
    - Topical minoxidil and oral retinoids reported to improve hair growth but no specific tx

Pili Annulati

- Characteristic alternating light and dark bands in hair shaft on clinical and microscopic exam
- Thought to be due to abnormal air cavities in hair shaft
- Appears at birth or in infancy
- Hair is NOT brittle – growth of scalp hair usually normal
- May affect axillae, beard, pubic regions
- No treatment necessary

Pili Trianguli et Canaliculi

- Entire hair shaft is rigid with longitudinal grooving. Cross section = triangular shape
    1. **Uncombable Hair Syndrome** – "Spun glass hair". May be result of premature keratinization of triangular-shaped inner root sheath caused by abnormally shaped dermal papilla
        - Scalp has>50% involvement
        - Hair shafts not twisted as in pili torti
        - Usually manifests in childhood
        - Associated problems are rare → cataracts, anomalies in bone development, alopecia areata, pili torti, and lichen sclerosus
        - Hair manageability tends to improve with age
        - Tx – may respond to biotin

Woolly Hair

- Hairs are tightly curled; can also contain wide twists over several mm along its own longitudinal axis
- Increased hair fragility, trichorrhexis nodosa, trichoschisis, and pili annulati
- Hair growth is normal (1 cm/month) but hair shafts ovoid, flattened, or irregular

- Dominant form
  - Usually affects entire scalp; seen at birth or in first few months
  - Can have pili torti, pili annulati, ocular problems, keratosis pilaris
- Recessive form
  - Fragile and fine hair which is light/blond in color at birth
  - Hair may not grow beyond few cm – likely due to shortened anagen phase
- With Cardiac disease
  1. **Naxos disease** – AR, plakoglobin
     - Woolly hair usually presents at birth
     - Palmoplantar keratoderma develops during childhood
     - Right ventricular cardiomyopathy (arrhythmogenic) – presents in adolescence or early adulthood
  2. **Carvajal syndrome** – AR, desmoplakin
     - Biventricular dilated cardiomyopathy
     - Palmoplantar keratoderma
     - Woolly hair
  3. **Naxos-like disease** – AR
     - Right ventricular cardiomyopathy (arrhythmogenic)
     - Woolly hair
     - Early-onset blistering on knees/palms/soles and dry skin
     - Skin biopsy of blister sites look like pemphigus foliaceus
- Without Cardiac disease
  1. **Woolly hair and skin fragility syndrome**
     - Similar to Naxos-like disease but NO cardiac problems
     - Recurrent *Staph aureus* on palms and soles
     - Dystrophic nails, woolly hair, focal and diffuse PPK, early onset blistering
  2. **Diffuse partial woolly hair** – AD
     - Hair is short, fine, kinky
     - Ocular problems reported
  3. **Woolly hair nevus**
     - Affects localized part of the scalp and typically presents in first 2 years of life
     - Hair is usually thinner and lighter compared to adjacent hairs
     - 50% of cases associated with epidermal or congenital nevus, usually located ipsilaterally on neck or arm
     - Also reported – bone abnormalities, precocious puberty, speech and dental anomalies

Other Hair Shaft Disorders

- **Loose anagen syndrome**
  - Anagen hairs lack inner root sheath and external root sheath
  - Ruffled cuticles that are easily pulled from scalp

- ○ Clinical – most patients are blond girls (older than 2) who never need a haircut. May persist into adulthood. Hair is not typically brittle and of normal strength
- **Mitochondrial disorders**
  - ○ May see trichorrhexis nodosa, trichorrhexis, longitudinal grooving, trichoschisis, pili torti
- **Marie Unna Hypotrichosis** – AD
  - ○ Have normal to coarse sparse hair and eyebrows
  - ○ Develop coarsening within first few years
  - ○ Eyebrows, eyelashes, axillary hair also affected
  - ○ Scalp – hair loss starts in parietal and vertex. Partial sparing of occipital scalp

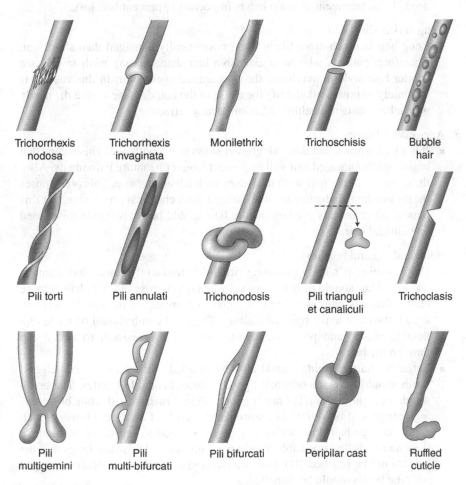

Trichorrhexis nodosa   Trichorrhexis invaginata   Monilethrix   Trichoschisis   Bubble hair

Pili torti   Pili annulati   Trichonodosis   Pili trianguli et canaliculi   Trichoclasis

Pili multigemini   Pili multi-bifurcati   Pili bifurcati   Peripilar cast   Ruffled cuticle

Fig. 1 Hair shaft anomalies

Hair Tips

(From Dr. Zoe Draelos)

There are many causes of hair loss including disease and genetic predisposition. Yet, the most common reason men and women experience hair loss is due to poor cosmetic grooming practices.

1. Scalp scratching
   - Even though mild-to-moderate seborrheic dermatitis does not cause hair loss, the scratching associated with the scalp pruritus can definitely predispose to hair loss. It is possible to remove all of the cuticular scale off of a hair shaft with only 90 min of continuous scratching by the fingernails. This loss of cuticle leaves the hair shaft weakened and permanently cosmetically damaged. Thus, treatment of scalp itch is important to prevent hair loss.

2. Long versus short hair
   - Long hair is much more likely to be cosmetically damaged than short hair. Therefore, patients who have extensive hair damage may wish to select a shorter hair style to maximize the appearance of the hair. In this case, it is extremely important to identify the cause of the hair damage so that the newly grown hair remains healthy and cosmetically attractive.

3. Age-related factors
   - It is a well-known fact that hair growth slows down with age. This means that cosmetically damaged hair will be present longer on mature individuals. Also, the diameter of the hair shaft decreases with advancing age. This predisposes the thinner hair shafts to chemical damage from chemical processing. For this reason, all chemicals used on mature hair should be weaker than those used on youthful hair.

4. Hair combing and brushing
   - Hair combing is a daily grooming ritual that frequently causes hair damage and loss. Hair should only be combed when dry, if possible. Wet hair is more elastic than dry hair, meaning that vigorous combing of the moist fibers can stretch the shaft to the point of fracture. The ideal comb should be made of a flexible plastic and possess smooth, rounded, coarse teeth to easily slip through the hair.
   - Extensive hair brushing should also be avoided while hair is wet. A good brush should have smooth, ball-tipped, coarse, bendable bristles. The brush should not tear the hair, but rather gently glide. Brushes used while blow drying hair should be vented to prevent increased heat along the brush, which could damage hair. Patients should be encouraged to brush and manipulate their hair as little as possible to minimize breakage. Older teachings that the hair should be brushed 100 strokes a day and the scalp vigorously massaged with the brush should be dispelled.

5. Hair clasps
   - Common sense applies to the selection of appropriate hair pins and clasps. Rubber bands should never be used; hair pins should have a smooth, ball-tipped surface; and hair clasps should have a spongy rubber padding where they contact the hair. Loose-fitting clasps also minimize breakage. The fact remains, however, that all hair pins or clasps break some hair since they must hold the hair tightly to stay in place. To minimize this problem, the patient should be encouraged to vary the clasp placement so that hair break-age is not localized to one scalp area. This problem is particularly apparent in women who wear a ponytail. These women frequently state that their hair is no longer growing when in actuality it is repeatedly broken at the same distance from the scalp due to hair clasp trauma. Pulling the hair tightly with clasps or braids can also precipitate traction alopecia.

6. Hair shaft architecture
   - It is important to remember that curlier hair tends to fracture more readily than straight hair. For this reason, hair shaft architecture can determine how aggressively the hair can be groomed. The kinky hair of African-American patients should be gently groomed with a wide-toothed comb or hair pick. Only Asian hair can be combed with minimal friction and hair shaft damage.

7. Hair cutting techniques
   - The hair should always be cut with sharp scissors. Any defect in the scissor blade will crush and damage the hair shaft. Crushing the end of the hair shaft predisposes to split ends.

8. Hair styling product use
   - Hair styling products are an important way to improve the cosmetic appear-ance of the hair shaft, but should always leave the hair shaft flexible. High hold stiff styling products can actually precipitate hair breakage when trying to restyle the hair with combing.

9. Hair styling techniques
   - In general, the less that is done to the hair, the healthier it will be. There is no hair style or procedure that can reverse hair damage, even though many salon owners would disagree. Hair is basically a textile. It works the best when new and degrades with age and use.

10. Hair coloring and bleaching
   - Hair coloring and bleaching are universally damaging to the hair shaft. It is sometimes said that chemical processing adds body to the hair. This means that the dyeing procedure allows the hair to stand away from the scalp with greater ease. This is not due to better hair health, but rather due to hair damage that makes the hair frizzy and more susceptible to static electric-ity. The basic rules of hair dyeing are always stay within your color group, preferably dyeing the hair no more than three shades from the natural color.

11. Hair relaxing
    ▪ Hair relaxing is weakening to the hair shaft, but can actually facilitate hair length in patients with kinky hair. This is due to decreased hair breakage during combing. The relaxing procedure straightens the hair and makes it easier to groom, but the grooming should be done gently to avoid hair shaft fracture.

12. Hair permanent waving
    ▪ Lastly, hair permanent waving is also damaging. The curls should be as loose as possible with the interval between procedures as long as possible. For patients with damaged hair, the perming solution should be weak and left in contact with the hair for as short a period as possible.

Shampoos and Hair Products

- Telogen Effluvium
  ○ Focus on hairspray for body and not stiffness
  ○ Gel
- Seborrheic Dermatitis
  ○ Head and shoulders – good for mild seb derm, good for prolonging disease-free episodes. Good technology
  ○ Nizoral 2% – effective, but can be very drying. Use with conditioners
- Women of Color
  ○ Pantene brown bottle
  ○ Keracare
- Colored hair
  ○ A color protectant shampoo and conditioner such as L'Oreal Vive
  ○ L'Oreal Vive (shampoo and conditioner) or other UV protectant
- Fine hair
  ○ AVOID Pantene
  ○ Use dimethicone-based products → will smooth cuticle, hair is shiny, looks more voluminous

Hypertrichosis

Etiology and Pathogenesis

- May be congenital or acquired, generalized or localized
- Other causes – medications, malignancy

Clinical Presentation

- Excessive amount of hair on any part of the body
- **Acquired Generalized** – the presence of lanugo hair, excessive vellus hair or terminal hair on much of the body. May sometimes see transformation of terminal hairs into lanugo hair
  - ○ Lanugo hair = nonpigmented, nonmedullated fine hair that covers the fetus. Normally shed in utero or in first few weeks of life. Replaced by vellus hair on the body and terminal hair on the scalp
  - ○ **Acquired hypertrichosis lanuginosa** (paraneoplastic)
    - ▪ Variety of malignancies – lung, colon, breast
    - ▪ Lanugo hair develops over body in short period of time
    - ▪ May be associated with burning tongue pain and other paraneoplastic dermatoses
  - ○ **Prepubertal hypertrichosis**
    - ▪ Relatively common in otherwise healthy children – usually Mediterranean or South Asian descent
    - ▪ Bushy eyebrows, low anterior hairline, hair on forehead, temples, preauricular area, proximal extremities, and back
    - ▪ Some have slightly elevated androgen levels
  - ○ **Acquired generalized hypertrichosis**
    - ▪ Often related to drug ingestion and typically reversible if drug stopped. Slow growth of terminal hair. Most evident on forehead, temples, flexoral extremities and trunk
      - □ Drugs often associated – acetazolamide, ACTH, anabolic steroids, benoxaprofen, cetuximab, **cyclosporine**, danazol, diazoxide, fenoterol, glucocorticosteroids, hexachlorobenzene, IFN-α, methoxypsoralen, **minoxidil,** penicillamine, **phenytoin**, prostaglandin E1, streptomycin, testosterone, trimethylpsoralen
      - □ Other etiologies – CNS disorder (traumatic brain disorder), POEMS syndrome, juvenile hypothyroidism, juvenile dermatomyositis, acrodynia, malnutrition, advanced HIV
- **Acquired Localized**
  - ○ **Trichomegaly** HIV, medications (cyclosporine, topiramate, latanoprost, bimatoprost, IFN- α, cetuximab, gefitinib), hypothyroidism, porphyrias, dermatomyositis, SLE, malnutrition, anorexia nervosa, kala-azar

- ○ **Other** – trauma, friction, irritation, vaccination sites, overlying lipoatrophy, healing psoriasis and morphea, PUVA, topical steroids or tacrolimus, anthralin, creams with mercury or iodine
- **Congenital Generalized**, evaluate for:

  - ○ Maternal drug/alcohol intake
  - ○ Family history of hypertrichosis
  - ○ Orofacial, skeletal, ocular or neurologic abnormalities

Table 6 Congenital conditions associated with generalized hypertrichosis

Acromegaly + hypertrichosis	AD, acromegaloid facies, hypertrichosis
Amaurosis congenital, cone-rod type + hypertrichosis	AR, photophobia, visual impairment due to retinal dystrophy, hypertrichosis
Ambras syndrome	AD. Fine, silky, long hair (>10 cm) uniformly distributed on face (including nose), ears, and shoulders. Persists for life. Minor facial dysmorphism, dental anomalies, supernumerary nipples
Barber-Say syndrome	AD, Hypertrichosis especially of the back, skin hyperlaxity and redundancy, facial dysmorphism, hypoplastic nipples
Beradinelli-Seip syndrome	Lipodystrophy, high TG, insulin resistance, fatty liver, cardiomyopathy, muscular appearance, hypertrichosis. Two types
CAHMR syndrome	AR, Cataracts, Hypertrichosis, MR
Cantu syndrome	AD, Hypertrichosis, cardiac anomalies, wide ribs, gingival hyperplasia, coarse facies, macrosomia at birth
Coffin Siris syndrome	Hypoplasia/aplasis of fifth phalanx and fifth fingernails, MR, generalized hypertrichosis, scalp hypotrichosis
Congenital hypertrichosis lanuginosa	AD, fine, downy, silvery-gray lanugo hair. May be shed over first year of life. Occasional dental anomalies. Can lead to "dog face" or "monkey face"
Cornelia de Lange	Hypertrichosis, synophrys, low-set ears, microcephaly, hearing loss, short stature, problems with digestive tract, skeletal problems
Craniofacial dysostoses	Various types. Hypertrichosis may be assoc
Donohue syndrome	AKA – Leprechaunism. Lipodystrophy, hypertrichosis, insulin resistance, acanthosis nigricans, endocrine problems
Erythropoietic porphyria	Ferrochelatase defect, photosensitivity in childhood and hepatobiliary disease. Hyper-trichosis may occur, waxy scarring on sun-exposed areas
Familial porphyria cutanea tarda	Hypertrichosis common on face, blisters, milia
Fetal alcohol syndrome	Failure to thrive, decreased muscle tone, heart defects, hypertrichosis, structural issues (face)
Fetal hydantoin syndrome	Caused by phenytoin, skull and facial abnormalities, underdeveloped nails, cleft lip and palate, developmental delays

(continued)

Table 6 (continued)

Gingival fibromatosis with hypertrichosis	AD, dark terminal hairs on peripheral face, central back and extremities. Have gingival hyperplasia, coarse facies, MR, seizures
Hemimaxillofacial dysplasia	Unilateral enlargement of the maxillary alveolar bone and the gingiva associated with hypoplastic teeth, facial asymmetry, and hypertrichosis of the facial skin on the ipsilateral side
Hepatoerythropoietic porphyria	Severe photosensitivity, hemolytic anemia, hypertrichosis on arms, splenomegaly, dark urine at birth
Hunter syndrome	Mucopolysaccharidosis. Lack iduronate sulfatase. Spasticity, MR, aggressive behavior, hypertrichosis, coarse facial features
Hurler syndrome	Mucopolysaccharidosis. Lack lysosomal alpha-L-iduronidase. Heart problems, cloudy cornea, hypertrichosis, MR, coarse facial features
MELAS syndrome	Mitochondrial myopathy, encephalopathy, lactic acidosis, and stroke (MELAS)=progressive neurodegenerative disorder. Lactic acidosis, cardiac issues, hypertrichosis, diabetes and endocrinopathies, short stature
Rubinstein-Taybi syndrome	Broad thumbs and toes, constipation, hypertrichosis, heart defects, slow motor skills
Sanfilippo syndrome	Mucopolysaccharidosis. Most common MPS. Types A-D. Coarse facial features, synophrys, MR, full lips, sleep difficulties, walking problems
Schinzel-Giedion syndrome	*SETBP1* gene defect. Midface retraction, hypertrichosis, multiple skeletal anomalies, cardiac and renal problems (hydronephrosis)
Stiff skin syndrome	Scleroderma-like disorder that presents in infancy or early childhood with rock-hard skin, limited joint mobility, mild hypertrichosis in the absence of visceral or muscle involvement, immunologic abnormalities, or vascular hyperreactivity
Universal Hypertrichosis	AD. Thicker, longer hair on frontal, temporal and preauricular areas of face, back and lower extremities. Increases during infancy and tends to persist
Winchester syndrome	Dwarfism (resulting from disturbances of the skeletal–articular system), corneal opacities, coarsening of facial features, leathery skin, hypertrichosis
X-linked Hypertrichosis	XR. Curly, shorter, dark hair most prominent on face and upper body. Anteverted nostrils, prognathism, occasional dental anomalies, deafness
Zimmerman-Laband syndrome	AD, gingival hyperplasia, coarse facies, hypoplastic nails and distal phalanges, joint hyperextensibility, macrosomia at birth, MR, hepatosplenomegaly, hypertrichosis

- **Congenital localized hypertrichosis**
  - Can affect specific anatomic sites – elbows, palms/soles, auricle, eyebrows, eyelashes, nasal tip, anterior cervical, posterior cervical
  - **Synophrys**
    - Isolated trait, Waardenburg syndrome, Cornelia de Lange, Zimmerman-Laband, Amaurosis congenital (cone-rod type), mucopolysaccharidoses
  - **Trichomegaly**
    - Isolated trait, Oliver-McFarlane, Cornelia de Lange, Rubinstein-Taybi, Ambras, congenital hypertrichosis lanuginosa, Cantu, Coffin-Siris, Barber-Say, Amaurosis congenital (cone-rod type), Hermansky-Pudlak, Kabuki and floating harbor syndromes, fetal alcohol syndrome
  - **Distichiasis (double row of eyelashes)**
    - Lymphedema-distichiasis syndrome, Setleis syndrome (double upper and absent lower eyelashes)
  - **Other –** Congenital nevi, Plexiform neurofibromas, Becker's nevus, Nevoid Hypertrichosis, Spinal dysraphism
  - **"Hair collar sign"** – ring of hypertrichosis surrounding aplasia cutis or ectopic neural tissue in scalp reflect incomplete neural tube defects

Labs – dependent on potential etiologies. Usually not necessary for hypertrichosis, but can be useful in hirsutism

DDx – Hirsutism

Treatment

- Depilatory creams – especially those containing barium sulfate
- Electrolysis
- Hair removal via laser – ruby, Nd:YAG, diode and alexandrite lasers
- Shaving
- Plucking
- Eflornithine cream 13.9% (Vaniqa) – inhibits ornithine decarboxylase and slows hair growth

Pearls and Pitfalls

- Depilatory creams containing barium sulfate are more effective than those containing calcium thioglycolate but also tend to be more irritating. Test a small area first
- Laser treatment and creams not typically covered by insurance plans

Hirsutism

Etiology and Pathogenesis

- Women with excessive growth of terminal hairs in a *"male pattern"* due to androgen overproduction (ovaries or adrenal glands) or increased sensitivity to androgens
- Ethnic differences – Asian women tend to have little body and facial hair, while Middle Eastern, Mediterranean, and East Indian women have moderate amounts
- **Ovarian origin** – PCOS, insulin resistance, HAIR-AN, hyperthecosis, ovarian tumors
  - ↑progesterone, Δ-4-androstenedione, and testosterone
- **Pituitary origin** – Cushing's disease, acromegaly, hyperprolactinemia, pituitary adenoma (secreting prolactin), psychogenic drugs (dopamine inhibits prolactin), and contraceptive pills (stimulate adrenal androgen production)
  - ↑ACTH → stimulates adrenals to produce ↑ androgens and cortisol
- **Adrenal origin** – Classic congenital adrenal hyperplasia, nonclassical (late-onset) congenital adrenal hyperplasia, Cushing's syndrome, adrenal tumors (adenomas and CA)
  - ↑ DHEA and DHEA-S
  - **Constitutional hirsutism** – May reflect familial ↑ response to normal levels of androgens
  - **Hepatic hirsutism** – SHBG made in liver. Liver disease → ↓ SHBG available → ↑ free testosterone and thus conversion to DHT may also be greater
- **Hirsutism due to ectopic hormone production** – ectopic ACTH secretion by tumors such as lung CA (especially small-cell) and carcinoids or production of β-HCG by choriocarcinomas
- **Drug-induced hirsutism**
  - Androgenic medications – testosterone, danazole, ACTH, metyrapone, phenothiazine,
  - Anabolic steroids
  - Androgenic progestins – levonorgestrel, norgestrel, norethindrone
  - Valproic acid – ↑ plasma testosterone
- **Hirsutism due to peripheral failure in converting androgens into estrogens**
- **Pregnancy** – aromatase deficiency in fetus, luteoma of pregnancy, hyperreactio luteinalis

Clinical Features

- Increased amount of hair in male pattern; may be accompanied by acne, seborrhea, androgenetic alopecia
- **Proposed diagnostic criteria for PCOS (Need two of three for diagnosis)**
  - ○ Oligo- or anovulation (< eight menses/year or cycles > 35 days)
  - ○ Clinical and/or biochemical signs of hyperandrogenism
  - ○ Polycystic ovaries and exclusion of other etiologies (Cushing's syndrome, congenital adrenal hyperplasia, androgen-secreting tumors) Source = 2003 Rotterdam PCOS consensus. Fertil Steril 2004; 81:19–25.
- **PCOS features**
  - ○ **Skin** – SAHA – seborrhea, acne, hirsutism, alopecia (androgenetic)
  - ○ **Menstrual** – oligomenorrhea, amenorrhea, anovulation and infertility, polycystic ovaries in 80–100%, dysfunctional uterine bleeding, theoretical risk for endometrial CA
  - ○ **Metabolic** – obesity common (BMI > 30), impaired glucose tolerance, type II diabetes, hyperlipidemia, ↑ risk of CV disease, sleep apnea
  - ○ **Labs** – ↓SHBG, LH:FSH > 2 (suggestive but low sense and specificity), ↑ testosterone, ↑ free testosterone, ↑ DHEAS, abnormal glucose tolerance, ↑ TG and elevated LDL:HDL ratio

Table 7 Clinical and laboratory features of hirsutism

Cause of Hirsutism	Clinical Hx	Menstrual Hx	Testosterone	DHEAS	17-OHP	LH/FSH	Cortisol	Prolactin	Comments
Acromegaly	Coarse facies, large hands, ring size keeps changing, HA, visual disturbance		NL to ↑	NL	NL	NL	NL	NL to ↑ (in 40%)	**Tests**=Somatomedin-C (IGF-1) level, head MRI
CAH (late-onset) – CYP21A2	Acne, hirsutism, premature puberty, family history of infertility and hirsutism	Irregular, primary amenorrhea	NL to ↑	NL to ↑	↑	NL/NL	NL to ↑	NL	**Tests**=↑ 17-hydroxyprogesterone, consider ACTH stim test, wrist x-ray (accel bone age)
Cushing's Disease	Fatigue, recurrent infections, mood and sleep disturbance, acne, hirsutism, alopecia, striae, fat redistribution	Irregular	NL to ↑	NL to ↑	NL	NL	↑	NL	**Tests**=↑24-h urine cortisol and overnight dexamethasone suppression test, evening ACTH level, CRH stim test; **Risks** – CV dz, osteoporosis, hypokalemia
HAIR-AN	Acne, hirsutism, insulin resist, obesity, acanthosis nigricans, HTN	Irregular	NL to ↑ >200 ng/dL	NL to ↑	NL	NL to ↑ LH	NL	NL	**Risks**=CV dz, diabetes, HTN, infertility. **Tests**=lipids, glucose tolerance test
Idiopathic	Mild Hirsutism	Regular	NL or sl ↑	NL	NL	NL/NL	NL	NL	
Neoplasm – Adrenal	Sudden onset, older age, signs of virilization, palpable abdominal mass	May be menopausal (since likely in older patients), irregular	↑ >200 ng/dL	↑ >700 ug/dL	NL	NL/NL	NL to ↑	NL	**Tests**=transvaginal u/s, CT or MRI of abdomen and pelvis
Neoplasm – Ovarian			↑ >200 ng/dL	NL	NL	NL/NL	NL	NL	**Tests**=androstendione >100 ng/dL, Imaging, as above
PCOS	Seborrhea, acne, hirsutism (variable), alopecia, acanthosis nigricans, obesity (some), HTN	Irregular	NL to ↑	NL to ↑	NL	NL to >2:1 ratio	NL	NL to ↑	**Risks**=CV, diabetes, HTN, infertility, endometrial CA; **Tests**=transvaginal u/s, ↓ SHBG, glucose tolerance, lipids
Prolactinemia	Galactorrhea	Amenorrhea	NL to ↑	NL to ↑	NL	NL	NL	NL to ↑	**Test**=Head MRI
Thyroid	Alopecia, weight change, heat or cold intol	May be irregular	NL	NL	NL	NL	NL	NL to ↑	**Tests**=TSH, free T4, thyroid antimicrosomal Ab

Table 8 Useful screening labs for patients with hirsutism

Lab	Evaluate for …
Testosterone (free and total)	PCOS, nonclassical CAH, HAIR-AN, androgen-secreting neoplasms and hirsutism associated with hyperandrogenism
Sex hormone binding globulin (SHBG)	PCOS
Dehydroepiandrosterone-sulfate (DHEA-S)	Nonclassical CAH, PCOS, androgen-secreting adrenal tumors
Δ-4-androstenedione	Ovarian origin
3-α-androstanediol gluronide (metabolite of DHT)	
17-Hydroxyprogesterone	Nonclassical CAH
	* get in early AM between first day of menses and ovulation
Prolactin	Reason for anovulation
Thyroid	Reason for anovulation
LH, FSH	Ovarian
Somatomedin-c	acromegaly
Transvaginal ultrasound	PCOS
24-h urine cortisol	Cushing's syndrome
ACTH level, evening	Cushing's syndrome
ACTH stimulation test • Should be started between 0730 and 0930 in a fasting state and scheduled on day 3–8 after a spontaneous vaginal bleed or after induced withdrawal bleed • Three baseline samples of 17-hydroxyprogesterone should be obtained 15 min apart and pooled • Subsequently, 0.25 mg ACTH (cosyntropin) is administered IV over 60 s • 17-hydroxyprogesterone should be measured again 60 min later • If the 17-hydroxyprogesterone level is stimulated above 10 ng/ml, the diagnosis of C21-hydroxylase-deficient CAH is confirmed	Nonclassical CAH
Dexamethasone suppression test – overnight	Cushing's syndrome
CRH stimulation test	Cushing's syndrome

DDx – hypertrichosis

Treatment

Table 9 Medications commonly used for hirsutism

Drug type	Active ingredient	Major mechanism	Indication	Contraindication	Dose
Cell-cycle Inhibitor – *Vaniqa*	Eflornithine hydrochloride, 13.9%	Irreversible inhibition of ornithine decarboxylase	Focal hirsutism	Pregnancy, lactating	Topical, BID
Oral contraceptives – *Yasmin* – *Yaz* – *Orthocyclen* – *Demulen 1–50*	Ethinyl estradiol 30 μg + drospirenone 35 μg + norgestimate 50 μg + ethynodiol diacetate	Suppresses ovarian fxn	Generalized hirsutism	Breast cancer, smoking (absolutely if age >35 year), CVD, uncontrolled HTN	1 tablet PO QHS (larger estrogen doses may be necessary in heavier women for menstrual regularity)
Anti-androgens (need reliable birth control)	Spironolactone	Competitive inhibitor of androgen receptor binding	Moderate or severe hirsutism	Lack of contraception, kidney or liver failure	50–200 mg/day by mouth, × 6 months
	Cyproterone acetate	Competitive inhibitor of androgen receptor binding	Moderate or severe hirsutism	Lack of contraception	*Induction:* 50–100 mg PO QHS, days 5–15 *Maintenance:* 5 mg PO QHS, days 5–15
	Flutamide	Nonsteroidal competitive inhibitor of androgen receptor binding	Severe hirsutism	Lack of contraception, liver disease	125–500 mg BID for 6–9 months. Low doses of 62.5–125 mg can be used
Glucocorticoids *Prednisone*	Glucocorticoid	Suppresses adrenal function	Congenital adrenal hyperplasia	Uncontrolled diabetes, obesity	Prednisone 7.5 mg QD × 2 months, 5 mg QD × 2 months, 2.5 mg QD × 6 months Dexamethasone 0.5 mg QHS × 3 months then q other night × 3 months
Gonadotropin-releasing agents *Lupron Depot*	Leuprolide acetate, depot suspension	Suppresses gonadotropins	Reserved for severe cases and HAIR-AN	Osteoporosis	7.5 mg monthly IM, with 25–50 μg transdermal estradiol or 3.75 mg q 28 days × 6 months

Reference: Used with permission from Elsevier. Rosenfield RL. Hirsutism. N Engl J Med 2005; 353: 2578–88

Pearls and Pitfalls

– If hirsutism appears rapidly, suspect and rule out a tumor (ovarian, adrenal, pituitary)
– Suspect ovarian source if → hirsutism mainly on areola, lateral face, and neck
– Suspect adrenal source if → hirsutism mainly distributed from pubic triangle to upper abdomen and from presternal region to neck and chin
– Suspect iatrogenic source if → hair on lateral face and on back (but can spread with time)
– Suspect Androgen-secreting tumor if …
  ○ Total testosterone > 200 ng/dl or DHEA-S of > 700 ug/dl
  ○ Imaging studies should be performed to localize the neoplasm
– Refer to endocrinology and/or gynecology if workup is significantly abnormal

Nail Disorders

Clubbing

Etiology and Pathogenesis

- Caused by enlargement of the soft tissue of the distal digit

Table 10 Conditions associated with clubbing

Congenital	Congenital heart disease (usually cyanotic)
	Cystic fibrosis
	Pachydermoperiostosis
	Pulmonary AV malformation (often in setting of hereditary hemorrhagic telangiectasia)
Acquired	Asthma complicated by lung infections
	Bronchiectasis
	Chronic infection (abscesses of lungs, tuberculosis)
	Cirrhosis
	Congestive heart failure
	Diamond's syndrome (myxedema, exophthalmos, clubbing)
	Endocarditis (bacterial)
	HIV infection
	Hypervitaminosis A
	Inflammatory bowel disease
	Laxative abuse
	Malignant neoplasm (primary or metastatic to lungs)
	Malnutrition
	Parasites (GI) – amebiasis, ascariasis
	POEMS syndrome
	Pulmonary fibrosis
	Sarcoidosis
	Secondary hyperparathyroidism
	Thyroid disease (especially hyperthyroidism)

(continued)

Table 10   (continued)

Limited to one or more digits	Aneurysm or dialysis fistula (unilateral)
	Arterial graft sepsis (clubbing limited to perfused extremities)
	Brachial plexus injury
	Gout
	Hemiplegia (unilateral)
	Maffucci's syndrome
	Sarcoidosis
	Severe herpetic whitlow
	Trauma

Clinical Presentation

- Nail plate is enlarged, excessively curved, with a >180 widening of the angle between the proximal nail fold and nail plate

Treatment

- Treat underlying cause

Pearls and Pitfalls

- Pseudoclubbing seen in Apert's syndrome, Pfeifer's syndrome, Rubinstein-Taybi syndrome

Drug-Induced Nail Changes

Table 11   Nail changes induced by medications

Nail finding	Medications implicated
Apparent leukonychia (e.g., Muehrcke's nails)	Chemotherapeutic agents (especially anthracyclines, vincristine)
Beau's line	Chemotherapeutic agents
Discoloration (non-melanin)	Minocycline, antimalarials, gold
Ischemic changes	Beta-blockers, bleomycin
Melanonychia	Chemotherapeutic agents (doxorubicin, daunorubicin, 5-FU), psoralens, zidovudine (AZT)
Nail thinning and brittleness	Chemotherapeutic agents, retinoids
Onycholysis/photo-onycholysis	Chemotherapeutic agents, taxanes, tetracyclines, psoralens, NSAIDs
Onychomadesis	Chemotherapeutic agents
Paronychia and periungual pyogenic granuloma	Retinoids, indinavir, lamivudine, methotrexate, cetuximab, gefitinib
True leukonychia	Chemotherapeutic agents

Longitudinal Erythronychia

Etiology and Pathogenesis

- Two Types – Localized and Polydactylous

Table 12   Localized longitudinal erythronychia

Longitudinal Erythronychia		
Localized	More Common	Bowen's disease Glomus tumor **Onychopapilloma** = most common Verrucae vulgares
	Less Common	Basal cell carcinoma Benign vascular proliferation Lichen planus (isolated lesion) Nail melanoma
Polydactylous	Acantholytic epidermolysis bullosa Amyloidosis, primary Darier disease Graft-versus-host disease Hemiplegia Idiopathic Lichen planus Multiple myeloma	

Clinical Presentation

- **Localized** – Linear erythematous band on one nail. Most common on thumbs in middle-aged patient. Toenail involvement is unusual. May or may not be painful. Onycholytic edge catches on clothing
- **Polydactylous** – Linear erythematous band on more than one nail. Commonly presents in adulthood

Treatment

- **Localized Longitudinal Erythronychia**
  - **Painful** – explore and excise surgically
  - **Asymptomatic**
    - If changing/evolving → Biopsy
    - Stable, patient is good historian → Measure, photograph, follow patient
- **Polydactylous Longitudinal Erythronychia**
  - Assess if patient has known diagnosis of → lichen planus, amyloidosis, Darier's disease, GVHD, hemiplegia
  - If no known associated disease → consider biopsy to diagnose underlying disease

Longitudinal Melanonychia

Table 13 Etiology of longitudinal melanonychia

Activation of melanocytes (multiple bands usually due to this)	Racial
	Trauma (especially toenails) – manicures, nail biting, onychotillomania, frictional)
	Drugs – chemo (doxorubicin, 5-FU), zidovudine (AZT), psoralens
	Pregnancy
	Laugier-Hunziker syndrome
	Peutz-Jegher syndrome
	Addison's disease
	HIV infection
	Postinflammatory – lichen planus, psoriasis, onychomadesis, radiation
Non-melanocytic tumors	SCC in situ, verrucae, BCC, subungal keratosis, myxoid cyst
Melanocyte hyperplasia Nevus (nail matrix) Melanoma	

Clinical Presentation

- Longitudinal brown or black band on nail plate. Extends from proximal nail fold to distal margin

Treatment/Management

- Look for cause
- If Hutchinson's sign present → concern for melanoma. Biopsy required
  - Pigmentation of the proximal nail fold or the hyponychium in association with longitudinal melanonychia

Pearls and Pitfalls

- Very common in African-Americans (90% have one or more pigmented bands)

Nail Terminology

Table 14 Nail terminology

Beau's lines	Horizontal ridges in nail plate (slow matrix proliferation during acute illness)
Bilobed nails	Only a few reported cases
Blue nails	Seen in – Wilson's disease, argyria, AZT, HIV, antimalarials, busulfan
Brachyonychia	Short, wide nails ("racquet nails" in Rubenstein-Taybi)
Chromonychia	Presence of abnormal nail color. May be from external or internal etiology
Clubbing	Increased curvature of the nail in the horizontal axis and bulbous overgrowth of the digital tip
Habit tic deformity	Parallel horizontal grooves in the nail plate, as the result of repetitive minor trauma to the proximal nail plate and lunula. Resembles washboard. Often grows normally once picking ceases
Half-and-Half nails	(Lindsay's nails) Transverse white lines associated with renal disease (transverse white line in nail bed at halfway point in nail)
Hapalonychia	Thinning of nail plate
Koilonychia	Spoon nails (iron deficiency; Plummer-Vinson; hyperthyroidism; hemochromotosis)
Leukonychia	White nails. May be congenital, acquired, complete or incomplete
Longitudinal nail grooves	Can occur in the nail as a result of a space-occupying lesion (myxoid cyst, fibroma) in the nail fold overlying the matrix
Macronychia	Large nails. Can be seen in congenital syndromes such as Proteus syndrome, Maffucci's syndrome. Also seen in tumors of the distal phalanx
Median nail dystrophy	Linear deformity and split in the midline of the nail, usually of the thumb. Resembles fir-tree. Etiology unknown. May be self-healing and/or recurrent
Mee's lines	Associated with heavy metals and some chemotherapy
Melanonychia striata	AKA – longitudinal melanonychia. Longitudinal pigmented bands in nail. Etiology – nevi, lentigines, medications, trauma, melanoma
Micronychia	Small nails. Usually secondary to congenital etiology – COIF syndrome (Congenital onychodystrophy of index finger)
Muehrcke's nails	Pale bands on nail bed associated with hypoalbuminemia
Nail pitting	Psoriasis vulgaris, alopecia areata, trachyonychia
Onychatrophy	Atrophic loss of nails, often following scarring process that irreversibly scars the nail matrix to prevent growth of nail plate
Onychauxis	Thick nail
Onychocryptosis	Ingrown nail
Onychogryphosis	Grossly thickened and hyperkeratotic nail which tends to curve as it thickens ("ram's horn" appearance)
Onycholysis	Separation of distal nail plate from nail bed. Associated with psoriasis, onychomycosis, yellow nail syndrome, contact dermatitis, meds, endocrine disorders, environmental causes. Can also be caused by phototoxicity
Onychomadesis	Separation of entire nail plate beginning proximally

(continued)

Table 14 (continued)

Onychomalacia	Softening of nails
Onychorrhexis	Longitudinal ridging of nails – seen in lichen planus, Darier's disease, circulatory disorders. Often see chips in the free edge in troughs where nail is fragile
Onychoschizia	Splitting of nails into layers parallel to surface at distal nail plate. Often caused by alternating wetting and dehydration on a continual basis. Moisturization may help
Onychotillomania	Habitual picking of the nails (coined by Dr. Elewski)
Pachyonychia	Thick nails seen in Pachyonychia congenita
Paronychia	Inflammation and/or infection of the proximal and lateral nail folds (paronychium). May be acute (Staph) or chronic (candida, pseudomonas, etc.)
Pincer nails	Exaggerated transverse overcurvature of nail plate along longitudinal axis. Usually acquired but may be congenital. Often have enlargement of underlying bony phalanx. May see pain, infection. Tx = remove lateral portion of nail matrix surgically or chemically
Pitting of nails	Small, round depressions in nail plate. Seen in psoriasis, alopecia areata, eczema
Platonychia	Flattened nails
Psoriasis	Nail pitting, oil spots, onycholysis
Pterygium	**Dorsal** – thinning and atrophy of nail plate with eventual growth of proximal nail fold onto the nail bed. Seen in – lichen planus, peripheral vascular disease, injury of nail **Ventral (inverse)** – hyponychium tissue grows and attaches to ventral surface of nail plate. Seen in CTD – scleroderma, SLE. May be familial, idiopathic
Red lunulae	Carbon monoxide, cardiovascular disease, lupus, alopecia areata, tamoxifen, LGV
Shoreline nails	Drug-induced exfoliative dermatitis (alternating bands of nail plate discontinuity and leukonychia)
Splinter hemorrhages	Thin, longitudinal, red-brown lines that resemble splinters in nail plate. Etiology – trauma (most common), psoriasis, other medical and vascular events
Terry's nails	Transverse lines associated with liver disease – occurs in distal third of nail (whitening of nail bed)
Trachyonychia	Rough nails composed of small irregular pitting, which gives nail roughened, lusterless surface. Seen in "20-nail dystrophy of childhood" but misnomer b/c can occur in less than 20 nails and in adults. Etiology – alopecia areata, psoriasis, lichen planus, chronic eczema, ichthyosis vulgaris, others
Yellow mottling of lunulae	Alopecia areata
Yellow nails	Yellow nail syndrome, Candida, carotenemia, MTX, AZT

Nail Pathology – Anatomic Region Affected

Table 15 Clinical features of abnormal nails and the corresponding location of pathology in the nail unit

Clinical Feature of Nail	Location in Nail Unit
Pitting Beau's lines Longitudinal ridging Longitudinal fissuring Trachyonychia Red spots in lunula	Proximal nail matrix
True leukonychia	Distal nail matrix
Onychomadesis Koilonychia Nail thinning	Proximal + distal matrix
"Oil drop" (salmon patches) Onycholysis Subungual hyperkeratosis Apparent leukonychia – fades with pressure Splinter hemorrhages	Nail bed
Cutaneous psoriasis	Proximal nail fold
Hyperkeratosis	Hyponychium

Pearls and Pitfalls

- Conditions with accelerated nail growth – psoriasis, pityriasis rubra pilaris (PRP), hyperthyroidism, AV shunts, itraconazole, L-dopa, calcium and vitamin D
- Thickness of the nail plate directly related to the size of the matrix
- Nail plate formed from the matrix
  - Distal matrix – more ventral, deeper plate
  - Proximal matrix – superficial plate
- Fingernails – grow 0.1 mm/day (2–3 mm per month)

Nail Tumors

Table 16 Features of benign and malignant nail tumors

Nail tumor	Clinical	Management
Benign		
Koenen's tumor	Asymptomatic, associated with tuberous sclerosis. Often multiple and can cause depressions in nail plate	Surgery for bothersome lesions
Acquired digital fibrokeratoma	Small growths that appear around the nail and are fleshy, asymptomatic. May have keratotic distal tip	Surgical removal
Subungual exostosis	Not a true tumor → bony outgrowth that occurs under nail and elevates nail plate. Often on toes. Exostoses have triad of bony growth under nail, x-ray changes, and pain	X-ray mandatory Surgical excision by orthopedics
Glomus tumor	Pinpoint throbbing (painful) lesion in nail bed. Pain exacerbated by pressure, cold. Usually visible through nail plate as red or blue macule. May not be visible if it involves matrix. Overlying nail plate may be thin. Hx of trauma	Surgical removal
Pyogenic granuloma	Benign tumor consisting of exuberant granulation tissue that is typically red and bleeds easily. May be friable, eroded, crusted. Often occurs after injury. DDx – amelanotic melanoma	Surgical removal
Onychomatricoma	Nail tumor characterized by longitudinal yellow bands and ridging. Consists of a group of hollow channels in a funnel-shaped configuration	Surgical removal
Myxoid pseudocyst	AKA – digital mucous cysts or synovial cysts. Common on distal fingers and rarely on toes. Non-inflamed, solitary, skin-colored or bluish nodules <1 cm. Usually not painful. May have assoc groove in nail plate	1. Clean well with betadine or chlorhexidine 2. Puncture and express myxoid material 3. Fill lesion with Kenalog 5 mg/mL 4. Compression with bandage
Malignant		
Squamous cell carcinoma	May present with paronychia, onycholysis with hyperkeratosis. Can be associated with HPV – especially types 16, 18, 34, 35	Mohs surgery
Keratoacanthoma	Rapidly growing painful, subungual tumor which can erode the bone and cause radiolucency on x-ray. Men > Women, age 30–60	Mohs surgery. If advanced bone invasion, amputation sometimes required

(continued)

Table 16 (continued)

Nail tumor	Clinical	Management
Benign		
Melanoma	A: Age. Peak incidence is fifth to seventh decade B: Brown, black, breadth > 3 mm in width of band C: Change in morphology of nail or lack of change after treatment D: Digit most commonly involved = thumb and great toenail E: Extension of pigment onto nail fold (Hutchinson's sign) F: Family hx or personal hx of melanoma or dysplastic nevus	Surgical treatment. Amputation often required

References: (1) Levit EK et al. The ABC rule for clinical detection of subungal melanoma. J Am Acad Dermatol 2000; 42:269–74. (2) Rich P. and Scher RK. An Atlas of Diseases of the Nail. Parthenon publishing, New York: NY 2003, pg. 83–89

Onycholysis

Etiology and Pathogenesis

Table 17 Causes of onycholysis

Chemical	Cosmetics, especially those with formaldehyde
	Depilatories
	Detergents
	Nail polish remover (with acetone)
	Organic solvents
Inflammatory	Alopecia areata
	Atopic dermatitis
	Contact dermatitis
	Lichen planus
	Psoriasis
Infectious	Bacterial paronychia
	Candidiasis
	Herpes simplex (whitlow)
	Onychomycosis
	Verrucae
Medications	Anticonvulsants (valproic acid)
	Chemotherapeutic agents
	Psoralens
	Retinoids (isotretinoin)
	Tetracyclines (photo-onycholysis)
	Thiazides
Systemic Diseases	Iron-deficiency anemia
	Rheumatic disease
	Thyroid disease – hypothyroidism or hyperthyroidism
	Yellow Nail syndrome
Trauma	Compulsive subungal cleaning
	Running – "Runners' toes"

Clinical Presentation

- Separation of distal nail plate from nail bed or from surrounding nail folds. Detached nail looks yellow-white

Treatment

- Look for a cause
- Keep nails short. Nail will act as a lever – small force distally
- Culture – rule out candida and fungal infections. Treat concomitant infections
- Strict irritant cosmetic avoidance during and at least 1 month after resolution
- Topical antifungal (many have mild anti-inflammatory effect)
- Consider PO Diflucan 150 mg q week in recalcitrant cases

Pearls and Pitfalls

- Often see concomitant candida infection. Unclear if this is causative or if it is secondary infection after onycholysis occurs
- The longer the onycholysis is present, the more difficult it is to reattach (especially in toenails)

Onychomycosis (OM)

Etiology and Pathogenesis

- The dermatophyte Trichophyton rubrum is the major cause of tinea pedis and onychomycosis. The pathogen is sequestered between the nail bed and the nail plate which allows it to grow and makes it difficult for topical agents to reach this area.
- "Onychomycosis" traditionally referred to a nondermatophytic infection of the nail but is now used as a general term to denote any fungal nail infection (tinea unguium specifically describes a dermatophytic invasion of the nail plate)
- Prevalence of onychomycosis increases with age

Clinical Presentation

- Approximately 80% of onychomycosis occurs on the feet, especially on the great toes. It is uncommon to have both toe- and fingernail involvement.
- Subtypes: (Patients may have a combination of these subtypes)
  - **Distal lateral subungual** OM (DLSO) – most common
    - *T. rubrum* is the most common pathogen in DLSO and PSO
  - **White superficial** OM (WSO)
    - Most often, *T. mentagrophytes* and, more rarely, species of nondermatophyte molds cause WSO
    - HIV patients – more commonly caused by *T. rubrum,* rather than *T. mentagrophytes,* in this population
  - **Proximal subungual** OM (PSO) – least common
  - **Endonyx** OM (EO)
  - **Candidal** OM
  - **Total dystrophic** OM refers to the most advanced form of any subtype
- Risk factors for OM include: family history, increasing age, poor health, prior trauma, warm climate, participation in fitness activities, immunosuppression (e.g., HIV, drug-induced), communal bathing, and occlusive footwear
- Approximately 80% of onychomycosis occurs on the feet, especially on the great toes. It is uncommon to have both toe- and fingernail involvement

Labs

- Fungal culture of nail
- Histology of nail clipping - PAS stain will detect fungal elements
- Direct microscopy - potassium hydroxide (KOH) may be used. Material is placed on glass slide and covered with glass coverslip. KOH is added and gently heated

- **DDx** – psoriasis, irritant contact dermatitis, lichen planus, malignant melanoma, bacterial paronychia, Darier disease, drug reaction (onycholysis), pachyonychia congenita, thyroid disease, yellow nail syndrome, melanonychia, periodic nail shedding

Treatment and Management

- Important to **document** fungal infection (nail culture or PAS or H&E) prior to Rx

Topical medications for Onychomycosis

Table 18 Topical medications used in the treatment of onychomycosis

Generic name	Trade name	Treatment regimen	Monitoring	Comments
Ciclopirox	Penlac Nail Lacquer	Apply to nails QHS × 48 weeks	None	For patients with *T. rubrum* without lunula involvement
Thymol 4% in alcohol	–	Apply to nails BID	None	
Composed of phenol, resorcinol, basic fuchsine, boric acid, and acetone	Castellani's Paint	Apply to nails, toe webs BID – (BEST for toe web infection)	None	– Better for fungal infections of skin – May be used to reduce secondary bacterial contamination in onycholysis and in chronic paronychia

Oral medications for Onychomycosis

Table 19 Oral medications used for the treatment of onychomycosis

Generic name	Trade name	Treatment regimen	Monitoring	Comments
Note – no oral antifungals are FDA-approved for the treatment of onychomycosis in children				
Terbinafine 250 mg tablets *Inhibits squalene epoxidase, which decreases ergosterol synthesis, causing fungal cell death	Lamisil	<20 kg – 62.5 mg QD 20–40 kg – 125 mg QD >40 kg – 250 mg QD **Duration:** Fingernails – 6 weeks Toenails – 12 weeks	CBC, LFTs, BUN/Cr at baseline and 6 weeks if plan on using the med for more than 6 weeks	Contraindicated in patients with hepatic or renal disease SE – ↓ WBC, pancytopenia, ↑ LFTs, taste changes

(continued)

Table 19 (continued)

Generic name	Trade name	Treatment regimen	Monitoring	Comments
Itraconazole 100 mg capsule 10 mg/mL (150 mL) soln *Fungistatic activity. Synthetic triazole antifungal agent that slows fungal cell growth by inhibiting CYP-450-dependent synthesis of ergosterol, a vital component of fungal cell membranes	Sporanox	<20 kg – 5 mg/kg/day for 1 week/month 20–40 kg – 100 mg/day for 1 week/month 40–50 kg – 200 mg/day for 1 week/month > 50 kg – 200 mg BID for 1 week/month **Duration:** Fingernails – 2 pulses/2 months Toenails – 3 pulses/3 months	CBC, LFTs, BUN/Cr	**Black box warning:** May aggravate CHF (negative inotropic effect), drug interactions (P450) Increased gastric pH may decrease absorption. Take with a full meal or 8 oz cola
Fluconazole 50 mg tablet 100 mg 150 mg 200 mg 10 mg/mL (35 mL per bottle) 40 mg/mL *selectively inhibits fungal CYP-450 and sterol C-14 alpha-demethylation, which prevents conversion of lanosterol to ergosterol, thereby disrupting cellular membranes	Diflucan	<50 kg – 3–6 mg/kg/day once weekly > 50 kg – 200 mg PO once weekly **Duration:** Fingernails – 12–16 weeks Toenails – 18–26 weeks	No monitoring necessary but consider Cr, LFTs at baseline	

Pearls and Pitfalls

- Clinical impression is never adequate to make the diagnosis of onychomycosis as many nail disorders can mimic this condition. Clinical findings must be confirmed by further testing (as mentioned under Labs)
- Despite the worry of many patients and some physicians, the oral treatments for onychomycosis are quite safe, although it is important to follow the FDA recommendations for monitoring
- Debridement of thick, dystrophic nails can be of added benefit when treating onychomycosis. Urea cream may be of benefit to some
- Topical lacquers are often ineffective unless there is only superficial involvement
- Always review prevention strategies with patient to avoid recurrence

Fungal Isolates and Their Significance

Courtesy of Judy Warner

At the UAB Fungal Reference Laboratory, protocols dictate that for a nail speci-men, only the dermatophytes and the non-dermatophyte causes of Onychomycosis will be reported. For skin specimens, all organisms will be reported since the labo-ratory has no knowledge of the patients' immunocompetency. If you ever question if the organism is the "real" cause, repeat the culture and see if the same organism is isolated.

Here are some of the most common isolates and pathogens. This list includes the most common isolates that might be reported to you that may or may not be the pathogen in the case. The true pathogens such as all the dermatophytes and dimor-phic molds have not been included.

Table 20 Common fungal isolates and their significance

Organism	Clinical significance
Acremonium sp.	Is a non-dermatophyte cause of onychomycosis but is a common contaminant
Aspergillus sp.	There are several species all important in the immunocompro-mised patient but only Aspergillus flavus, Aspergillus terreus, and Aspergillus versicolor are considered causes of onychomycosis
Aureobasidium pullulans	Will occasionally cause a cutaneous infection but is a common contaminate
Bipolaris sp.	A common contaminate but maybe important in the immuno-compromised patient
Candida albicans	Most common cause of candidiasis but can be found as normal flora of the skin and mouth and vaginal mucosa
Candida krusei	Causes infections in immunocompromised patients and is resistant to fluconazole
Candida parapsilosis	Common cause of paronychia. But is normal flora on the skin
Candida tropicalis	Can cause disease in immunocompromised patients but is normal skin flora
Chaetomium sp.	Occasionally, a cause of onychomycosis; isolated from dirt
Cladophialophora sp.	Nonpathogenic sp are called Cladosporium sp. Can cause chromoblastomycosis. But are a common contaminant
Curvularia sp.	Rarely a cause of infection. But a very common contaminant
Epicoccum sp.	Contaminant
Exophiala sp.	Can cause phaeohyphomycoses and tinea nigra. But can be contaminant
Fonsecaea sp.	Agent of chromoblastomycosis – will make sclerotic cells. But is also a common contaminant from soil and plants
Fusarium sp.	A non-dermatophyte cause of onychomycosis – it can be a common contaminant

(continued)

Table 20 (continued)

Organism	Clinical significance
Malassezia furfur	Causes tinea versicolor and Seb derm. This organism is seen on KOH/Calcofluor but will only grow in culture with an oil overlay
Nigrospora sp.	Common contaminant
Paecilomyces lilacinus	A common contaminant now thought to be a non-dermatophyte cause of Onychomycosis
Penicillium sp.	Usually nonpathogenic
Phialophora sp.	A cause of chromoblastomycosis, and yet can be a contaminant
Phoma sp.	A common plant pathogen that makes large pycnidia. Rare cases of subcutaneous phaeohyphomycosis have been seen
Pithomyces sp.	No infections reported. A common saprophytic mold
Rhodotorula sp.	Is a common contaminant but can colonize immunocompromised patients
Scedosporium apiospermum	**Scedosporium apiospermum** is the asexual stage of **Pseudallescheria boydii.** Systemic infections are most common maybe subcutaneous of cutaneous
Scopulariopsis sp.	A non-dermatophyte cause of Onychomycosis
Scytalidium sp.	A non-dermatophyte cause of Onychomycosis and skin infections
Trichosporon sp.	Causes white piedra and can be invasion and cause superficial and subcutaneous infections. Can also be a contaminant
Wangiella dermatitidis	Causes phaeohyphomycoses and can be disseminated in some patients. Is also isolated from soil and plant material
Zygomycetes: Mucor sp. Rhizopus sp. Rhizomucor sp.	Are all causes of zygomycosis but are very common contaminants

Paronychia

Etiology and Pathogenesis

- **Acute** – often from *Staphylococcus aureus* or *Streptococcus pyogenes*. Follows minor trauma to the nail. Occasionally due to herpes simplex virus infection
- **Chronic** – often from chronic inflammation from environmental factors. Leads to superinfection by *Candida* and *Pseudomonas aeruginosa*

Clinical Presentation

- **Acute** – affected digit becomes swollen, red, and painful. Compression of the nail fold may produce pus
- **Chronic** – commonly seen in women. Inflammation of the proximal nail fold with erythema, edema, and absence of cuticle. One or several fingernails affected (especially the thumb and second or third fingers of dominant hand). Often a prolonged course with superimposed recurrent episodes of acute exacerbation

Labs

- Bacterial culture
- Fungal/yeast culture
- Consider – viral culture, PCR, and/or direct fluorescent antibody (DFA)

Treatment

- Drain abscesses, if present
- Systemic antibiotics or antifungals according to culture results
- Topical antifungal (many have mild anti-inflammatory effect)
- Combination of topical antifungal and corticosteroid helpful in paronychia
- Keep nails short and do NOT remove cuticles, cut cuticles or push back cuticles
- Irritant avoidance
  - Strict irritant cosmetic avoidance during and at least 1 month after resolution
  - White cotton gloves under vinyl gloves (not latex – can have contact irritant)
  - Give handout to patient

Pearls and Pitfalls

- Nail biting can lead to paronychia
- Consider HSV infection in recurrent episodes of acute paronychia

Pediatric Dermatology

Acrodermatitis Enteropathica

Etiology and Pathogenesis

- Inherited form – AR disorder that typically presents in early infancy. Caused by mutations in SLC39A, which encodes intestinal zinc transporter
- Acquired form
  - Breastfed babies – from inadequate secretion of zinc in maternal milk
  - Premature infants with low zinc storage – especially those fed exclusively human milk
  - Adults with bowel bypass
  - Patients on total parental nutrition (TPN) with inadequate zinc supplementation
  - Complication of Crohn's disease or ulcerative colitis
  - HIV infection and diarrhea (causing inadequate absorption of zinc)
  - Cystic fibrosis patients with poor zinc absorption – noted at 3–5 months before any evidence of pulmonary disease
  - Chronic alcoholics
  - Anorexia nervosa
  - Tuberculosis of the GI tract
  - Vegetarian diets or fad diets containing low zinc levels

Clinical Presentation

- Triad of acral and periorificial skin lesions (vesiculobullous, pustular, and eczematous), diarrhea, and alopecia
  - Skin lesions usually develop around the mouth, nose and perineum. Lesions often symmetrically located on buttocks and extensor surfaces of major joints, scalp, fingers, and toes

83

- ○ Secondary infection with *Candida albicans* is common
- ○ Commonly are – listless, anorexic, apathetic, irritability, failure to thrive
- ○ Frothy, bulky, foul-smelling diarrheal stools present during exacerbations
- ○ Other potential findings – conjunctivitis, photophobia, stomatitis, perleche, nail dystrophy, alopecia of scalp/eyelashes/eyebrows
- Bottle-fed babies → manifests days to weeks after birth
- Breastfed babies → manifests shortly after being weaned

Labs

- Abnormal sweat test and low serum albumin level → confirms diagnosis of cystic fibrosis
- Low serum zinc levels (50 µg/dl or lower)
- May see:
  - ○ Low serum alkaline phosphatase (even when zinc level normal)
  - ○ Low serum lipid levels
  - ○ Defective chemotaxis

DDx – biotin deficiency (genetic or by ingesting large quantities of egg whites), kwashiorkor (low albumin, edematous, flaky paint scale, weight may be stable b/c of edema), essential fatty acid deficiency, pellagra, Hartnup's disease

Histology – Skin biopsy not diagnostic and same histology seen in other nutritional deficiencies:

- Psoriasiform hyperplasia with pale epidermis
- Spongiosis with superficial perivascular lymphocytic infiltrate

Treatment

- If untreated, will see progressive course of general disability, infection which often leads to death
- Zinc supplementation
  - ○ Zinc sulfate (5 mg/kg/day divided BID or TID) – dosage may differ with other formulations of zinc
  - ○ Older children – 150–200 mg per day
  - ○ Give 1–2 h before meals since some foods can affect the absorption of zinc
- After stabilizing zinc levels, check levels about 6- to 12-month intervals and adjust supplementation of zinc accordingly

Pearls and Pitfalls

- Note – Zinc contamination of glass tubes and rubber stoppers often occurs. Blood samples should be collected in acid-washed sterile plastic tubes with the use of acid-washed plastic syringes
- Will usually see improvement in irritability in 1–2 days. Diarrhea and skin lesions start responding in 2–3 days after initiating therapy. Hair growth begins 2–3 weeks after therapy. General growth begins in 2–3 weeks
- Excessive zinc intake can induce a copper deficiency and nephrosis. Don't overdo it

Aplasia Cutis Congenita (ACC)

Etiology and Pathogenesis

- Congenital defect characterized by absence of the epidermis, dermis, and some-times the subcutaneous tissue
- Most cases are sporadic, occasionally a family history. Some associations:
  - Teratogens, limb abnormalities
  - Epidermal nevus or nevus sebaceous – usually in close proximity to ACC
  - Underlying embryologic malformations – cleft lip, cleft palate, eye defects, cardiac anomalies, GI anomalies, spinal dysraphism, hydrocephalus, underly-ing skull defects, spastic paralysis, seizures, mental retardation, and vascular anomalies
  - Epidermolysis bullosa
  - Infections – HSV, varicella
  - Medications – methimazole (propylthiouracil recommended in pregnancy), carbimazole, misoprostol, low-molecular-weight heparin, valproic acid
  - Maternal antiphospholipid syndrome

Clinical Presentation

- Solitary or multiple, sharply demarcated, weeping or granulating, oval to circular ulcerations ranging from 1 to 3 cm in diameter. Lesions are usually on the scalp (80% occur near hair whorl) but sometimes on the face, trunk, or extremities.
- At birth, lesion can vary from a well-healed scar to an ulcer with a granulating base to a translucent glistening membrane ("membranous aplasia cutis")
- Some have the "hair collar sign" where the around is surrounded by long, dark hair (simulating a neural tube defect)
- End result is a smooth, hairless scar
- Diagnosis is usually a clinical one, and histology varies

Syndromes with ACC

- **Adams–Oliver syndrome**
  - AD malformation syndrome consisting of aplasia cutis congenita, transverse limb defects (usually hypoplastic limbs or absent distal phalanges) and car-diac and CNS abnormalities
  - Other anomalies may include cutis marmorata telangiectatica congenita, hemangiomas, cranial arteriovenous malformation, skin tags, supernumerary nipples, and woolly hair

- **Oculocerebrocutaneous (Delleman) syndrome**
  - Orbital cysts, cerebral malformations, focal skin defects including ACC-like lesions and skin tags
  - CNS malformations, clefting, and microphthalmia/anophthalmia
- **Bart syndrome**
  - A phenotypic pattern that neonates with all major forms of EB may demonstrate at birth, although most common in dystrophic EB
  - Localized absence of skin, usually on lower extremities. Usually see blistering elsewhere on skin, mucous membranes. Often see nail dystrophy
- **Johanson–Blizzard syndrome**
  - AR, stellate or membranous ACC. UBRI gene, dwarfism, hypoplastic nasal alae, hypodontia, deafness, microcephaly, hypothyroidism, pancreatic insufficiency
- **Finlay–Marks syndrome**
  - AD, ACC may heal with hypertrophic scarring. Nipple/breast hypoplasia or aplasia. Abnormal ears, teeth, nails. Syndactyly, reduced apocrine secretion
- **Trisomy 13 (Patau syndrome)**
  - Sporadic, membranous or large ACC defects. Ocular abnormalities, deafness, cleft lip/palate, cardiac malformations, polydactyly, narrow/convex nails, early death
- **4p- (Wolf–Hirschhorn syndrome)**
  - Sporadic, midline ACC. Microcephaly, ocular abnormalities, cleft lip/palate, periauricular pits and tags. Often early death
- **Microphthalmia with linear skin defects syndrome (MIDAS, Xp22 microdeletion syndrome)**
  - X-linked dominant, Facial ACC. HCCS gene. Microphthalmia, sclerocornea, agenesis of corpus callosum, genital anomalies, short stature
- **Seitleis syndrome**
  - AD with variable penetrance. ACC-like atrophic lesions on bilateral temples (from lateral eyebrows to hairline. Abnormal eyelashes, upward slanting of eyes, leonine facies
- **Brauer lines**
  - Looks like Seitleis syndrome (bitemporal ACC) but normal eyelashes, no leonine facies

DDx – forcep injury, congenital herpes simplex infection or congenital varicella, congenital syphilis, epidermolysis bullosa, focal dermal hypoplasia (Goltz syndrome

Histology – nonspecific

- Epidermal atrophy with superficial or deep ulcer
- Dermal atrophy, fibrosis with absent adnexal structures
- Lymphocytes and neutrophils associated with ulcer

Treatment and Management

- Thorough history (including obstetric history and family history) and physical exam
  - ○ Consider viral culture (and/or PCR, Tzanck, DFA) to rule out HSV, varicella
  - ○ Consider genetic workup based on history and physical
    - ■ Any patient presenting with scalp ACC and congenital anomalies warrants chromosomal evaluation
- Supportive care in most cases as area heals – gentle care to prevent extension and prevent infection. Most will heal in first few weeks to months
- Larger areas (>4 cm) may require surgical grafting to prevent hemorrhage, venous thrombosis, and meningitis

Pearls and Pitfalls

- With aging, most scars become relatively inconspicuous but surgical correction can be performed

Atopic Dermatitis

Etiology and Pathogenesis

- Pathogenesis still poorly understood but appears to be complex interaction between immune dysregulation, epidermal barrier dysfunction, and environment. Has T_H2 predominance → IL-4, -5, -13. These interleukins trigger B cells which produce IgE → peripheral eosinophilia. Mechanical trauma from scratching and rubbing causes epidermal cells to release proinflammatory cytokines which perpetuate the inflammation
- Atopic patients have decreased level of ceramides in the epidermis – likely affects both barrier function and inflammatory responses
- Abnormal barrier makes patients prone to secondary infection
- The prevalence rate is 10–12% in children and 0.9% in adults. 30% develop asthma and 35% have nasal allergies

Clinical Presentation

- Essential features = pruritus and eczematous changes
  - Pattern in infants and children → face, neck, extensor surfaces
  - Pattern in older children and adolescents → flexural areas, sparing groin and axillae
  - Pattern in adults → flexural areas, eyelids, face, hands
- Important features (usually seen)
  - Early age of onset
  - Atopy (IgE reactivity)
  - Xerosis
- Associated features (may or may not be seen but common in atopic patients)
  - Keratosis pilaris/ichythosis vulgaris/palmar hyperlinearity
  - Atypical vascular responses
  - Perifollicular changes
  - Ocular/periorbital changes
    - Atopic pleat – seen just below lower lid of both eyes. Referred to as Dennie–Morgan fold/lines
  - Perioral/periauricular lesions
- Lymphadenopathy may be seen in severe atopic dermatitis and erythroderma
- Infectious complications common, especially with *Staphylococcus aureus*, molloscum contagiosum, and sometimes herpes (Kaposi varicelliform eruption, AKA eczema herpeticum)
- Aeroallergens and environmental allergies can aggravate skin lesions
- Urticaria and acute anaphylactic reactions to food more common in AD patients – peanuts, eggs, milk, soy, fish, and seafood. Latex allergy more common

Labs – Rarely helpful

- Consider checking platelets if concerned about Wiskott–Aldrich
- Consider checking for immunodeficiency (such as in Job Syndrome)
- KOH if tinea suspected
- Allergy and RAST testing rarely helpful

DDx – irritant dermatitis, allergic contact dermatitis, nummular eczema, lichen simplex chronicus, psoriasis, scabies, seborrheic dermatitis, tinea corporis, underlying immunodeficiency, acrodermatitis enteropathica, Langerhans cell histiocytosis

Histology

- Superficial perivascular lymphocytes, occasional eosinophils
- Focal parakeratosis, sometimes with crusting
- Neutrophils in the stratum corneum if secondarily impetiginized
- Acanthosis or hyperkeratosis in chronic lesions
- Spongiosis, sometimes spongiotic vesicles (if more acute)

Treatment

- Topical corticosteroids – limit the number of refills and specify the tube size. Parents often will use liberally on children – can lead to striae, increased absorption, etc. Ointments preferred – work better and are less likely to cause burning (less preservatives)
- Protopic ointment 0.1%, Elidel cream
  - A black box warning has been issued in the United States based on research that has shown an increase in malignancy in associated with the calcineurin inhibitors. While these claims are being investigated further, the medication should likely only be used as indicated (i.e., for AD in persons older than 2 years and only when first-line therapy had failed)
- NbUVB, UVA therapies
- Methotrexate
- Azathioprine
- Cyclosporine
  - 3–5 mg/kg/day PO divided bid; if no improvement within 1 month, may be increased gradually; not to exceed 5 mg/kg/day
  - As skin lesions improve, reduce dose by 0.5–1 mg/kg/day/month; lowest effective dose for maintenance
  - Discontinue if no improvement in 6 weeks
- Other – probiotics, ABX as need for coinfection

- Nonmedical Efforts
  - Dry skin care essential
    - Vaseline, Aquaphor (may irritate some b/c contains Lanolin), CeraVe, Cetaphil, Vanicream. Ointments may be less irritating for some
    - No dryer sheets or fabric softener
    - Fragrance-free detergent
    - Lukewarm water with fragrance-free soap (such as Dove, Cetaphil) only to areas that need it. Pat dry, don't rub dry
    - Moisturize within 2–3 min of getting out of shower
  - Clothing should be soft next to the skin. Cotton (100%) is comfortable and can be layered in the winter. Avoid wool products – can irritate the skin
  - Cool temperatures better because sweating causes irritation and itch
  - Advise patients to apply a barrier of petroleum jelly around the mouth prior to eating to prevent irritation from tomatoes, oranges, and other irritating foods
  - A humidifier (cool mist) prevents excess drying and should be used in both winter, when the heating dries the atmosphere, and in the summer, when the air conditioning absorbs the moisture from the air
  - Clothes should be washed in a mild, fragrance-free detergent (such as All Free and Clear or Dreft) with no fabric softener
  - No dryer sheets

Table 21 Dosing information for commonly prescribed pediatric medications

Drug name		Liquid form	Tablet form	Dosing
Antihistamines	Benedryl	12.5 mg/5 mL	25, 50 mg	2 mg/kg/day divided q 6–8 h
	Atarax	10 mg/5 mL	10, 25, 500, 100 mg	2 mg/kg/day divided q 6–8 h
	Zyrtec	1 mg/1 mL or 5 mg/5 mL	5, 10 mg chew tablets	<2 years old – ½ tsp >2 years old – 1 tsp
	Doxepin	10 mg/1 mL	10, 25, 50, 75, 100, 150 mg	Start **0.5 mL** and work up slowly as tolerated. Dispense with dropper
	Singulair		4, 5 mg chew tab 4, 10 mg granule packet	Granule packet to be mixed with ice cream, applesauce, carrots or rice 2–5 years old – 4 mg/day 6–14 years old – 5 mg/day >15 years old – 10 mg/day
	Claritin	5 mg/5 mL	10 mg	2–5 years old – 5 mg/day >5 years old – 10 mg/day

Pearls and Pitfalls

- It is important to review good skin care in detail with the parents (and child). Remind them that this condition is often chronic with a relapsing/remitting nature or they may jump from physician to physician because the patient is "not cured"
- Addition of low concentrations of chlorine bleach to bathwater (1/4 cup – ½ cup per full tub) can decrease *Staph* infections
- If writing for Doxepin, always write weight of child on prescription to allow for double-checking of dosage by the pharmacist since **0.5 mL** is often mistaken for 5 mL

Collodian Baby

Etiology and Pathogenesis

- Causes
  - **Nonbullous congenital ichthyosiform erythroderma**
  - **Classical lamellar ichthyosis**
  - Conradi syndrome
  - Trichothiodystrophy
  - Recessive X-linked ichthyosis
  - Self-healing collodian babies (5%)

Clinical Presentation

- Breaking and shedding of the collodian membrane leads to thermoregulatory issues and increased risk of infection
- Collodian membrane may be the intial presentation of any number of conditions (see causes)
- Infant born with cellophane or oiled parchment-like membrane covering the body – can distort features
- Not a disease entity but a phenotype common to several disorders
- Often premature
- At risk for …
  - Inability to suck properly
  - Respiratory difficulties due to restriction of chest expansion
  - Systemic infection
  - Aspiration pneumonia
  - Excessive transcutaneous fluid loss and electrolytes loss
  - Hypernatremic dehydration
  - Increased metabolic requirements
  - Temperature instability

DDx – Harlequin fetus

Treatment and Management

- Management
  - Humidified incubator
  - Special attention given to prevention of temperature instability, sepsis, fluid, and electrolyte imbalance
  - Desquamation is encouraged by the application of emollients, rather than manual debridement
  - Given the poor cutaneous barrier and potential toxicity, use of keratolytics agents should be avoided

Diaper Dermatitis

Table 22 Diaper dermatitis – potential etiologies and symptoms

Type	Symptoms
Irritant dermatitis	Diaper-covered surfaces, spares folds
	Chronic wetness, increased pH, diarrhea
Candidal dermatitis	**Bright red**, moist patches with satellite pustules
	Intertriginous involvement of thrush
Seborrheic dermatitis	Groin, scalp, intertriginous areas
	Salmon colored, waxy scaling patches, and plaques
Psoriasis	Well-demarcated, pink plaques with minimal scale, creases involved
	Most common presentation of psoriasis in infants
Acrodermatitis Enteropathica/zinc deficiency	Brown, orange crusted plaques with vesicles and bullae
	Perineal, perioral areas, and distal extremities
	2° to low serum zinc level
	1.) <u>Premature infants</u>: poor absorption, inadequate stores, and ↑ zinc requirement
	2.) <u>Healthy infants</u>: low breast milk zinc levels with normal maternal serum zinc level
	3.) <u>Acquired form</u>: malabsorption and/or inadequate nutritional intake (i.e., TPN)
	4.) <u>Autosomal recessive inherited form</u>: defect in intestinal zinc-specific transporter SLC39A4 that manifests when infant is weaned off breast milk (due to greater availability of zinc maternal breast milk than non-maternal source)
	Alkaline phosphatase (zinc-dependent enzyme) also low
	Make sure lab uses non-zinc containing tube (special collection tube).
Langerhans cell histiocytosis (Letterer–Siwe Disease)	Yellowish-brown, crusted papules with **petechiae** in a seborrheic distribution
	CD1+, S100+ Langerhans cells with comma-shaped or reniform nuclei.
	Multisystem involvement may be present
Jacquet's erosive dermatitis	Severe erosive papules, nodules. May cause pain with urination
	Multifactorial etiology: yeast, irritant dermatitis, and moisture
Granuloma gluteale infantum	Red-purple, granulomatous nodules
	2° local irritation, maceration and *Candida* (multifactorial)
Allergic contact dermatitis	Topical preparations or foods
Cystic fibrosis	Resembles zinc deficiency
	Pedal edema common
	Failure to thrive, hepatosplenomegaly, infections, malabsorption

(continued)

Table 22 (continued)

Type	Symptoms
Biotin deficiency/multiple carboxylase deficiency	Resembles zinc deficiency but affects all biotin-dependent enzymes *Neonatal form*: AR holocarboxylase synthetase – vomiting *Juvenile form*: AR biotinidase – optic atrophy and hearing loss *All*: seizures (6 months of age), hypotonia, ataxia, lactic acidosis/ketosis, hyperammonemia, alopecia Treatment → biotin lifelong
Perianal streptococcal Disease	**Bright red**, well-defined erythema perianally and in creases
MRSA	Increasingly common – may see nodules/abscess
Bullous impetigo	Flaccid bullae with honey-colored crusts
Miliaria	Blocked eccrine ducts secondary to heat and humidity of diaper area. May be superficial, small, clear vesicles (miliaria crystalline) or small, erythematous papules/pustules (miliaria rubra/miliaria pustulosa)
Scabies	Lesions tend to be more nodular under the diaper
Kawasaki's Disease	2/3 of patients present with **confluent, tender erythema in perineum**. Later → desquamates
Congenital syphilis	Condyloma lata or generalized papulosquamous eruption of secondary syphilis may be present in diaper area
Perianal pseudoverrucous Papules and Nodules	Erythematous flat-topped papules and nodules in children with chronic fecal incontinence
Human immunodeficiency virus (HIV)	Very severe erosive diaper dermatitis. May be complicated by secondary bacterial and viral infections

Epidermolysis Bullosa

Table 23 Classification of epidermolysis bullosa

Major EB type	Major EB subtypes	Targeted protein(s)
EB simplex (EBS)	Suprabasal subtypes	
	• Lethal acantholytic EBS	Desmoplakin
	• Plakophilin-1 deficiency	Plakophilin-1
	• EBS superficialis (EBSS)	unknown
	Basal subtypes	
	• EBS, localized (Weber–Cockayne)	K5, K14
	• EBS, Dowling–Meara	K5, K14 – clumped tonofilaments on EM
	• EBS, other generalized (Koebner)	K5, K14
	• EBS with mottled pigmentation	K5
	• EBS with muscular dystrophy	Plectin
	• EBS with pyloric atresia (MC with JEB)	Plectin, α6β4 integrin
	• EBS, autosomal recessive	K14
	• EBS, Ogna variant	Plectin
	• EBS, migratory circinate	K5
Junctional EB(JEB)	JEB, Herlitz type	Laminin-332
	JEB, generalized non-Herlitz	Laminin-332; type XVII collagen
	JEB, localized non-Herlitz	Type XVII collagen
	JEB with pyloric atresia	α6β4 integrin
	JEB, inversa	Laminin-332
	JEB, late onset	unknown
	LOC (*l*aryngo-*o*nycho-*c*utaneous) syndrome (AKA -Shabbir's syndrome)	Laminin-332 (α3 chain)
Dominant dystrophic EB (DDEB)	DDEB, generalized	Type VII collagen
	DDEB, acral	
	DDEB, pretibial	
	DDEB, pruriginosa	
	DDEB, nails only	
	DDEB, bullous dermolysis of newborn (not always transient)	
Recessive dystrophic EB (RDEB)	RDEB, severe generalized (Hallopeau–Siemens)	Type VII collagen
	RDEB, generalized other (non-HS)	
	RDEB, inversa	
	RDEB, pretibial	
	RDEB, pruriginosa	
	RDEB, centripetalis	
	RDEB, bullous dermolysis of newborn (not always transient)	
Kindler syndrome		Kindlin-1

Genodermatoses Predisposing to Malignancy

Table 24 Genodermatoses predisposing to malignancy

Genetic skin disease	Tumor susceptibility	Inheritance
Albinism	Squamous cell carcinoma, basal cell carcinoma, melanoma	Mainly AR
Ataxia telangiectasia	Lymphoma, leukemia, epithelial carcinomas	AR
Bazex Dupré–Christol syndrome	Basal cell carcinoma	AD
Beckwith–Wiedemann syndrome	Wilms' tumor, adrenal carcinoma, hepatoblastomas	AD
Bloom's syndrome	Leukemia, lymphoma, carcinoma of the GI tract, cervix, and larynx; Wilms' tumor	AR
Cowden's syndrome	Carcinoma of the breast, uterus and thyroid	AD
Dyskeratosis congenita	Leukoplakia, squamous cell carcinoma	XLR
Epidermolysis bullosa dystrophica	Squamous cell carcinoma	AR
Epidermolysis verruciformis	Squamous cell carcinoma	?AR
Familial atypical mole-malignant melanoma (FAMMM) – AKA Dysplastic nevus syndrome	Melanoma	AD
Fanconi's anemia	Leukemia, hepatic carcinoma	AR
Gardner's syndrome	Adenocarcinoma of the colon	AD
Gorlin syndrome (Basal cell nevus syndrome)	Medulloblastoma, ovarian fibrosarcoma	AD
KID syndrome (keratitis, ichthyosis, and deafness)	Squamous cell carcinoma	AD
Maffucci's syndrome	Chondrosarcoma; ovarian tumors; gliomas	?AD
Muir–Torre syndrome	Sebaceous tumors, keratoacanthomas; adenocarcinoma of colon and breasts	AD
Neurofibromatosis types 1 and 2	CNS tumors; neurofibrosarcoma, Wilms' tumor	AD
Peutz–Jeghers syndrome	Adenocarcinoma of the bowel; increased frequency ovarian, breast, pancreatic and testicular cancer	AD
Porokeratosis of Mibelli	Squamous cell carcinoma, basal cell carcinoma	AD
Rothmund–Thomson syndrome	Squamous cell carcinoma, osteosarcoma	AR
Sclerotylosis	Squamous cell carcinoma of the skin, tongue and tonsil; bowel carcinoma	AD
Tuberous sclerosis	CNS, renal and cardiac tumors	AD
Turcot's syndrome	Adenocarcinoma of the colon; CNS tumors	AR
Tylosis	Esophageal carcinoma	AD
Von-Hippel–Lindau disease	Renal cell carcinoma	AD
Werner's syndrome	Tumors of connective tissue or mesenchymal origin	AR
Wiskott–Aldrich syndrome	Lymphoma, leukemia	XLR
Xeroderma pigmentosum, several forms (types A-G)	Squamous cell carcinoma, basal cell carcinoma, melanoma, other internal malignancies	AR

Genoderm Buzzwords

Table 25   Buzzwords for genodermatoses

Buzzword	Genoderm
Eye buzzwords	
Blue grey sclera	Alkaptonuria
Corneal opacities in whorl-like configuration	Fabry disease
Congenital hypertrophy of the retinal pigment epithelium (CHRPE)	Gardner syndrome
Downward lens displacement	Homocystinuria
Upward lens displacement	Marfan syndrome
Optic atrophy	Multiple carboxylase deficiency
Lester iris (hyperpigmentation of papillary margin of iris)	Nail patella syndrome
Lisch nodules (iris hamartoma)	Neurofibromatosis Type I
Optic gliomas	Neurofibromatosis Type I
Juvenile posterior subcapsular lenticular opacities	Neurofibromatosis Type II
Cherry red spot	Niemann–Pick Disease
Blue sclera	Osteogenesis imperfecta (Type I, III, IV)
	Ehlers–Danlos Syndrome
Angioid streaks	Pseudoxanthoma elasticum
Retinitis pigmentosa with salt and pepper retinal pigmentation	Refsum disease
	Cockayne syndrome
Dendritic keratitis with corneal ulceration	Richner–Hanhart
Tyrosine crystals on slit-lamp examination	Richner–Hanhart
Perifoveal glistening white dots	Sjögren–Larsson syndrome
Retinal hamartoma	Tuberous sclerosis
Retinal hemangioblastoma	Von-Hippel–Lindau
Heterochromia irides	Waardenburg syndrome
Dystopia canthorum	Waardenburg syndrome (Type I, III, IV)
Kayser–Fleischer Ring (calcium deposition in Decemet's Membrane of the cornea)	Wilson disease
Comma-shaped corneal opacities	X-linked ichthyosis
Oral buzzwords	
Cobblestoned oral mucosa	Cowden syndrome
Hypodontia/Anodontia	Ankyloblepharon–Ectodermal Dysplasia–Cleft lip/palate
	Ectrodactyly–Ectodermal Dysplasia–Cleft lip/palate
	Hypomelanosis of Ito
	Incontinentia Pigmenti
Jaw cysts	Gorlin syndrome
Retained primary teeth (double row of teeth)	Hyper IgE syndrome
Peg teeth/Conical teeth	Hypohidrotic ectodermal dysplasia
	Incontinentia pigmenti

(continued)

Table 25 (continued)

Buzzword	Genoderm
Enamel pits	Junctional epidermolysis bullosa
	Tuberous sclerosis
Wooden tongue	Lipoid proteinosis
Thickened lips	Ascher syndrome (double lip)
	Multiple endocrine neoplasia syndrome Type IIb
Oral leukoplakia	Dyskeratosis congenita (premalignant)
	Pachyonychia congenita Type I (not premalignant)
Natal teeth	Pachyonychia congenita Type II
Grimacing smile	Rubinstein–Taybi syndrome
Gingival fibroma	Tuberous sclerosis
Musculoskeletal buzzwords	
Hemihypertrophy	Beckwith–Wiedermann syndrome
Osteopoikilosis	Buschke–Ollendorff syndrome
Stippled epiphysis	Conradi–Hunermann syndrome
Lobster claw deformity	Ectrodactyly–Ectodermal Dysplasia–Cleft lip/palate
	Goltz syndrome (Focal Dermal Hypoplasia)
Ehrlenmeyer flask deformity	Gaucher disease
Osteopathia striata	Goltz syndrome (Focal Dermal Hypoplasia)
Bifid Ribs	Gorlin syndrome
Acro-osteolysis	Haim–Munk disease
Tufted terminal phalanges	Hydrotic ectodermal dysplasia
Multiple enchrondromas	Maffucci syndrome
Polyostotic fibrous dysplasia	McCune–Albright syndrome
Metaphyseal widening	Menkes disease
Wormian bones in sagittal and lambdoid sutures	Menkes disease
Dysostosis multiplex	Mucopolysaccharidoses (Hurler's, Scheie's, Hunter's, Maroteaux–Lamy's)
Posterior iliac horns	Nail patella syndrome
Absent/hypoplastic patella	Nail patella syndrome
Occipital horns (exostosis at insertion of trapezius and sternocleidomastoid muscles)	Occipital horn syndrome
Radial ray defects (absent/hypoplastic radius and thumbs)	Rothmund–Thompson syndrome
	Fanconi anemia
Broad thumbs	Rubinstein–Taybi syndrome
Scissor gait	Sjögren–Larrson syndrome
CNS buzzwords	
Basal ganglia calcification	Cockayne syndrome
Frontal bossing	Conradi–Hunerman syndrome
	Gorlin syndrome
	Hypohidrotic ectodermal dysplasia
	Progeria syndrome
	Rothman–Thompson syndrome
Falx cerebri calcification	Gorlin syndrome
Temporal and hippocampal calcification	Lipoid proteinosis
Sphenoid wing dysplasia	Neurofibromatosis I

(continued)

Table 25 (continued)

Buzzword	Genoderm
Dural calcification	Papillon–Lefevre syndrome
Tram-track calcifications beneath leptomeningeal lesions	Sturge–Weber syndrome
Urine buzzwords	
Dark urine	Alkaptonuria
Maltese cross under polarized light	Fabry disease
Mousy odor	Phenylketonuria (PKU)
Sexual buzzwords	
Calcifying sertoli-cell (testicular) tumor	Carney complex
Precocious puberty	McCune–Albright syndrome
	Russell–Silver syndrome
Heme buzzwords	
NBT (nitroblue tetrazolium) reduction assay	Chronic granulomatous disease
Crumpled tissue paper macrophages	Gaucher disease
Cold abscesses	Hyper IgE syndrome
Foam cells on bone marrow biopsy	Niemann–Pick disease
Absent thymic shadow	Severe combined immunodeficiency
Other buzzwords	
Linear earlobe crease	Beckwith–Wiedermann syndrome
Left-sided cardiomyopathy	Carvajal syndrome
Low-pitched cry at birth	Cornelia de Lange syndrome
Exuberant granulation tissue	Junctional epidermolysis bullosa, herlitz type
Pain insensitivity	Lesch–Nyhan syndrome
	Riley–Day syndrome
Hoarse cry at birth	Lipoid proteinosis
Eyelid string of pearls	Lipoid proteinosis
Right-sided cardiomyopathy	Naxos disease

Hemangiomas

Etiology and Pathogenesis

- Hemangiomas are a result of a localized proliferative process of angioblastic mesenchyme. Represents a clonal expansion of endothelial cells

Clinical Presentation

- **Infantile hemangioma** most common (1–2% of newborns)
  - More common in – female infants (3x > males), premature infants
  - Less common in African-American infants and Asian infants
  - Location – head and neck more common
  - Usually present in first 2–3 weeks of life with continued growth until 9–12 month of age
  - GLUT1 + (absent in other vascular lesions)
  - Superficial, deep or mixed lesions
  - Natural history – proliferative phase, plateau phase and spontaneous regression
    - 30% gone by age 3
    - 50% gone by age 5
    - 70% gone by age 7, etc. …
  - *Worrisome* – Life-threatening (CHF), function-threatening, periocular, nasal tip, ear (extensive), lips, genitalia and perineum, airway, hepatic, large facial and/or "Beard distribution", ulcerating, lumbosacral, multiple
- **Diffuse neonatal hemangiomatosis** – patients with multiple cutaneous lesions in conjunction with extracutaneous organ involvement.
  - **Thorough physical exam and history**
- **Benign neonatal hemangiomatosis** – infant has multiple cutaneous lesions without any symptomatic visceral lesions or complications. May have only a few – up to hundreds. No standard "cutoff" for number of cutaneous lesions. Need to rule out systemic involvement
- **Congenital hemangioma** – fully formed at birth. May involve in accelerated fashion (RICH – rapidly involuting congenital hemangioma, often gone by 14 months) or may persist unchanged (NICH – noninvoluting congenital hemangioma, GLUT1 neg)

Table 26 Manifestations of PHACES

	Manifestation(s)	Comment
P	Posterior fossa malformations	Dandy–Walker malformation; hypoplasia or agenesis of various CNS structures
H	Hemangioma	Extensive facial; plaque-like; segmental; occ airway involvement
A	Arterial anomalies	Mainly head and neck; aneurysms, anomalous branches, stenosis
C	Cardiac anomalies and aortic coarctation	Patent ductus arteriosus (PDA) , ventricular septal defect (VSD), atrial septal defect (ASD), pulmonary stenosis, teratology of fallot, etc.
E	Eye abnormalities	Horner syndrome, ↑ retinal vascularity, microphthalmia, optic atrophy, cataracts, coloboma, others
S	Sternal clefting and supraumbilical abdominal raphe	Ventral developmental defects

Labs

Consider the following workup in babies with diffuse neonatal hemangiomatosis
- Liver ultrasound
- CBC – anemia, thrombocytopenia occasionally present
- LFTs
- Stool exam for occult blood
- Coagulation studies
- Urinalysis
- Echo/EKG
- CNS imaging

Treatment and Management

- Each lesion must be judged individually and treatment will be based on size, location and complicating factors
- Hemangiomas that are located on the nose, around the eyes or mouth, ears, or genital area can be particularly problematic and should be followed closely
- Propranolol is emerging as a preferred treatment for complicated hemangiomas, but there is no accepted treatment protocol to date (see table below)

Treatments for infantile hemangioma	
Treatment	Comment
Active non-intervention	Active emotional support and guidance
Local wound care	When ulcerated; topical antibiotic, nonstick wound dressings, compresses
Oral antibiotics	When 2° infection present
Pain control	When ulcerated
Topical corticosteroids	Potent formulations; may be useful for localized, superficial lesions
Intralesional corticosteroids	Usually Kenalog; localized lesions; caution w/periocular lesions
Oral corticosteroids	Mainstay of therapy; prednisone or prednisolone, 2–4 mg/kg/day
Interferon alfa 2a or 2b	Subcutaneous injection; for life-threatening lesions; risk of spastic diplegia
Laser therapy	Usually PDL; mainly useful for ulcerated lesions
Vincristine	Severe or life-threatening lesions
Surgical excision	Useful only in select situations, i.e., incomplete resolution
Propranolol	Becoming more of a mainstay tx; clinical trials underway for most ideal dosing regimen. Initial report in NEJM.

Propranolol Protocol (optimal protocol for infantile hemangiomas is not known)
Propranolol 20 mg/5 ml *Baseline*: EKG/rhythm strip, BP, HR, whole blood glucose Day 1: 0.17 mg/kg/dose TID Day 2: 0.34 mg/kg/dose TID Day 3: 0.67 mg/kg/dose TID *Monitoring*: BP/HR – 1 h after first dose and then 1 h after each dose increase on day 2 and day 3 *Caution*: babies with segmental facial hemangiomas or multiple hemangiomas *Pearls and Pitfalls* 1. Contraindicated in uncompensated congestive heart failure, heart block, asthma or hyperactive airway disease 2. Give with feeds. Have the child feed every 4 hours to prevent hypoglycemia (applies more to infants 3 months of age and under). Hold medication if child unable to eat or has a upper respiratory tract infection complicated by wheezing

Pearls and Pitfalls

– Hemangiomas should not be surgically treated in the proliferative phase, as they will commonly recur. Surgery is NOT recommended unless the hemangioma has completely burnt out and there is redundant, lax skin present

– The hemangiomas can cause significant stress for the parents and much of the visit is often spent educating parents about the natural course of these benign tumors, what to expect and what to do if things go awry. Recommend that they call the office if ulceration is present since more aggressive treatment will be necessary

- Occasionally these hemangiomas can bleed profusely. If 20-30 minutes of constant pressure does not stop the bleeding, advise parents to take the child to the emergency department
- Topical timolol can occasionally help for small hemangiomas, but results have been inconsistent

Henoch–Schönlein Purpura (HSP)

Etiology and Pathogenesis

- Form of small-vessel vasculitis (IgA) that occurs primarily in children (especially boys)
- Etiology unclear but has been linked to group A beta-hemolytic streptococci, *Bartonella henselae*, other bacterial or viral organisms, immunizations, drugs, neoplasm
- Frequency of preceding upper respiratory tract infection suggests a hypersensitivity phenomenon
- Immunoglobulin deposition in vessels results in complement activation and vessel damage

Clinical Presentation

- Seen often between the ages of 2 and 11
- Classic presentation – palpable purpura in dependent areas, arthritis, abdominal pain, and glomerulonephritis (although many do not present with this tetrad)
  - Lesions primarily on buttocks and lower legs but may involve upper extremities, trunk, and face. Skin lesions are presenting sign in approximately 50%
  - Petechiae or ecchymoses may predominate in some patients
  - Other morphologies may occur – vesicles, bullae, erosions or ulcers, necrosis, gangrene, even erythema multiforme-like lesions
- Marked edema of hands, feet, scalp or face may be seen
- Males – vasculitis of scrotal vessels may lead to acute scrotal swelling, with or without purpura and can be quite painful (mimicking testicular torsion)
- Rarely, can see recurrent attacks at intervals for weeks to months
- Systemic involvement – seen in up to 80% and usually involves kidneys, GI tract, joints

- ○ **Renal disease** most frequent and is the most significant correlate of long-term prognosis
  - ■ Renal involvement may not be apparent for several weeks
  - ■ If renal involvement is going to occur, usually does within 3 months of disease onset
  - ■ Potential correlates of renal disease in HSP → age > 4, persistent purpura, severe abdominal pain, depressed coagulation factor XIII activity < 80%
- ○ **Gastrointestinal disease** – colicky abdominal pain, hematochezia, hematemesis
  - ■ Intussusception seen in up to 2% and more likely in boys
  - ■ If intussusception seen in children > age 2, consider HSP. (Non-HSP-Intussusception usually occurs before age 2.)
  - ■ Colitis
- ○ **Rheumatologic disease**
  - ■ Tender joints with periarticular swelling
  - ■ Ankles and knees most frequently but elbows, hands, and feet may also be involved
  - ■ Symptoms usually transient – rarely result in permanent deformity
- ○ Other organ involvement – CNS, respiratory

Labs

- Approximately 1/3 of patients have elevated serum IgA levels
- Stool guaiac may be positive – vasculitis can affect gut and cause GI bleeding
- Urinalysis – microscopic hematuria. Nephritic and nephrotic syndromes may occur
- Serum chemistry
- CBC + differential
- Coagulation studies
- Consider checking antistreptolysin O (ASLO) titers

Imaging

- If testicular involvement, ultrasound, and/or radionuclide scans can help differentiate testicular torsion from HSP

DDx – erythema multiforme, drug reaction, urticaria, other types of vasculitis (DIF and biopsy can help distinguish in conjunction with the clinical)

Histology

- **Renal histology** – can distinguish from IgA nephropathy (Berger disease), although latter tends to involve older patients
- **Cutaneous histology** – leukocytoclastic vasculitis of the small vessels. DIF shows granular IgA immune complexes in superficial dermal blood vessels, along with C3 and fibrin deposits. Other immunoglobulins may be seen but not as predominant as IgA

Treatment and Management

- Overall prognosis is excellent. Disease runs its course in 4–6 weeks
- Renal disease is most important prognostic factor
  - Serial urinalysis and serum chemistries helpful in monitoring
  - ESRD may occur in up to 2–5% of children. Adults more likely to have long-term renal disease
  - Long-term follow-up needed for those with renal involvement
- Supportive care
  - NSAIDs – use conservatively, particularly if renal involvement
  - Systemic corticosteroids may be helpful if severe involvement of kidneys, GI tract, joints, scrotum but not generally recommended
  - Cytotoxic medications (especially cyclophosphamide or azathioprine) are often used to treat severe renal disease
  - Smaller studies and reports have shown benefit from – plasmapheresis, aminocaproic acid, IVIG
  - Factor XIII infusions were shown to improve both arthralgias in GI bleeding in one study

Pearls and Pitfalls

- Children and young adults with a history of HSP may be at increased risk for pregnancy-induced hypertension and/or proteinuria. Proper counseling and evaluation is recommended

Ichthyoses

Table 27   Features and inheritance patterns of ichthyoses

Disease	Inheritance	Gene (protein)	Clinical
Primary forms of ichthyosis			
Ichthyosis vulgaris	AD	(fillagrin)	Fine scale on extensor surfaces, hyperlinearity of palms. Flexures spared. Face usually spared. Associated with atopy, keratosis pilaris. *Histology* – retention hyperkeratosis with ↓/absent granular layer. EM: abnormal keratohyaline granules
X-linked ichthyosis	XR	**ARSC1** (Steroid sulfatase or arylsulfatase C)	Brown scales, "dried mud". Not present at birth – appears within few weeks of life. Neck involvement prominent. Face/palms/soles spared. *Assoc* – corneal opacities (50%), cryptochordism (20%) with ↑ testicular CA, prolonged labor in mothers of affected sons. *Histology* – compact hyperkeratosis with normal granular layer
Epidermolytic hyperkeratosis (Bullous congenital ichthyosiform Erythroderma)	AD	**KRT1 KERT 10** (Keratin 1, 10)	Bullae at birth with evolution into odorous verrucous plaques, ridge-like skin markings > flexural involvement, dystrophic nails. **Mauserung sign** – scales shed in full thickness leaving denuded base. *Histology* – hyperkeratosis with upper dermal vacuolar and clumped keratin proteins. EM – clumped keratin filaments
Classic lamellar ichthyosis	AR	**TGM1** (transglutami-nase 1)	Coarse dark scales, thick palms/soles, prominent flexural involve-ment. **Collodian baby**, ectropion, eclabion, alopecia. Note: Other type of lamellar ichthyosis is CIE phenotype – TGM1, ALOXE3, ALOX1
Nonbullous congenital ichthyosi-form erythroderma	AR	**ALOX12B** (transglutami-nase 1 or 12R lipoxygenase) **ALOXE3** (lipoxygenase 3)	Fine scaling overlying generalized erythema with flexures involved, hyperkeratotic palms and soles, hair and nails may be affected. Loss of eyebrows/eyelashes. Mental and growth retardation. Neurologic abnormalities may be present. Decreased life expectancy. **Collodian baby** (90% present as collodian baby).

(continued)

Table 27 (continued)

Disease	Inheritance	Gene (protein)	Clinical
Ichthyosiform Disorders			
Neutral lipid storage Disease (Dorfman–Chanarin syndrome)	AR	**CCI-58**	Fine scaling on erythroderma. May present as **collodian baby**. Ectropion, cataracts, myopathy, and central neuropathy. Fatty liver/HSM. No fasting ketonemia. *Histology* – lipid laden vacuoles in keratinocytes and granulocytes – **"Jordan's anomaly"**
CHIME syndrome (Zunich neuroecto-dermal syndrome)	AR	?	Coloboma (usu retinal), heart defects, ichthyosiform dermatosis, mental retardation, ear abnormalities *Facies* – hypertelorism, broad nasal root, upslanting palpebral fissures, long columnella but short philtrum, macrostomia, full lips, cupped ears *Assoc* – heart defects, brachydactyly. Hair may be fine, trichorrhexis nodosa
Neu–Laxova syndrome	AR	?	Severe intrauterine growth retarda-tion, edematous appearance, microcephaly, abnormal brain development with lissencephaly and agenesis of corpus callosum. Ichthyosis often present at birth – ranges in severity to mild to severe. X-rays → commonly show poor bone mineralization *Facies* – protuberant eyes, flattened nose, slanted forehead, micrognathia, deformed ears, short neck. Syndactyly, limb or digital hypopla-sia common.
KID syndrome (Keratitis, ichthyosis, deafness)	AD	GJB2 – connexin 26	Progressive vascularized keratitis, congenital hearing loss, hyperkera-totic skin lesions. ↑ SCC and skin infections
Erythrokeratoderma variabilis (Mendes da Costa syndrome)	AD	**GJB3** – connex-ins 31, 30.3 **GJB4** – EKV + erythema gyratum repens	Hyperkeratotic plaques on face, extremities, transient erythematous migratory patches (hour to hour), hypertrichosis
Progressive symmetric erythrokeratoderma	AD	**Loricrin**	Erythematous and hyperkeratotic plaques develop shortly after birth. Distributed symmetrically over body, especially on extremities, buttocks, and sometimes the face, together with PPK

(continued)

Table 27   (continued)

Disease	Inheritance	Gene (protein)	Clinical
Netherton syndrome	AR (almost all female)	**SPINK5** (encodes serine protease inhibitor, LEKT1)	*Triad* – ichthyosis linearis circumflexa, trichorrhexis invaginata, atopy. Also – failure to thrive, **hypernatremic dehydration**, recurrent infections *Histology* – ↓ granular and spinous layers (↑ drug absorption)
Refsum disease	AR	**PAHX** (Phytanoyl-CoA alpha-hydroxylase) **PEX7** (peroxin 7)	Mild ichthyosis, cerebellar **ataxia**, peripheral **neuropathy**, **retinitis pigmentosa** (salt and pepper), and deafness *Tx* – diet low in green vegetable, dairy and ruminant fats
Sjögren–Larsson syndrome	AR	Gene encoding fatty aldehyde dehydrogenase	Pruritic velvety ichthyosis as infant Hair/nails normal Mental retardation by age 2–3. Spasticity, retinal "**glistening white dots**", photophobia, dental enamel dysplasia.
Gaucher syndrome	AR	Absence of lysosomal β-glucocerebrosidase	Neonate with type 2 may present as **collodian baby**, neurologic signs, HSM. Absence of glucocerebrosidase leads to abnormal skin thickening and ↑ transepidermal water loss.
Conradi syndrome	XLR ⟶ XLD ⟶ AR ⟶	**Arylsulfatase E** **EBP** **PEX7**	Peroxisomal biogenesis disorder. Ichthyosiform erythroderma in lines of Blaschko, follicular atrophoderma, stippled epiphyses. Patchy alopecia, cataracts, asymmetric limb shortening.
CHILD syndrome	XLD (lethal in males)	**NSDHL** (NADPH steroid dehydrogenase-like protein)	Unilateral ichthyosiform erythroderma, limb/visceral hypoplasia, and stippled epiphyses. Severe nail dystrophy – claw-like. Intertriginous lesions persist *Histology* – infilt of papillary dermis of histiocytes with foamy cytoplasm ("verrucous xanthoma")
Peeling skin syndrome (Keratolysis exfoliativa congenita)	AR	?	Lifelong, superficial peeling of the skin. Nikolsky sign tends to be "+" *Histology* – thickened stratum corneum w/separation b/n SC and granular layer Type A – onset at birth, but common to present b/n ages 3–6 Type B – always begins at birth. Inflammation, pruritus. Short stature, easily removable anagen hairs Acral form – life-long, painless peeling. Exacerbated by water, sweating.

Immunodeficiencies

Table 28 Screening lab tests for a patient with recurrent cutaneous infections

Test	Finding	Immunodeficiency Identified
CBC with differential, platelet count, and examination of smear	• Giant granules within neutrophils, +/– neutropenia • Neutrophilia • Small platelets, thrombocytopenia	Chédiak–Higashi syndrome Leukocyte adhesion deficiency Wiskott–Aldrich syndrome
Hair shaft examination	• Small, regular clumps of melanin • Large, irregular clumps of melanin	Chédiak–Higashi syndrome Griscelli syndrome (type 2; *RAB27A*)
Quantitative immunoglobulins	• All Ig ↓ • IgA ↓, IgG ↓, +/– IgM ↓ • IgA ↓ or IgM ↓ • IgM ↑, all other Ig ↓ • IgM ↑, +/– IgA ↑, +/– IgG ↓ • IgA ↓, IgE ↓, IgG ↓ • IgE ↑↑ • IgM ↓, +/– IgG ↓, IgA ↑, IgE ↑	X-linked agammaglobulinemia Common variable immunodeficiency Selective IgA or IgM deficiency Hyper-IgM syndrome Hypohidrotic ectodermal dysplasia with immunodeficiency Ataxia telangiectasia Hyper-IgE syndrome Wiskott–Aldrich syndrome
Total hemolytic complement (CH50)	• Marked ↓	Various complement deficiencies
Nitroblue tetrazolium (NBT) reduction assay	• < 10% of normal NBT reduction	Chronic granulomatous disease
T- and B-cell analysis by flow cytometry	• Lack of T cells +/– B cells	Severe combined immunodeficiency

Reference: Used with permission from Elsevier. Schaffer JV and Paller AS. Primary Immunodeficiencies. In: Dermatology. Eds: Bolognia JL, Jorizzo JL, Rapini RP. 2nd ed, 2008. Mosby: New York; 803

Incontinentia Pigmenti (IP)

Etiology and Pathogenesis

- AKA – **Bloch–Sulzberger syndrome**
- X-linked dominant; mutation in NEMO (NF-κβessential modulator) → found mostly in females. Thought to be mostly lethal in males, but reports in Klinefelter patients (XXY) and as a mosaic condition
- Affected females have functional mosaicism because of random inactivation of one of the X chromosomes (lionization). As a result, skin lesions follow lines of Blaschko, resulting in clonal growth of cells that express the affected allele
  ○ Variable severity and expression of clinical involvement of other organs reflects the random inactivation of the affected X allele in these tissues

Clinical Presentation and Types

- Usually appears at birth or within first 2 weeks of life and > 95% have onset before 6 weeks of age

Table 29 Four distinct stages of incontinentia pigmenti

Stage	Clinical Manifestations	Histology
1. **Inflammatory or vesiculobullous**	Inflammatory vesicles, pustules, or bullae that develop in crops over the trunk and extremities Presents at birth to 1–2 weeks. Persist for months	– Eosinophilic spongiosis and intraepidermal vesicles containing eosinophils – Dyskeratotic keratinocytes – Perivascular infiltrate of lymphocytes and eosinophils
2. **Verrucous**	Irregular, linearly arrayed warty papules on one or more extremities and often on hands/feet Presents at 2–6 weeks. Resolves spontaneously usually within 2 years	– Hyperkeratosis and acanthosis – Pale glassy keratinocytes forming squamous eddies – Minimal perivascular lymphocytic infiltrate – Melanin incontinence
3. **Streaks of hyperpigmenta-tion**	During or shortly after the verrucous stage, the pigmentary phase will occur in 80%. See thin bands of slate-brown to blue-gray discoloration arranged in lines and swirls on trunk and extremities. May appear purpuric at onset Presents at 3–6 months. Lesions persist for years. Fade in adolescence and disappear in 2/3	Melanin incontinence
4. **Streaks of hypopigmentation and atrophy**	Atrophic streaks that are often hypopigmented. Common on arms, thighs, trunk, and especially calves. Areas show diminished hair, eccrine glands, sweat pores. May be subtle – Wood's light can highlight Presents in second to third decade	

- **Hair** – Cicatricial alopecia seen in up to 65% of patients. Most common near vertex and doesn't necessarily relate to sites of skin involvement
- **Nails** – Nail dystrophy in up to 50%. Painful, grayish-white verrucous or keratotic subungual tumors seen in up to 10%, usually during second to third decade
- **Dental** – delayed dentition, partial anodontia, pegged or conical teeth (looks like hypohidrotic ectodermal dysplasia)
- **CNS** – involvement seen in about 30%. Seizures common and are attributed to acute microvascular hemorrhagic infarcts. About 8% have severe neurologic problems – MR, frequent seizures, and/or spastic abnormalities
- **Eyes** – seen in 35% and include strabismus, cataracts, optic nerve atrophy, retinal neovascularization or detachment, blindness
- **Cardiac, skeletal** (microcephaly, syndactyly) anomalies occasionally reported

Labs – CBC in infancy → may see a peripheral eosinophilia

DDx – Goltz syndrome, lichen striatus, pigmentary mosacism, congenital herpes or varicella (especially when vesiculopustules present in combination with seizures), EB in vesicular stage, congenital syphilis

Treatment and Management

- Derm – diagnosis and topical skin care
- Ophthalmologist – Early and serial eye exams
- Neurology evaluation if seizures or evidence of neurologic delay
- Dental consultation
- Let clinical exam dictate the workup of other organ systems
- Normal life span

Pearls and Pitfalls

- Careful history and exam of mother as she may be a carrier – important for genetic counseling. May see subtle manifestations such as a patch of cicatricial alopecia, conical incisor, nail dystrophy, atrophic streak seen on side lighting. Mom may have a difficult time conceiving and an increased rate of miscarriages
- In stage 3 of IP, the bands may appear purpuric at onset and can be mistaken for child abuse
- Refer patient to the Incontinentia Pigmenti International Foundation (www. imgen.bcm.tmc.edu/IPIF)

Juvenile Xanthogranuloma (JXG)

Etiology and Pathogenesis

- A common form of non-langerhans cell histiocytosis. May be derived from dermal dendrocytes
- Generally a benign, self-limited disease of infants, children, and occasionally adults
- No association with hyperlipidemia or metabolic disturbances despite having "xantho" in its name

Clinical Presentation

- Firm, round, papule or nodule ranging from 5 mm to 2 cm
- Early lesions are red, orange, or tan. With time, they become more yellow in color
- Lesions may be solitary or multiple
- Lesions occur most often on the skin, although extracutaneous disease occasionally occurs
  - Eye is most common organ of involvement (iris)
    - Potential complications of ocular JXG – hyphema, glaucoma, or blindness
    - Patients may experience eye redness, irritation, photophobia
    - Risk factors – those with multiple skin lesions and those < age 2
  - Intramuscular JXG
    - Deep, soft tissue lesion that may have imaging features similar to malignant tumors
    - Tends to affect infants and toddlers as solitary lesion in skeletal muscles of trunk
  - Other sites → lung, liver, testis, pericardium, spleen, CNS, bone, kidney, adrenal glands, larynx

- Location – head, neck, trunk most common. May occur on mucosal surfaces or at mucocutaneous junction (mouth, vaginal orifices, perineal area)
  - Oral lesions may appear verrucous, pedunculated, umbilicated or fibroma-like
  - Oral lesions occur on lateral tongue, gingiva, buccal mucosa, and midline hard palate
- Lesions may be present at birth (20%) or appear in first 6–9 months of life. May persist or continue to erupt for years

DDx – Spitz nevus, solitary mastocytoma, dermatofibroma, xanthomas, nevus sebaceous (if yellow coloration prominent), sarcoid

Histology

- Dense dermal infiltrate of foamy histiocytes, foreign body cells, and Touton giant cells (virtually pathognomonic for this condition)
  - ○ Touton giant cell – giant cell with central wreath of nuclei and a peripheral rim of eosinophilic cytoplasm
- Lymphocytes and eosinophils are often seen
- Histiocytes in JXG are S100- and CD1a-

Treatment and Management

- JXG usually run a fairly benign course, with spontaneous regression occurring over 3–6 years. Rarely lasts into adulthood
  - ○ Skin lesions do not need to be treated, although surgical excision occasionally performed for diagnosis or cosmetic purposes
  - ○ Pigmentary alteration, atrophy, or anetoderma-like changes may occur at sites of involvement
- Rule out ocular involvement, as risk of complications is fairly high
  - ○ Ophthalmology may treat intraocular lesions with IL or systemic steroids, radiation therapy, or excision
- Systemic treatment recommended only for the rare cases where lesions impair organ function

Pearls and Pitfalls

- Association of JXG and childhood leukemia, especially juvenile chronic myelogenous leukemia which is seen with increased frequency in patients with multiple JXG lesions. In reported cases, there is family history of NF1 and patients had café-au-lait macules. Vast majority of kids with multiple JXG, however, do not develop JCML

Kawasaki Disease (KD)

Etiology and Pathogenesis

- Acute febrile disease leading to acquired cardiac disease, primarily seen in children. Kawasaki disease is a vasculitis affecting small- and medium-sized vessels, with a predilection for the coronary vessels
- Genetics may play role in susceptibility. Etiology otherwise not clear but possibly viral etiology since higher incidence in winter and early spring

Clinical Presentation

- Majority of cases are in children < age 5 with a peak incidence in those aged 2 and younger
- Boys > Girls and siblings have a tenfold higher risk than the general population
- Fevers usually abrupt and are quite high (> 39°C), minimal response to antipyretic meds
- Rash – typically nonspecific morbilliform rash but may resemble scarlet fever sandpaper rash, pustules on urticarial erythema (may mimic pustular psoriasis)
  - o Usually see accentuation of eruption in fold areas, especially the groin
  - o Perianal desquamation very common
- Irritability
- May also see CNS and GI involvement, lethargy, urethritis with sterile pyuria, anterior uveitis, musculoskeletal complaints, and peripheral gangrene
- Cardiac involvement is the most concerning complication of KD
  - o Early →pericardial effusions, myocarditis, congestive heart failure, arrhythmias, and valvular regurgitation
  - o Coronary artery aneurysms may occur
  - o Death can occur 3–8 weeks after the onset of the disease

Table 30 Diagnostic criteria for Kawasaki disease

Fever for 5 days or more plus at least 4/5 of the following clinical signs:
▪ Bilateral conjunctival injection – halo of sparing around iris (perilimbal sparing)
▪ Oral mucous membrane changes: injected pharynx, injected or fissured lips, strawberry tongue
▪ Peripheral extremity changes: erythema or edema (acute), periungal desquamation (late finding)
▪ Polymorphous rash
▪ Cervical lymphadenopathy (at least 1.5 cm)

Labs

- Increasing ESR in light of clinical improvement
- CBC – ↑ WBC, ↓ Hgb/Hct
  - o ↓ platelets (Thrombocytopenia) – associated with severe coronary disease
  - o ↑ platelets (thrombocytosis) – in subacute stage

- Lipids – Abnormal – ↓ HDL, total cholesterol, ↑ triglycerides, LDL
- Liver – ↓ albumin, ↑ transaminases, bilirubin – secondary to gallbladder hydrops
- Urine – Sterile pyuria, occasional mild proteinuria

DDx – toxin-mediated bacterial infections (scarlet fever, toxic shock syndrome), Rocky Mountain spotted fever, viral exanthems, drug reactions (including Stevens–Johnson syndrome and toxic epidermal necrolysis), pustular psoriasis

Histology – features are nonspecific

Treatment and Management

- No reliable diagnostic test to confirm KD, so diagnosis rests on clinical vigilance and the overall picture of the patient
- Goals of therapy = reduce inflammation and thus the potential for damage to the arterial wall
  - IVIG – 2 g/kg (in one IV infusion)
    - Steroid pulse therapy may be useful for KD patients with IVIG-resistant disease and persistent fever, although transient coronary artery dilatation may be noted during this treatment
  - Aspirin started with IVIG at 80–100 mg/kg/day until fever subsides
    - Then 3–5 mg/kg/day – primarily for antiplatelet effect
    - Risks = hepatitis, hearing loss, Reye syndrome (usually occurs in setting of acute varicella or influenza)
- Baseline echocardiogram/EKG
- Long-term follow-up:
  - Echocardiogram once a month × 2 months after illness onset
  - Children whose coronary arteries are normal at 2 months following the diagnosis are considered free of cardiac disease
  - Some consider a history of KD to be a risk factor for the later development of coronary artery disease

Pearls and Pitfalls

- A Kawasaki-like syndrome has also been observed in adults infected with HIV
- Missed diagnosis of KD is among the most common malpractice verdicts against child health practitioners. Consider the diagnosis in any infant with prolonged, unexplained fever.

Keratodermas

Table 31   Inherited palmar plantar keratodermas (PPK)

Name	Gene(s)	Inheritance	Clinical Manifestations
Acrokeratoelastoidosis	Unknown	AD	Yellow, hyperkeratotic papules (appearing umbilicated) on border of palms/soles
Brunauer–Fuhs–Siemens syndrome (Striate PPK)	Desmoglein 1	AD	Linear hyperkeratotic streaks on volar surface of finger and palms, with no systemic association
Clouston syndrome (hidrotic ectodermal dysplasia)	Connexin 30	AD	Diffuse transgredient PPK, alopecia, nail dystrophy, and other anomalies (cataracts, strabismus, tufted terminal phalanges)
Darier's disease	ATP2A2	AD	Hyperkeratotic papules in seborrheic distribution; white and red longitudinal bands, pterygium and V notch on nails
Epidermolysis bullosa simplex associated with PPK	Keratin 5/14	AD	PPK with traumatic palmoplantar and mucocutaneous blistering
Epidermolytic PPK with polycyclic psoriasiform plaques	Keratin 1	AD	Chronic diffuse PPK with flares of psoriasiform plaques
Erythrokeratoderma variabilis	Connexin 31 and 30.3	AD	Transient areas of figurate erythema, hyperhidrosis, PPK with transgrediens, hyperkeratotic plaques
Focal acral hyperkeratosis	Unknown	AD	Crateriform papules showing no elastorrhexis
Focal epidermolytic PPK	Unknown	AD	Focal and painful keratotic lesions, mainly on plantar pressure points
Focal non-epidermolytic PPK	Unknown	AD	Focal keratosis, often localized to pressure points on palms and soles
Focal palmoplantar keratoderma with oral mucosa hyperkeratosis	Keratin 16	AD	Focal PPK, oral hyperkeratosis, subungual hyperkeratosis
Greither disease (progressive PPK)	Keratin 9	AD	PPK with transgrediens, involvement of Achilles tendon
Howel–Evans Syndrome	Envoplakin	AD	PPK at pressure sites associated with esophageal cancer and oral leukoplakia
Huriez syndrome	Unknown	AD	PPK with sclerodactyly, hypohidrosis
Ichthyosis hystrix of Curth–Macklin	Keratin 1	AD	Spiky, verrucous hyperkeratotic plaques often associated with PPK
Keratosis palmoplantaris punctata (Bushke–Fischer–Bauer)	Unknown	AD	Multiple punctate keratoses on palmoplantar surface

(continued)

Table 31 (continued)

Name	Gene(s)	Inheritance	Clinical Manifestations
Olmsted syndrome	Unknown	AD	PPK infancy, oral leukoplakia, ainhum
Pachyonychia congenita type I (Jadassohn–Lewandowsky)	Keratin 6a/16	AD	PPK, hyperhidrosis, mucosal leukokeratosis
Pachyonychia congenita type II (Jackson–Sertoli)	Keratin 6b/17	AD	PPK, steatocyst multiplex, natal teeth
Pachyonychia congenita type III (Schafer–Branauer)	Keratin 6a/17	AD	PPK with corneal leukokeratosis
Pachyonychia congenita type IV (Tarda)	Unknown	AD	PPK, hyperpigmented flexures
Progressive symmetric erythrokeratoderma	Loricrin	AD	Fixed, symmetric, erythematous hyperkeratotic plaques – extremities, buttocks, and face
Vohwinkel's (Classical) Syndrome	Connexin 26	AD	PPK– honeycomb surface, juxta-articular "star-fish" keratotic papules, pseudo-ainhum and high-frequency deafness
Vohwinkel's syndrome, ichthyotic variant	Loricrin	AD	Classic Vohwinkel's syndrome, but NOT associated with deafness
Vorner syndrome (Diffuse epidermolytic PPK)	Keratin 9	AD	Non-transgrediens, symmetric hyperkeratosis of palms and soles, knuckle pads
Unna–Thost (Diffuse non-epidermolytic PPK)	Keratin 1	AD	Non-transgrediens, hyperhidrosis, knuckle pads
Bart–Pumphrey syndrome	GJB6	AD	Non-mutilating PPK with deafness, knuckle pads, and leukonychia
Carvajal syndrome	Desmoplakin	AR	Generalized PPK with woolly hair and dilated left ventricular cardiomyopathy
Ectodermal dysplasia/ skin fragility syndrome	Plakophilin	AR	Painful PPK, trauma-induced skin erosions, dystrophic nails, sparse hair
Haim–Munk syndrome	Cathepsin C	AR	PPK with severe periodontitis, arachnodactyly, acro-osteolysis, onychogryphosis, and radiographic deformity of fingers
KID syndrome	Connexin 26	AR	Keratitis, ichthyosis, deafness and stippled PPK (moth-eaten)
Lamellar ichthyosis	Transglutaminase 1	AR	Generalized ichthyosis with large scales, hypohidrosis, ectropion, and PPK
Mal de Meleda	SLURP-1	AR	Transgrediens, glove-and-stocking malodorous PPK, palmoplantar hyperhidrosis, hyperkeratotic plaques over joints, nail dystrophy, and perioral erythema

(continued)

Table 31   (continued)

Name	Gene(s)	Inheritance	Clinical Manifestations
Naxos disease	Plakoglobin	AR	PPK, congenital woolly hair, right ventricular cardiomyopathy
Papillon–Lefevre syndrome	Cathepsin C	AR	Symmetric, diffuse transgrediens PPK, periodontitis and loss of deciduous/permanent teeth and calcification of tentorial falx
Richner–Hanhart syndrome	Tyrosine transaminase	AR	Corneal ulcers, mental retardation, painful punctate keratoses on palms/soles, increased serum and urinary tyrosine levels

Langerhans Cell Histiocytosis (LCH)

Etiology and Pathogenesis

- LCH is term used to describe a disorder characterized by infiltration of Langerhans cells into various organs of the body
  - Older terms now obsolete → histiocytosis X, eosinophilic granuloma, Letterer–Siwe disease, Hand–Schuller–Christian syndrome, Hashimoto–Pritzker syndrome (older system based on spectrum of organ involvement)
- Langerhans cells are a type of dendritic cell found primarily in the epidermis and in mucosal epithelia, thymus, esophagus, and lung
- Pathogenesis unknown. Theories – somatic mutations, infection (viral), immune dysregulation, and apoptosis. Unclear whether LCH is neoplastic. Monoclonality is present

Clinical Presentation and Classification

- May occur at any age, from newborn to elderly, but peak incidence is between ages 1 and 4
- Cutaneous involvement common and is often the presenting complaint
  - Seborrheic dermatitis-like eruption common → prominent involvement of scalp, posterior auricular regions, perineum, and axillae. Resistant to therapy
  - Red-brown papules often seen (scalp and flexural areas common) → may have secondary erosion, hemorrhage, or crusting
  - Crusted papules on palms/soles, especially in infants in whom scabies has been excluded
  - Vesiculopustular lesions may predominate in neonates → may be misdiagnosed as congenital varicella or herpes. May become crusted or hemorrhagic
  - Nodules, ulcerative lesions are common
  - Granulomatous plaques
- Other clues
  - Gingival erythema, erosions, hemorrhage
  - Premature eruption of teeth or loosening of teeth as a result of severe gingivitis
  - Chronic otitis media from involvement of external auditory canals
    - Middle ear extension may cause destructive changes with resultant deafness
  - Bone lesions
  - Lymphadenopathy may be present

- Previous Classification (no longer used)
  - **Hand–Schuller–Christian** – triad of skull lesions, diabetes insipidus, exophthalmos. Prototype for multifocal LCH
  - **Letterer–Siwe** – "disseminated LCH" is most serious form with extensive involvement: Lymph node involvement (often cervical), hepatosplenomegaly, biliary cirrhosis, liver dysfunction, pulmonary involvement, GI involvement, thymus, bone marrow involvement, constitutional symptoms, CNS (resulting in diabetes insipidus), neuropsych deficits
  - **Congenital Self-Healing Reticulohistiocytosis** – aka "Hashimoto–Pritzker" or "Congenital Self-Healing LCH". Congenital presence of LCH lesions, usually papules and nodules, break down → ulcers. Usually no systemic signs. Lesions involute over a few months and are usually gone by 12 months. Workup for systemic involvement still needed and reports of cutaneous and systemic relapse, so need long-term f/u. Favorable prognosis

Labs and Imaging

- X-ray → "punched out" appearance to bone lesions (single or multiple lytic lesions)
- Orbital wall involvement – can radiographically simulate mastoiditis
- Vertebral involvement – may result in compression with radiographic findings of vertebra plana
- Pulmonary involvement – CXR shows diffuse micronodular or reticular pattern and pneumothoraces may result
- Posterior pituitary infiltration – can be seen on MRI as absence of a normally bright signal or thickening of the pituitary stalk. (Clinically → diabetes insipidus)
- Thymus involvement – enlargement on CXR
- PET scan has been useful in identifying areas with altered metabolism due to CNS LCH and can be useful in following the response to treatment

DDx – may depend somewhat on presentation. Seb derm, scabies, intertrigo, herpes, varicella

Histology

- Routine H&E specimens show infiltrate of typical Langerhans cells (S100+, CD1a+)
- EM reveals Birbeck granules in cytoplasm of cells, but this is rarely performed

Treatment

- Tx depends on extent of disease. Patients usually treated by pediatric oncologist
- Limited cutaneous involvement (after workup to rule out systemic involvement)
  - Close follow-up with observation alone since lesions may resolve spontaneously
  - Topical corticosteroids are only sometimes helpful
  - Painful lesions may be treated with curettage, surgical excision or intralesional steroids, or occasionally localized radiation therapy
- Severe cutaneous involvement
  - Topical nitrogen mustard
- Systemic LCH
  - Systemic chemotherapy – most commonly vinblastine or etoposide
  - Prednisone or methylprednisolone often used during the induction phase
  - Reports of cyclosporine A, 2-chlorodeoxyadenosine, interferon-α, allogenic bone marrow, or cord blood transplantation

Prognosis

- Potentially fatal disorder and prognosis is quite variable. Depends on extent of organ involvement, response to therapy
- Morbidity and mortality may be related to progressive disease or late sequelae

Pearls and Pitfalls

- Refer all patients to oncology, even if you think only limited cutaneous involvement
- Arnold–Chiari malformation (basilar invagination with associated hydrocephalus) reported in long-term survivors of LCH (in addition to other conditions such as Osteogenesis Imperfecta)
- Clues to LCH (especially if these are in combination with lymphadenopathy):
  - Recalcitrant seb derm-like eruption
  - Rash localized to scalp, posterior auricular regions, perineum, axillae
  - Eroded papules in flexural areas
  - Crusted papules on palms/soles and scabies prep is negative

Molloscum Contagiosum

Etiology and Pathogenesis

- Common cutaneous infection caused by molloscum contagiosum virus, which is a poxvirus
- Virus spreads through skin-to-skin contact and via fomites

Clinical Presentation

- Typically seen in healthy kids, often in school-age children
  - Can be sexually transmitted or associated with immunodeficiency (especially HIV)
- Pearly, flesh-colored to pink, umbilicated papules that often appear translucent
  - Range in size from 2 to 8 mm
  - Central dell may or may not be evident
  - Lesions often cluster and are common around sites of eczema
  - Common in sites of rubbing or in moist areas – axillae, popliteal fossae, groin
  - Lesions may become very erythematous, which typically represents a host immune response against the molloscum. Lesions typically heal with spontaneous involution thereafter
  - Children can occasionally have large lesions or very high numbers of lesions
  - Infectious part of lesion is the central core
- Often see dermatitis surrounding the molloscum – called "molloscum dermatitis". These areas are itchy → patient scratches → cycle perpetuated → can get secondary impetiginization
- Lesions around eyes can be problematic and lead to chronic conjunctivitis, superficial punctate keratitis
- Spontaneous clearing occurs but varies between weeks, months, and years

DDx – verrucae vulgares, adnexal tumors, condyloma accuminata, basal cell carcinoma, Spitz nevus. In immunocompromised host, consider disseminated cryptococcis, histoplasmosis, coccidiomycosis

Histology

- Epidermal hyperplasia producing a crater filled with Henderson–Patterson bodies (large basophilic intracytoplasmic inclusions that push the nucleus and numerous keratohyaline granules aside)
- Intact lesions show little or no inflammation
- Ruptured lesions have dense inflammatory infiltrate consisting of mononuclear cells, neutrophils and multinucleated giant cells

Treatment

- Treatment usually sought for – cosmetic significance, pruritus, or epidemiologic concerns of other parents/teachers/school nurses. Additionally, kids with underlying eczema tend to spread the molloscum by scratching their eczema (autoinoculation)
- Cantharidin (0.7 or 0.9%) – extract from blister beetle, *Cantharis vesicatoria*
  - With appropriate application and patient education, can be a well-tolerated treatment Apply medication very *carefully* to lesions – use single drop and avoid painting
  - Wash off in 4 h (sooner if vesiculation or discomfort occurs)
  - Avoid treating facial, mucosal, occluded areas
  - Treat a max of 20–30 lesions per treatment session
  - Use blunt end of a wooden cotton-tipped applicator
  - Let areas dry for 2 min before child puts clothes on
  - Do not occlude treated areas
- Cimetidine 40 mg/kg/day – can be useful if extensive involvement, facial involvement
- Imiquimod 3.75% or 5%
  - Can be extremely irritating. Start by using small amount 3x/week. Educate parents that mild irritation is ok and may be beneficial, but hold medication if area becomes very red and inflamed
- Tretinoin cream 0.025% – can be a helpful alternative for facial lesions. Apply QHS, as sunlight can inactivate the generic product
- Salicylic acid
- Tape stripping

Pearls and Pitfalls

- If applying cantharidin, give handout to parents with the time the medication was placed and the time the medication needs to be washed off.
  - Educate parents that lesions will look worse before they look better
- Curettage and cryotherapy are sometimes used in adults. Do not recommend this treatment in children, as it is painful and very traumatic
- Some advocate having parents gently remove the infectious core, although many parents do not feel comfortable doing this
- Molloscum are caused by a poxvirus, which in and of itself can cause mild scarring
- If adult presents with molloscum, recommend checking for HIV-1 and -2
- In immunocompromised host, consider disseminated infection with Cryptococcis, histoplasmosis, coccidiomycosis, penicillium marneffei (if person has been in southeast Asia)

Neurofibromatosis I (von Recklinghausen disease)

Etiology and Pathogenesis

- AD disorder; spontaneous mutation in 50%
- 1:3000, M=F
- Most common type of neurofibromatosis – 85% of all cases

Clinical Presentation

- **NIH Consensus Criteria for Diagnosis (1987) – Need two or more features**
  - Six or more café au lait macules over 5 mm in greatest diameter in prepubertal individuals and over 15 mm in greatest diameter in postpubertal individuals
  - Two or more neurofibromas of any type **or** one plexiform neurofibromas
  - Freckling in the axillary or inguinal regions
  - Optic glioma
  - Two or more Lisch nodules
  - A distinctive osseous lesion such as sphenoid dysplasia or thinning of long bone cortex with or without pseudoarthrosis
  - A first-degree relative with NF-1 by the above criteria

Treatment and Management

- Always evaluate other family members for the presence of cutaneous lesions to consider if a sporadic mutation or if a parent is affected – genetic counseling
- Ophthalmologic exams
  - Annual eye exams
  - Can help if the diagnosis is equivocal
- Always check blood pressure
  - If ↑ in child – consider renal artery stenosis
  - If ↑ in adult – consider pheochromocytoma
- Optional – can offer baseline MRI
- Precocious puberty may suggest CNS tumor
- Multiple juvenile xanthogranuloma (JXG) may be associated with nonlymphocytic leukemia in a child with CALM
  - If xanthogranulomas present → CBC, but likelihood of leukemia is small
- Follow serial head circumference in children → risk of hydrocephalus and the frequency of macrocephaly without hydrocephalus
- Refer to NF support group

Pearls and Pitfalls

- May have shortened life span due to neurofibrosarcoma, pheochromocytoma, vascular disease complications, CNS tumor complications, Tumors (optic gliomas, astrocytomas, meningiomas, acoustic neuroma, ependymoma, Wilms' tumor, nonlymphocytic leukemia, visceral neurofibromas)
- Great variation in severity of disease

Neurofibromatosis II (Bilateral acoustic neurofibromatosis)

Etiology and Pathogenesis

- AD; mutation in SCH gene. Leads to a defect in schwannomin/merlin, the NF-2 gene product, and may affect tumor suppressor activity at the cell membrane level
- 1:35,000, M = F

Clinical Presentation

- Symptoms frequently appear at 15–25 years of life
- Normal intelligence
- Skin – neurofibromas (less common than in NF-1), café au lait macules
- CNS – bilateral vestibular schwannomas and of other nerves, meningiomas, astrocytomas, CNS tumors
- Eye – juvenile posterior subcapsular lenticular opacity
- **NIH Consensus Criteria for Diagnosis (1987) –**
  - Bilateral 8th nerve masses (visualized with CT or MRI) **– or –**
  - First-degree relative with NF-2 **– and either-**
  - Unilateral 8th nerve mass **– or –**
  - Any two of the following: neurofibromas, meningioma, spinal glioma, schwannoma, juvenile posterior subcapsular lenticular opacity

Treatment and Management

- Refer to neurologist/neurosurgeon – surgical debulking of tumors
- Refer to ENT specialist/audiologist, ophthalmologist
- Examine first-degree relatives
- Pt must never swim alone; avoid going under water – can get underwater

Pearls and Pitfalls

- Progressive deterioration with loss of hearing, ambulation, and sight
- Death resulting from CNS tumors approximately 20 years after onset of symptoms
- Offspring of affected individuals should have an eye exam at birth because cataracts may be present very early on

Nevus Sebaceus (of Jadassohn)

Etiology and Pathogenesis

- A hamartoma that is typically sporadic consisting of epidermal, follicular, sebaceous, and apocrine elements

Clinical Presentation

- Common congenital lesion that occurs mainly on the face and scalp
- Hairless, yellow-orange plaque. Surface may be verrucous or velvety. Hyperpigmentation may be prominent in some, causing lesion to look like epidermal nevus
- Lesion often linear or oval
- Size – few millimeters to several centimeters in length
- Lesions enlarge proportionally with child's growth
- At puberty – they tend to become significantly thicker, more verrucous and greasy (result of hormonal stimulation of the sebaceous glands). Papillomatous projections may occur and simulate a verruca vulgaris
- Can develop benign and malignant growths within the nevus sebaceous later in life
  - o Syringocystadenoma papilliferum (most common secondary benign neoplasm), BCCs, tricholemmomas, apocrine cystadenoma, spiradenoma, and trichoblastoma
  - o More aggressive malignant neoplasms can occur including apocrine carcinoma with metastases, adnexal carcinomas, and squamous cell carcinoma

- **Schimmelpenning Syndrome**
  - o Multiple nevi sebaceous may occur in association with cerebral, ocular, and skeletal abnormalities as part of the epidermal nevus syndrome

DDx – epidermal nevus, verruca vulgaris, aplasia cutis congenital, seborrheic keratosis (in older patient)

Histology

- Epidermal hyperplasia that may range from slight to prominent – simple, verrucous, seborrheic keratosis-like, and acrochordon types
- Hair follicles may be normal in number, absent, few in number, and embryonic or normal in development
- Sebaceous glands may be absent or present, immature, and normal or hyperplastic. Apocrine glands are either present or absent

Treatment and Management

- Surgical excision
  - Timing of surgery is controversial, but recommend complete removal prior to onset of puberty
  - Provide objective data and allow parents to make the decision
- Alternatives to surgery include photodynamic therapy, carbon dioxide laser resurfacing, and dermabrasion. None of these treatment modalities completely removes the lesion, and there is therefore a risk of recurrence or the potential for the development of tumors in the residual lesion. These alternatives not currently recommended

Pearls and Pitfalls

- Timing of removal of a nevus sebaceous is controversial, but many parents desire to have it removed prior to the child's enrollment in school

Pediatric Medication Dosing

Table 32 Pediatric medication dosing

	Drug name	Liquid form	Tablet form	Dosing
Antibiotics	Cephalexin	125 or 250 mg/5 mL	250 mg 500 mg	30–50 mg/kg divided BID-TID × 10 – 14 days
	Bactrim	40 mg TMP/200 mg SMX/5 mL	80/400 160/800	6–10 mg TMP/kg/day divided BID × 10 days
	Clindamycin	75 mg/5 mL	75 mg 150 mg 300 mg	10–30 mg/kg/day divided TID
	Erythromycin EES (CYP450 3A4 substrate/inhibitor)	200 or 400/5 mL	400 mg	30–50 mg/kg/day divided BID *Try to stay closer to 30 mg/kg and almost always use the EES
	Doxycycline	25 mg/5 mL	20, 50, 75, 100 mg 75, 100 mg ER	2.2 mg/kg/day divided QD-BID Do not use in children < age 8
	Tetracycline	125 mg/5 mL	250, 500 mg	25–50 mg/kg PO QD div q 6 h for bacterial infection (max 3 g/day) Do not use in children < age 8
	Minocycline	None	50 mg 75 mg 100 mg	2–4 mg/kg/day divided QD-BID (200 mg max daily dose) Do not use in children < age 8
Antifungals Shampoos: – Nizoral 2% – Selsun 2.5%	Griseofulvin susp (microsize)	125 mg/5 mL	None	20–25 mg/kg/day divided QD-BID
	GrisPEG (ultramicrosize)		125 mg 250 mg	15 mg/kg/day
	Terbinafine	Granules: 125 mg 187.5 mg	250 mg	<20 kg – ¼ tab QD (62.5 mg) 20–40 kg – ½ tab QD (125 mg) >40 kg – 1 tab QD (250 mg)
	Fluconazole	10 mg/mL 40 mg/mL	50 mg 100 mg 150 mg 200 mg	6 mg/kg/day divided QD (6 weeks for tinea capitis) 6 mg/kg/week for onychomycosis (off-label)
	Itraconazole	Don't use the suspension (per Elewski)	100 mg	5 mg/kg/day divided QD-BID Divide dose BID if > 200 mg/day. Give caps with food < 60 lbs – 100 mg QOD > 60 lbs (27.3 kg) – 100 mg QD

(continued)

Table 32   (continued)

	Drug name	Liquid form	Tablet form	Dosing
Antihistamines	Benedryl	12.5 mg/5 mL	25, 50 mg	Take ½ tsp q 6 h or BID and double at HS (2 mg/kg/day q 6)
	Atarax	10 mg/5 mL	10, 25, 500, 100 mg	Same as above
	Zyrtec	1 mg/1 mL or 5 mg/5 mL	5, 10 mg chew tablets	<2 years old – ½ tsp >2 years old – 1 tsp
	Doxepin	10 mg/1 mL	10, 25, 50, 75, 100, 150 mg	Start **0.5 mL** and work up slowly as tolerated. Dispense with dropper.
	Singulair		4, 5 mg chew tab 4, 10 mg granule packet	Granule packet to be mixed with ice cream, applesauce, carrots or rice 2–5 years old – 4 mg/day 6–14 years old – 5 mg/day >15 years old – 10 mg/day
	Claritin	5 mg/5 mL	10 mg	2–5 years old – 5 mg/day > 5 years old – 10 mg/day
Miscellaneous	Tagamet	300 mg/5 mL	300, 400, 800 mg	40 mg/kg/day BID-TID Always check for drug interactions
	Orapred	15 mg/5 mL		Start 2 mg/kg/day If no improvement, can go up to 3 mg/kg/day. Can give high dose × 6 weeks. If no response seen at 6 weeks, start to taper by 1 mL every 2 weeks. If rebounds, can increase. Follow growth and blood pressure
	Squaric acid			Sensitize with 2% Start tx with 0.1% (30 mL). Can increase to 0.2% Start 0.1% for alopecia areata and 0.4% for warts
	IL Kenalog			3–5 mg/kg
	Enbrel			0.8 mg/kg twice weekly

Note: Always put the weight of the child in kg on the Rx to prevent medication overdoses

Phakomatosis Pigmentovascularis (PPV)

Etiology and Pathogenesis

- Term used to describe the association of a nevus flammeus (port wine stain) with a pigmented nevus or, in some cases, a nevus anemicus
  - Nevus anemicus = vascular birthmark characterized by blanching of cutaneous blood vessels and thus presents as a "white" patch on the skin. This white area represents vasoconstriction

Clinical Presentation and Types

Table 33 Classification of phakomatosis pigmentovascularis

Type	Description
I	Nevus flammeus + pigmented linear epidermal nevus
II	**Nevus flammeus + dermal melanocytosis ± nevus anemicus (MOST COMMON TYPE)**
III	Nevus flammeus + nevus spilus ± nevus anemicus
IV	Nevus flammeus + dermal melanocytosis + nevus spilus ± nevus anemicus
V	Cutis marmorata telangiectasia congenital + dermal melanocytosis
Further divided into: a – skin findings only b – skin findings and systemic abnormalities Dermal melanocytosis = Mongolian spots, nevus of Ota, etc.	

- **Systemic involvement** – estimated that 50% have this and most are **type IIb**
  - Changes mimic those seen in Sturge–Weber syndrome or Klippel–Trenaunay syndrome. Involvement usually related to the body surface area affected by the vascular lesion
  - **Neurologic abnormalities** – seizures, cortical atrophy, spinal dysraphism, Arnold–Chiari type I malformation, bilateral deafness, idiopathic facial paralysis, hydrocephalus, diabetes insipidus, plexiform neurofibroma, psychomotor delay, EEG alterations
  - **Ocular abnormalities** – melanosis oculi (most common eye finding), iris mammilations, iris hamartomas, glaucoma, prominent vessels in sclera, chronic edema in cornea, pigmentary alterations in retina, cataracts
  - **Miscellaneous abnormalities** – leg-length discrepancies, scoliosis, hemihypertrophy, syndactyly, macrocephaly, renal agenesis, hepatosplenomegaly, pyogenic granuloma, cavernous hemangioma, hypoplasia of leg veins, umbilical hernia, IgA deficiency, Hyper IgE syndrome, premature eruption of teeth

Treatment

- PPV without systemic complications is benign and requires no treatment
  - ○ Quality of life may be improved by treating nevus flammeus with pulsed dye laser and by treating pigmentary nevus with Q-switched lasers
- Lesions of dermal melanocytosis may or may not fade with time

Pearls and Pitfalls

- Neurologic abnormalities, if present, usually seen in first few months of life

Reference:

Fernández-Guarino M, et al. Phakomatosis pigmentovascularis: clinical findings in 15 patients and review of the literature. J Am Acad Derm 2008; 58(1): 88–93.

Pigmentary Mosaicism

Etiology and Pathogenesis

- Term used to describe group of disorders with patterned streaks of hyper- or hypopigmentation
  - AKA – patterned dyspigmentation
  - Group includes – Hypomelanosis of Ito, linear and whorled nevoid hypermelanosis (LWNH) and the segmental form of nevus depigmentosus
  - Likely reflects gene mosaicism in affected area
- Chromosomal abnormalities have been described in 60% of affected pediatric patients with more extensive pigmentary mosaicism
- Does not tend to be hereditary

Clinical Presentation

- Linear hyper- or hypopigmented streaks which tend to follow lines of Blaschko or a phylloid pattern of mosaic distribution
- Associated abnormalities seen in about 30% and may include:
  - **CNS** – developmental delay, seizures, microcephaly, hydrocephalus, hypotonia
  - **Bone** – syndactyly, polydactyly, clinodactyly, short stature, scoliosis, coarse facies ·
  - **Eyes** – congenital cataracts
  - **Cardiac** – congenital heart defects (ventricular septal defect, patent ductus artery, tetralogy of Fallot)
  - **Dental** – second molar agenesis, enamel defects
  - **Other** – choanal atresia, impaired hearing, inguinal hernia

DDx – incontinentia pigmenti, CHILD syndrome, Condradi–Hünermann syndrome, Goltz syndrome, lichen striatus

Treatment and Management

- Thorough history – including birth and family history of any pigmentary, skin, hair, or teeth anomalies to identify children with incontinentia pigmenti
- Thorough physical exam
- If widespread pigmentary mosaicism …
  - Refer to neurology for baseline exam to evaluate for subtle delays or motor defects
  - Baseline ophthalmologic exam
  - Genetic evaluation (including karyotype testing)

Pearls and Pitfalls

– **Most patients are normal**, but evidence of neurologic, ocular, and bony defects should be sought especially with more extensive pigmentary changes

Reference:

Treat J. Patterned pigmentation in children. Pediatr Clin North Am 2010; 57(5): 1121–9.

Pilomatricoma

Etiology and Pathogenesis

- AKA – calcifying epithelioma of Malherbe, pilomatrixoma
- Mutations in CTNNB1, the gene that encodes for β-catenin, are present in pilomatricomas
  - β-catenin is a signaling pathway that influences cell differentiation and proliferation

Clinical Presentation

- Usually a solitary skin-colored to faint blue nodule or papule. Rarely see multiple lesions
- Lesions are firm and reflect calcification that typically occurs in the lesions, along with fibrosis and inflammation
  - "Teeter-totter sign" – downward pressure on one end of the lesion causes the other end to spring upward in the skin
  - "Tent sign" – multiple facets and angles (resembling a tent) are seen when the overlying skin is stretched
- Size – ranges from 5 mm–5 cm
- May develop on any non-glabrous surface, but usually on head or upper trunk
- Usually seen in childhood or adolescence but can occur at any age
- Occasionally, the dermis overlying a pilomatricoma will develop anetoderma
- Variants
  - Cystic-appearing pilomatricomas where hemorrhage may result in blue-red translucent nodule with rapid enlargement
  - Extruding pilomatricoma – chalky material discharged spontaneously
  - Perforating pilomatricoma
- Multiple pilomatricomas may be seen in → Gardner syndrome, Rubinstein–Taybi syndrome, Trisomy 9
- Familial forms may be seen in association with → myotonic dystrophy (an uncommon AD disease associated with hypotonia, muscle wasting, cataracts, hypogonadism, progressive MR, frontal baldness.)

DDx – cyst, BCC (if seen in an older patient)

Histology

- Well-circumscribed nodule in the dermis, sometimes with a squamous epithelial lining at periphery. Keratinous debris, calcification, or ossification often present

- Basaloid cells in early lesions, especially at periphery of nodule
- Shadow (ghost) cells – pale, empty space where nucleus used to be, with abundant pink cytoplasm. Transitional cells may be present, with pyknotic nuclei – becoming shadow cells

Treatment

- Surgical excision
- If multiple recurrences are observed, complete excision (with negative margins) should be performed to exclude the possibility of pilomatrical carcinoma

Pearls and Pitfalls

- Patients with multiple lesions or familial disease should be examined and followed closely for associated disorders, especially myotonic dystrophy and Gardner syndrome
  - Myotonic dystrophy may not occur until adulthood; molecular diagnosis available

Pityriasis Amiantacea

Etiology and Pathogenesis

- Pityriasis amiantacea represents a reaction pattern rather than a specific diagnosis. This condition may be the end result of severe seborrheic dermatitis, tinea capitis, psoriasis, or atopic dermatitis. It may be idiopathic

Clinical Presentation

- Thick yellow scaly plaques which are adherent to tufts of hair and can cause pain if the affected area is manipulated
- Alopecia may occur
- There may be cutaneous signs to the etiology
  - If psoriasis – elbows, knees, nails, etc.
  - Atopic dermatitis – Dennie–Morgan lines, flexural involvement, allergies, etc.
  - Tinea capitis – cervical lymphadenopathy, pustules, kerion, etc.
- The scales may resemble asbestos, giving rise to the term amiantacea – the French word for asbestos is "amiante"

Labs – Fungal culture of scalp

DDx – head lice, lichen simplex chronicus

Treatment

- Treatment is aimed at treating the scale and addressing the underlying condition
- Mineral or vegetable oils, especially olive oil may help to loosen the adherent scales
- Washable leave-on creams or wash-off shampoos containing salicylic acid, coal tar and sulfur may be of help in reducing the scaling and inflammation
- Intermittent courses of topical steroids are useful for psoriasis and various types of dermatitis, often as lotions or gels or oils
- Antifungal shampoo (e.g., ketoconazole or ciclopirox) is often prescribed and may be helpful for underlying seborrheic dermatitis
- Oral antifungal agents are necessary for confirmed tinea capitis infection

Pearls and Pitfalls

- Always do a fungal culture to rule out tinea

Spitz Nevus

Etiology and Pathogenesis

- Formerly known as "benign juvenile melanoma"
- Etiology unclear

Clinical Presentation

- Smooth-surfaced, hairless papule or nodule with red-brown color
- Usually solitary, although can have multiple lesions and rarely, disseminated lesions
- Vary in size from few mm to 1 cm in diameter
- Presence of brown pigment (either clinical or by compressing with slide – "diascopy") may be useful in confirming the melanocytic nature of the lesion
- Surface telangiectasias may be prominent
- Distribution – most common on head and neck, but can occur on shoulders, trunk, legs
- Usually seen in children and young adults

DDx – pyogenic granuloma, early juvenile xanthogranuloma, amelanotic melanoma

Histology – All spitz nevi should be read by a trained dermatopathologist

- Symmetrical lesion with epidermal hyperplasia. Rete ridges often clutching melanocytic nests
- Melanocytic nests may be spindle-shaped or epithelioid, or both
- Clefts often around melanocytic nests, sometimes pagetoid
- Maturation of melanocytes deeper in lesion (cells become smaller with less atypia)
- HMB-45 and Ki-67 (MIB-1) staining often shows stratification → more likely to be positive in superficial portion
- Bizarre multinucleated or atypical melanocytes often in superficial portion of lesion, sometimes with mitoses limited to superficial portion. Often have angulated shape

Treatment and Management

- Most behave in a benign fashion and treatment is controversial
  - Atypical spitz nevi should be excised completely in a conservative fashion
  - Some recommend excising all spitz nevi on the basis of the uncertainty of their biologic behavior and occasional reports of aggressive potential

Pearls and Pitfalls

- Incompletely removed spitz nevi can recur and may be misread as malignant melanoma
- Histology may be difficult to distinguish from a spitzoid melanoma

Staphylococcal Scalded Skin Syndrome

Etiology and Pathogenesis

- AKA – Ritter's disease
- Blistering skin disease caused by the epidermolytic toxin-producing *Staph aureus*
  - Most cases caused by phage group II strains (types 3A, 3C, 55, 71) of *Staph aureus*. These exfoliative toxins (ETA and ETB) target desmoglein 1 in the stratum granulosum
    - Desmoglein 1 (DSG1) is a cell–cell adhesion molecule found in desmosomes of the superficial epidermis. (Same target as in pemphigus foliaceus)
- Disease preferentially affects neonates, children, and adults (latter usually have renal disease, diabetes, immunosuppression, malignancy, or heart disease). These patients seem to lack protection from antitoxin antibodies and have decreased renal excretion of the toxin
- Some reports of nosocomial spread

Clinical Presentation

- Begins as localized infection of conjunctivae, nares, perioral region, perineum or umbilicus
  - Other infections can serve as a nidus – pneumonia, septic arthritis, endocarditis, or pyomyositis
- Constitutional symptoms – fever, malaise, lethargy irritability, poor feeding and then skin eruption
- Skin – begins as erythema that progresses to large, superficial, fragile blisters that rupture easily and leave behind denuded, red, tender skin
  - Most marked in flexural areas but may involve entire surface of skin
  - Nikolsky sign + (progression of blister cleavage plane induced by gentle pressure on edge of bulla)
  - Widespread skin involvement can lead to decreased thermoregulatory ability, fluid losses, electrolyte imbalances
  - Get characteristic radial fissures around the mouth → "Sad man facies"
  - Mucosal involvement is lacking in SSSS, but may have perioral crusting
  - Risk for secondary infection and sepsis
  - Scaling and desquamation continue for 3–5 days. Reepithelialization occurs in 2 weeks. Affected skin heals without scarring

Labs

- Diagnosis is confirmed by isolation of *Staph aureus* (blisters are usually sterile so have to find the source). Most easily recovered from pyogenic areas on skin, nares, nasopharynx or conjunctivae

- Leukocyte count may or may not be elevated
- Biopsy can also be very helpful

DDx – Toxic epidermal necrolysis (this has mucosal involvement), scalding burns, epidermolysis bullosa, graft versus host disease, nutritional deficiency dermatosis, bullous ichthyosis in the neonate, drug reaction, Kawasaki disease, extensive bullous impetigo, toxic shock syndrome, pemphigus foliaceus

Histology

- Subcorneal blister containing only rare inflammatory cells and some acantholytic cells. Split is in the granular layer
- Minimal or absent perivascular neutrophils and lymphocytes
- Bacteria not present in the blister (since toxin-mediated)

Treatment

- Treatment aimed at eradicating toxin-producing staphylococci. Antibiotic choice should be either → β-lactamase-resistant penicillin (e.g., dicloxacillin, cloxacillin), first- or second-generation cephalosporin, or clindamycin. Modify antibiotic as needed once sensitivities return
- If MRSA etiology – parenteral vancomycin or other agents (as dictated by sensitivities)
- To hospitalize or not …
  - Older children – often a mild disease and may be able to do ambulatory therapy if they can take PO
  - Adults – would hospitalize since very high mortality (> 50%, almost 100% if underlying disease), and these patients are usually very sick
  - Neonates, infants, or children with severe involvement – hospitalize
    - Attention to fluid status and electrolyte imbalances
    - Infection control measures – including contact isolation
    - Pain management
    - Meticulous wound care – bland emollients (such as vaseline ointment) to decrease pruritus and tenderness
    - If very severe case, admit to burn unit. Do NOT actively debride areas

Pearls and Pitfalls

- Mortality rate is 3% for children and > 50% in adults (almost 100% if underlying disease)

Streptococcal Toxic Shock Syndrome

Etiology and Pathogenesis

- Thought to be caused by direct tissue invasion and destruction by bacteria
- By binding to the Class II MHC complex of antigen-presenting cells and the Vβ region of T-cell receptors, streptococcal antigens act as superantigens and can stimulate T cells → inflammatory mediators and cytokine release → shock
- *Strept pyogenes* strains, especially M types 1 and 3 – release streptococcal pyogenic exotoxins A, B, or both. These produce TNF-α and IL-1 which lead to fever, hypotension, and tissue destruction
- Disruption of the cutaneous barrier is usually the portal of entry, but up to 50% have no known source for their strept bacteremia

Clinical Presentation

- Mainly affects healthy adults between ages of 20 and 50, but varicella infection in children is important risk factor for invasive Group A beta-hemolytic strept (GABHS)
  - ○ In a child with varicella who becomes febrile after having been afebrile, or who has any fever beyond the fourth day of illness, GABHS should be considered
- Group A strept infection with early onset of shock and organ failure (within about 48–72 h)
- Disease begins insidiously with nonspecific flu-like symptoms
  - ○ Fever, chills, myalgias, diarrhea
  - ○ CNS symptoms are common – confusion, coma
- Most common initial symptom = severe localized pain in an extremity
  - ○ 50% show signs of underlying soft tissue infection – swelling, redness, tenderness
    - Development of violaceous hue, bullae, necrosis points to a deeper infection (such as necrotizing fasciitis), and has a poorer prognosis
  - ○ Some present with only pain and no physical findings
- Skin – generalized blanching macular erythema is seen much less than in staphylococcal TSS
  - ○ Desquamation of hands and feet in 20%
- Severe complications
  - ○ Renal failure
  - ○ Disseminated intravascular coagulation
  - ○ Adult respiratory distress syndrome

Labs

- Blood cultures – positive in about 50%
- Wound cultures
- CMP – serum creatinine rises early in course
- Creatine kinase – rises in setting of necrotizing fasciitis or myonecrosis
- CBC + diff – white count may be increased or normal, but profound left shift. Thrombocytopenia common
- Evidence of DIC may be seen

DDx – Staphylococcal TSS

Histology

- Spongiosis, subepidermal blister formation, neutrophilic invasion, necrotic keratinocytes, dermal lymphocytic perivascular infiltrate

Treatment

- Early antibiotics – Clindamycin thought to inhibit bacterial toxins (cause of shock) and is first-line treatment
  - ○ IVIG given once may be beneficial when used in combination with antibiotics for streptococcal TSS, although adequate controlled studies are lacking
- Early surgical intervention – debridement, fasciotomy, amputation in appropriate cases and can be life saving
- Hypotension – aggressive IV fluids, support with vasopressor agents

Pearls and Pitfalls

- NSAIDs, which lessen the fever and symptoms of infection, might delay the diagnosis
- Pain out of proportion to clinical findings – consider necrotizing fasciitis or myonecrosis. Call surgery immediately
- Mortality rate varies from 30% to 60%

Tinea Capitis

Etiology and Pathogenesis

- The most common dermatophytosis of childhood
  - *T. tonsurans* is also the most common cause in Canada, Mexico, and Central America
  - *T. tonsurans* accounts for greater than 90% of cases of infection in UK and USA
  - *Epidermophyton floccosum* and *T. concentricum* do not invade scalp hair
- **Ectothrix** (extending outside the hair shaft)
  - Fluorescent
    - *M. audouinii, M. canis, M. distortum, M. ferrugineum*
  - Nonfluorescent
    - *M. gypseum* (sometimes fluoresces), *M. nanum, T. megninii, T. mentagrophytes, T. rubrum, T. verrucosum*
- **Endothrix** (inside hair shaft)
  - *T. gourvilli, T. rubrum, T. tonsurans, T. soudanense, T. yaounde, T. violaceum*

Clinical Presentation

- Scaly, erythematous pruritic patches on the scalp, often with associated hair loss
  - Pustules may be present
  - Cervical lymphadenopathy (neck) often present
  - "Black dots" may be seen – represent hair shafts broken off at the surface of the skin
  - Kerion may be seen – boggy, tender plaque with pustules. Represents a vigorous host immune response
  - Favus – yellow, cup-shaved crusts around the hair. Usually caused by *T. schoenleinii* (sometimes fluoresces); also caused by *T. violaceum, M. gypseum*. Seen predominantly in Africa, Mediterranean, Middle East. Rare in North and South America
- Widespread "Id" reaction is common and presents as papular or papulovesicular eruption, usually more predominant on extremities. Can mimic a drug eruption

Labs – Fungal culture and KOH, bacterial culture

DDx – Alopecia areata, atopic dermatitis, drug reaction, id reaction, impetigo, SCLE, psoriasis (plaque and pustular), seborrheic dermatitis, syphilis, trichotillomania, bacterial folliculitis, dissecting cellulitis, abscess, neoplasia, pyoderma, secondary syphilis

Histology – Biopsy not usually performed unless diagnosis is in question

- PAS + fungal structures and spores in follicular epithelium
- Usually a surrounding abscess containing neutrophils, eosinophils, histiocytes, and lymphocytes
- Spongiosis or intraepidermal vesicles
- Psoriasiform epidermal changes (sometimes)
- Often see parakeratosis and neutrophils in stratum corneum
- Compact orthokeratosis rather than normal basket-weave pattern may be a sign of tinea

Treatment

- Griseofulvin for 6–8 weeks …
  - Microsize 20–25 mg/kg/day
  - Ultramicrosize 7.3 mg/kg/day
- Terbinafine for 2–4 weeks
  - Does not work for *M. canis*
  - >40 kg → 250 mg/day
  - 20–40 kg → 125 mg/day
  - 10–20 kg → 62.5 mg/day
- Fluconazole 6 mg/kg/day for 6 weeks
- Itraconazole 3–5 mg/kg/day for 4–6 weeks (endothrix)
  - Pulse regimen: 5 mg/kg/day for 1 week, skip 3 weeks → repeat × 3 pulses
  - Do not use liquid formulation in children
- Take with fatty meal; acid helps absorption
- Prevent shedding and spread to other family members:
  - Ketoconazole 2% shampoo (or 2.5% selenium sulfide shampoo)
- Re-swab for fungal culture in 6–8 weeks to make sure that fungus has been completely eliminated. Look at family members for possible infection/carrier state if patient appears to be "resistant" to therapy

Pearls and Pitfalls

- *M. canis* **does not respond to terbinafine** (why culture is important). If this is the culture result, recommend that all cats and dogs be evaluated by a veterinarian
- Fluorescence (under Woods Light) is due to pteridine production
- Always treat hair-bearing areas with oral antifungals since the fungus tracts down the hair follicle and cannot be treated with topicals alone

- Majocchi's granuloma – can lead to scarring.
  - Be aggressive in treatment with oral antifungals
  - Oral steroids (0.5–1 mg/kg/day for 2–4 weeks) may help reduce the risk for and extent of permanent alopecia in the treatment of Kerion. Avoid using topical steroids
- Oral ketoconazole not recommended due to risk of hepatotoxicity
- Longer duration of therapy may be required for ectothrix infection (e.g., *M. canis, M. audouinii*)
- If a child has had tinea capitis, consider washing their hair with Nizoral 2% shampoo immediately after returning from barber
- Do not share hair combs, brushes, hats, or hooded jackets with others when infection is present

Toxic Shock Syndrome (TSS)

Etiology and Pathogenesis

- Multisystem disease caused by an exotoxin produced by *Staph aureus*
- Has been associated with tampon use for menstruation → "menstrual TSS"
- Most cases are NOT associated with menstruation and tampons and usually seen in patients who have undergone surgical procedures.
- Due to infection or colonization with certain strains of *Staph aureus* that are able to produce a particular protein → Toxic shock syndrome toxin-1 (TSST-1). Can also be due to staphylococcal enterotoxins (SEA, SEB, SEC)
  - Major risk factor = absence of antibodies to TSST-1
  - This toxin isolated in > 90% of cases
  - Damage done by three mechanisms: (1) Direct toxic effects on multiple organ systems, (2) impaired clearance of endogenous endotoxins derived from gut flora, and (3) by acting as a "superantigen" which can cause stimulation of T cells → inflammatory mediators and cytokines

Clinical Presentation

- Characterized by sudden onset of high fever with myalgias, vomiting, diarrhea, headache, and pharyngitis. Can progress rapidly to shock
  - Illness can vary from fairly mild disease to shock/fatal
- Skin – manifestations are more extensive and predictable than in streptococcal TSS
  - Diffuse scarlatiniform exanthem that starts on trunk and spreads centripetally. Accentuation at skin folds is common
  - Erythema of palms and soles
  - Erythema of mucous membranes + strawberry tongue
  - Hyperemia of conjunctivae
  - Generalized non-pitting edema – hands, feet, face
  - Desquamation of hands and feet occurs 1–3 weeks after onset of symptoms
  - After recovery – Beau's lines in nails, nail shedding, telogen effluvium can occur
- Associated with focal cutaneous pyodermas, postpartum infections, deep abscesses, and infections associated with nasal packing or insulin pump infusion sites

Labs – Common findings include:

- Complete metabolic profile → elevated BUN/Cr, decreased renal function, elevated LFTs
- CBC + diff → low platelets

- Blood cultures may be + for *Staph aureus*. Also check throat and/or CSF
- Consider serologic tests for RMSF, leptospirosis, measles

DDx – Kawasaki's disease, scarlet fever, SSSS, early TEN, Rocky Mountain spotted fever, leptospirosis, atypical measles

Histology

- Superficial infiltrate with many neutrophils and lymphocytes in the upper dermis
- There may be edema of papillary dermis and epidermal spongiosis and exocytosis
- Similar findings seen around hair follicles and sweat glands

Treatment

- Intensive supportive therapy
  - Hypotension – IV fluids and vasopressor agents
  - Remove any foreign bodies (e.g., meshes, nasal packing, tampon)
  - ABX – β-lactamase-resistant antibiotic to eradicate any foci of toxin-producing staphylococci
    - Some advocate that antibiotics can suppress toxin production, particularly clindamycin, rifampin, or fluoroquinolones
  - In severe cases of shock not responding to antibiotics, low-dose corticosteroids have been used

Pearls and Pitfalls

- Patients typically complain of exquisite skin or muscle tenderness when they are touched or moved
- After recovery, can see complications including decreased renal function, protracted myalgias and fatigue, vocal cord paralysis, carpal tunnel, arthralgias, amenorrhea, gangrene, paresthesias in extremities
- Do not use clindamycin alone as resistance common
- Rifampin not meant to be used alone as resistance will occur quickly

Tzanck Smear – Neonatal Conditions

Table 34   Findings on Tzanck of blister scrapings and Wright/Gram Stains of blister fluid contents of neonatal conditions

Transient neonatal pustular melanosis	Many polymorphonuclear leukocytes
Pustular psoriasis	Many polymorphonuclear leukocytes
Acropustulosis of infancy	Many polymorphonuclear leukocytes
Incontinentia pigmenti	Many eosinophils
Erythema toxicum neonatorum	Many eosinophils
Eosinophilic pustular folliculitis	Many eosinophils
Toxic epidermal necrolysis	Cuboidal cells with high nuclear to cytoplasmic ratio; inflammatory cells present
Staphylococcal scalded skin syndrome	Broad epidermal cells without inflammation
Histiocytoses	Histiocytes with oval nuclei with longitudinal grooves or "kidney bean" shape
Varicella or herpes simplex	Multinucleated giant cells

Reference: Used with permission from Elsevier. Cunningham BB, Wagner AM. Diagnostic and Therapeutic Procedures. Textbook of Neonatal Dermatology, 2001, p. 76

Verrucae Vulgaris

Etiology and Pathogenesis

- Due to HPV infection, of which there are more than 60 subtypes
- General verrucae vulgares often due to HPV-2

Clinical Presentation

- Occur predominantly on the hands, periungal regions, and feet. May occur anywhere on skin
- Flesh-colored, verrucous papules which may present as single or multiple lesions
  - May be dome-shaped, filiform, exophytic
  - Individual lesions may coalesce into larger plaques
  - Oral lesions may present as small, pink to white, soft papules and plaques of the labial, lingual, buccal or gingival mucosa
  - Lesions near the nails can distort the nail plate
  - Gentle paring with #15 blade will reveal characteristic punctate black dots that represent thrombosed capillaries
  - A linear array of verrucous papules can occur from scratching → koebnerization
- **Verrucae plana** – (flat warts) – Commonly caused by HPV-3. Tend to occur mostly on the face, neck, arms, and legs. May be smooth, flesh-colored, or slightly pink to brown. Patient may have a few or hundreds and are commonly spread by shaving
- **Verrucae plantaris** – (plantar warts) – occur on plantar surfaces of feet and tend to be the most symptomatic and most difficult to treat. Lesions tend to develop an "endophytic" component because of the pressure of walking which is painful. Coalescence of lesions may result in mosaic warts
- **Myrmecia wart** – "Anthill wart" – see tremendous mounds of hypergranulosis, koilocytes resembling specks of dirt on an anthill. Usually HPV-1 or 63, usually on soles, toes
- **Heck's disease** – "Focal epithelial hyperplasia" usually due to HPV-13 or -32. Causes multiple verrucous papules on the mucosal lip or elsewhere in the mouth. Often seen in patients with native American heritage

DDx – punctate keratoderma, corns/calluses, talon noir, verrucous carcinoma, bowenoid papulosis

Histology

- Hyperkeratosis, papillomatosis, hypergranulosis. Columns of parakeratosis, especially over projecting dermal papillae
- Vacuolated superficial keratinocytes with koilocytes
- Rete riges often slow inward showing arborization – can give a "spread-fingers" appearance
- Dilated capillaries in dermal papillae
- Perivascular lymphocytes

Treatment

- Watching waiting, particularly in young children
- Topical salicylic acid
  - Available over-the-counter in 5–40%. Greater concentrations require prescription. May be more effective with occlusion or duct tape
- Cryotherapy
  - Can be traumatic in children. Can repeat treatment q 3–4 weeks. Pare thick lesions prior to treatment for improved efficacy
- Imiquimod 3.75% or 5% at bedtime
  - Use small amount
  - Lesions on feet or hands – can cover with bandaid to keep medication in place
  - Use 3x/week to lesions on face or in genitals to start with. Discuss side effects of erythema and irritation with parent/patient. Decrease frequency of application if area becoming too irritated
- *Candida* injections
  - 0.3 mL to warts q month × 3 months
- 5-FU + salicylic acid
  - Rotate every other day. Can use under occlusion
- Cantharidin + salicylic acid (Cantharone Plus)
  - Apply to wart, wash off in 6 h
- Laser
  - Pulsed dye, Nd:Yag, CO2 lasers. Targets blood vessels and can be effective. Somewhat painful
- Topical retinoids (tretinoin, adapalene)
  - Can be especially helpful with verruca plana or facial lesions
- Oral cimetidine
  - 25–40 mg/kg/day divided BID or TID. Do not exceed 2,400 mg/day
- Squaric acid
  - Sensitize with 2%
  - After 1 week, use very dilute form 0.1% daily or every other day

- Intralesional bleomycin – regimen courtesy of *Dr. Alexandra Zhang*
  - Rarely used in children. Contraindicated if patient has Raynaud's phenomenon, peripheral vascular disease
  - Informed consent. SE – Raynaud's, hyperpigmentation, pain, erythema, eschar formation
  - Dilute bleomycin to 1 mg/mL (1.0 –U/mL) solution with sterile saline
  - Give patient local anesthesia or digital nerve blocks before bleomycin injection
  - Inject 0.5–1 mL of diluted bleomycin soln. into each wart (depends on wart size)
- Trichloroacetic acid
  - Not recommended in children. Use 80% and apply very careful to wart after keratotic debris is pared off. Do not use on face or in genital area. May be helpful for palmoplantar warts
- Topical cidofovir – do not use on large body surface area as risk of systemic absorption → nephrotoxicity. Very expensive

Pearls and Pitfalls

- Best to have patient avoid shaving areas where warts are present (such as beard area, genital area, legs). Shaving will spread the lesions
- Cimetidine has a lot of drug interactions. Always tell patient/parents and always check for drug-interactions
- For periungual digital verrucae vulgares in HIV patients, consider an underlying SCC, especially if difficult to treat. Have a low threshold to biopsy

Procedural Dermatology

Anatomy

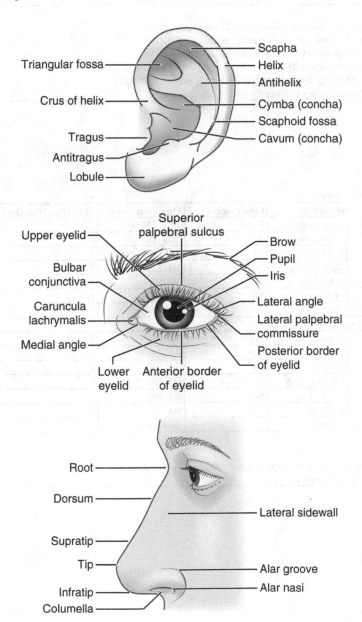

Scapha

Helix

Antihelix

Triangular fossa

Crus of helix

Cymba (concha)

Scaphoid fossa

Tragus

Cavum (concha)

Antitragus

Lobule

Upper eyelid

Superior palpebral sulcus

Brow

Pupil

Bulbar conjunctiva

Iris

Lateral angle

Caruncula lachrymalis

Lateral palpebral commissure

Medial angle

Posterior border of eyelid

Lower eyelid

Anterior border of eyelid

Root

Dorsum

Lateral sidewall

Supratip

Tip

Alar groove

Alar nasi

Infratip

Columella

Fig. 2 Facial Anatomy

Table 35   Anesthesia (Topical)

Anesthetic	Components	Vehicle	Onset (min)
EMLA	2.5% lidocaine 2.5% prilocaine	Oil in water	60–120
X 4	4% lidocaine	Liposomal	30–60
LMX 5	5% lidocaine	Liposomal	30–60
Notes: May achieve effective anesthesia with 25 min application Recommend 60 min application under occlusive dressing Depth of analgesia at 60 min approximates 3 mm Depth of analgesia at 120 min approximates 5 mm Risk of methemoglobinemia with prilocaine (caution in infants) Risk of alkaline injury to cornea with EMLA			

Anesthesia (local)

Without epinephrine		Onset (min)	Duration (min)	Max Dose[a] (mg/kg)
Amides	Bupivacaine	2–10	120–240	2.5
	Etidocaine	3–5	240–360	4.5
	Lidocaine	<1	30–120	5
	Mepivacaine	3–20	30–120	6
	Prilocaine	5–6	30–120	6
Esters	Procaine	5	15–30	10
	Tetracaine	7	120–240	2
With Epinephrine[b, c]				
Amides	Bupivacaine	2–10	240–480	3
	Etidocaine	3–5	240–360	6.5
	Lidocaine	<1	60–400	7
	Mepivacaine	3–20	60–400	8
	Prilocaine	5–6	60–400	10
Esters	Procaine	5	30–90	14
	Tetracaine	7	240–480	2
Notes: [a]Based on 70 kg patient [b]Full vasoconstriction with epinephrine requires 7–15 min [c]Epinephrine is category C				

Chemical Peels[*]

Table 36 Characteristics of chemical peels

Peel	Components	Depth	MOA/Strength	Comments
Jessner's	Resorcinol, Sal acid, lactic acid, ETOH	Very superficial	Keratolysis	Limited absorption of resorcinol in combination with TCA medium peel
TCA	Concentration: weight per volume	35% – medium 40% – deep	Protein precipitation/ coagulation No toxicity	Frost correlates with depth of peel. TCA concentration and amount applied determines depth of peel
Alpha-hydroxy acid: – Glycolic acid – Lactic acid	70% glycolic acid	Very superficial hydrophilic-water soluble	Keratinocyte discohesion and epidermolysis *Peel is time dependent; frosting is not an end point **Needs neutralization**	The amount of free acid determines depth of peel (pH and pKa are the most impt determinates) Increased photosensitivity
Beta-hydroxy acid: – Salicylic acid	20–30% salicylic acid	Very superficial	Localizes to pores given lipophilic nature	Often used for acne, milia, keratolysis Frost indicates peel complete
Resorcinol	Phenol derivative	Very superficial		Toxicity similar to phenol. Ochronosis. Anti-thyroid effect – myxedema Methemoglobinemia
Phenol	Phenol – component of Baker's Peel	Deep	Paradox: dilution increases penetration: "protein precipitation" prevents extension of peel	Myocardial, glomerulo-nephritis, hepatic toxicity. Phenol poisoning: Central depression, hypotension, HA, N/V
Baker's phenol	Phenol, Croton oil Septisol (soap)	Deep		
Monheit peel	Jessner's peel + TCA 35%			

Very superficial – stratum corneum and stratum granulosum
Superficial – basal layer and upper papillary dermis
Medium – through papillary dermis and upper reticular dermis
Deep – mid-reticular dermis

Chemical Peels*

Table 37   Chemical peel – procedure checklist*

[ ] Prophylactic antiviral medication
[ ] Informed consent signed
[ ] Photos taken
[ ] Preoperative medications given
[ ] Liquid nitrogen treatment to keratoses if needed
[ ] Apply septisol
[ ] Apply acetone
[ ] Turn on fan
[ ] Apply Jessner's
[ ] Apply TCA
[ ] Apply cool saline compresses
[ ] Postoperative instructions given
[ ] Procedure note documented in chart

Courtesy of Dr. Wade Foster

Chemical Peel Procedure (Medium-depth) – Postoperative Care*

Courtesy of Dr. Wade Foster

1. Starting tomorrow morning:
   o Soak the treated area for 15 min, four times a day using a solution of 1 tbsp white vinegar in 1 pint of cool water on a washcloth. Any scabs present should be gently soaked off if possible. DO NOT PICK TO REMOVE DEAD SKIN OR SCABS
   o After soaking, pat the skin dry with a towel and apply a layer of Eucerin® cream over the entire face. Reapply whenever the skin feels dry
2. Sleep on your back with your head elevated on a few pillows for the first few days if the face is swollen
3. Avoid strenuous exercise for 2 weeks to avoid irritating the skin
4. Do not expose the skin to the sun for 2 weeks. After complete healing, it will be able to tolerate sunscreens
5. Most chemical peels today are supplemented by the use of creams such as retinoic acid (Retin-A), which cause a constant turnover of the top layers of the skin, further improving its integrity. Your physician will instruct you when to resume the appropriate strength of Retin-A

   Do not use α-hydroxy acid or Retin-A products until directed by physician

Postoperative expectations

1. Mild/moderate redness is expected for 7 days after the procedure and will fade gradually over a 4- to 6-week period
2. Oozing of clear fluid from the surgical site may occur for 3–7 days
3. Mild-to-moderate swelling is normal and may last 3–7 days

Botox Cosmetic

- Botulinum toxin (BTX) cleaves proteins (collectively called the SNARE complex) in the presynaptic neuron, which are required for the release of acetylcholine. Injection into the muscles of facial expression results in a chemical denervation of these striated muscles and thus a temporary paralysis
- BTX-A (Botox) cleaves **SNAP-25** protein
- BTX-B (Myobloc) cleaves **synaptobrevin** (VAMP) protein of the SNARE complex
- Supplied in 100 U vials (contains 100 U *Clostridium botulinum* type A neurotoxin + 0.5 mg human albumin + 0.9 mg NaCl)
- BOTOX interferes with Ach release (permanent effect, however, nerves develop new synapses)
- H chain binds neurotoxin selectivity to cholinergic terminal
- L chain acts within cell to prevent Ach release

BOTOX Reconstitution

Botox can be diluted in a number of ratios depending on what it is used for:

- Examples of dilution are 4:1, 3:1, 2:1, and 1:1 (wherein 4:1, it means 4 cc saline added to one vial of dry Botox powder)
- For cosmetic uses, most dermatologists use 2:1 or 1:1 ratio
- For axillary/palmoplantar hyperhidrosis, many use a 4:1 ratio
- Each clinician will have their own technique

- Remember to always be aware of how many units you are giving a patient: you can only give a max of 200 units at any one time

When reconstituting:

- Use PRESERVED 0.9% NaCL (saline), the bottle will say this, and it will increase the longevity of the Botox
- DO NOT SHAKE THE VIAL OF BOTOX WHEN MIXING
- Use a 3 cc saline syringe to add the NaCL to the Botox Vial, DO NOT ATTEMPT TO REMOVE THE BOTOX POWDER FROM ITS ORIGINAL VIAL
- Add the saline slowly to Botox powder vial
- Each vial contains 100 units of botulinum toxin
- Use within 4 h (store at 2–8 °C)

- Example, in a 4:1 dilution, 1 cc of solution would contain 2.5 units of botulinum toxin

---

Fig. 3 BOTOX Reconstitution

Pearls and Pitfalls

– Avoid injection near levator palpebrae superioris
– Do not inject closer than 1 cm above central eyebrows

Cosmeceuticals

Table 38 Properties and uses of common cosmeceuticals

Type	Uses
Ascorbic acid (vitamin C)	Antioxidant and anti-inflammatory properties. Increases dermal production of collagen, reduces phototoxicity due to ultraviolet light, and lightens hyperpigmentation
Glycolic and lactic acids (alpha hydroxy acids)	Induce exfoliation of photodamaged skin and increase mucopolysaccharide and collagen synthesis which may improve appearance of fine wrinkles
Beta-hydroxy acids (salicyclic acids)	Promote exfoliation of the skin by increasing epidermal cell turnover. Do not penetrate the dermis and therefore their effects are confined to the epidermal layer
Alpha-lipoic acid	Potent antioxidant that protects intracellular vitamin C and vitamin E. It is absorbed to the level of the subcutaneous fat and has been shown to diminish fine lines presumably through induction of collagen synthesis
Human growth factors (topical)	Cause epidermal thickening and new collagen formation
Peptides (argireline and copper, etc)	Biologically play a role in wound healing and enzymatic processes. Are emerging as novel treatments for photoaged skin due to their ability to increase collagen and elastin production and potentially influence neurotransmitter release
Niacinamide	Reduces facial erythema, improves skin texture and hyperpigmentation. May diminish fine lines

Fillers

Table 39   Composition and uses of common fillers

Product name	Composition	Comments	Uses
Zyderm Zyplast	95% type I collagen, 5% type III collagen, saline, lidocaine	*Required*: Two skin tests performed at 6 weeks, then at 2 weeks prior to first collagen treatment	Superficial rhytides Deeper furrows
Artecoll	Nonbiodegradable polymethylmethacrylate microspheres suspended in bovine collagen	Permanent filler *Required*: Two skin tests performed at 6 weeks, then at 2 weeks prior to first collagen treatment	
CosmoDerm CosmoPlast	Bioengineered human-derived collagen products obtained from neonatal foreskin	No need for pretreatment hypersensitivity testing	Rhytides
Radiance	Calcium hydroxylapatite microspheres	Calcium hydroxylapatite is a normal constituent of bone and can be seen on radiographic imaging	
Restylane	Hyaluronic acid. Binds water to create volume and plump the skin	Granulomatous foreign body reactions can occur producing blue nodules in the skin	
Perlane		Acute angioedema-type hypersensitivity reaction has been reported	
		Duration of action 6–12 months (longer than collagen)	
Sculptra (*called New-Fill outside the US*)	Biodegradable polymer of poly-L-lactic acid	May have longer duration period than other currently available biodegradable fillers	Approved for treatment of HIV-associated lipoatrophy
Silicone	Synthetic, viscous compound composed of long polymers of dimethylsiloxanes	Hypersensitivity reactions, product migration, granuloma formation can occur – even many years posttreatment	Not currently FDA-approved for soft tissue augmentation
Juvederm	Hyaluronic acid	Can be used in the lips	Correction of moderate to severe facial wrinkles and folds (such as nasolabial folds)

Lasers

Table 40 Lasers (Light amplification by stimulated emission of radiation)

Laser type	Wavelength	Dermatologic application
Argon (continuous wave)	488, 514 nm	Vascular lesions
Argon-pumped tunable dye	577, 585 nm	Vascular lesions
Copper vapor/ bromide	510, 578 nm	Pigmented lesions, vascular lesions
Potassium-titanyl-phosphate (KTP)	532 nm	Pigmented lesions, vascular lesions
Nd:YAG (frequency doubled)	532 nm	Pigmented lesions, red/orange/yellow tattoos
Pulsed dye	510 nm	Pigmented lesions
	585–595 nm	Vascular lesions, hypertrophic and keloid scars, striae, verrucae, nonablative dermal remodeling
Ruby	694 nm	Pigmented lesions, blue/black/green tattoos
Q-switched		Hair removal
Normal mode		
Alexandrite	755 nm	Pigmented lesions, blue/black/green tattoos
Q-switched		Hair removal, leg veins
Normal mode		
Diode	800–810 nm	Hair removal, leg veins
Nd:YAG	1,064 nm	Pigmented lesions, blue/black tattoo
Q-switched		
Normal mode		Hair removal, leg veins, nonablative dermal remodeling
Nd:YAG (long-pulsed)	1,320 nm	Nonablative dermal remodeling
Diode (long-pulsed)	1,450 nm	Nonablative dermal remodeling
Erbium: glass	1,540 nm	Nonablative dermal remodeling
Erbium: YAG (pulsed)	2,940 nm	Ablative skin resurfacing, epidermal lesions
Carbon dioxide (continuous wave)	10,600 nm	Actinic cheilitis, verrucae, rhinophyma
Carbon dioxide (pulsed)	10,600 nm	Ablative skin resurfacing, epidermal/dermal lesions
Intense pulsed light source	515–1,200 nm	Superficial pigmented lesions, vascular lesions, hair removal, nonablative dermal remodeling

Reference: Used with permission from Elsevier. Tanzi EL, Lupton JR and Alster TS. Lasers in dermatology: Four decades of progress. J Am Acad Dermatol 2003; 49: 1–31

Sutures

Table 41 Absorption Times of commonly-used sutures

Suture Characteristics	
Absorbable	**Absorption (days)**
Surgical gut (fast-absorbing)	21–42
Surgical gut (plain)	70
Surgical gut (chromic)	70–90
Polyglytone 6211 • Caprosyn: Syneture	56

Polyglactin-910
  • Vicryl: Ethicon
  • Vicryl Rapide: Ethicon
	56–70

Lactomer • Polysorb: Syneture	56–70
Polyglycolic acid • Dexon S/II: Syneture	60–90
Glycomer 631 • Biosyn: Syneture	90–110
Poliglecaprone 25 • Monocryl: Ethicon	90–120
Polydioxanone • PDS II: Ethicon	180
Polyglyconate • Maxon: Syneture	180
Nonabsorbable	NA

Silk
  • Perma-Hand: Ethicon
  • Sofsilk: Syneture	

Nylon, monofilament
  • Ethilon: Ethicon
  • Monosof: Syneture	

Nylon, braided
  • Nurulon: Ethicon
  • Surgilon: Syneture	

Polybutester • Novafil: Syneture	

Polypropylene
  • Prolene: Ethicon
  • Surgipro: Syneture	

Polyester, braided
  • Mersilene: Ethicon
  • Dacron: Syneture	

Polyester, braided + Teflon coated
  • Ethibond: Ethicon
  • Ticron: Syneture	

Polyhexafluoropropylene-VDF • Pronova: Ethicon	

Med Toxicity Monitoring

Antimalarials

- Adverse reaction to one drug group (4-aminoquinolone → chloroquine and hydroxychloroquine) does not preclude use of the other drug group (quinacrine). No cross-reactivity

Mechanism of Action

- Not entirely clear
- ↑ Lysosome pH results in …
  - ↓protease activity
  - ↓ class II MHC assembly
  - ↓ TLR-9, -7, -8 and -3 activation
  - ↑loading of class I MHC
  - ↓ receptor recycling, membrane turnover
- Other
  - Act as anticoagulants
  - Lower lipids
    - Hydroxychloroquine has been associated with a 15–20% decrease in serum cholesterol, TG and LDL levels
  - May decrease insulin degradation and thus improve glucose intolerance
  - Vaccine adjunct – Can improve vaccination to hepatitis B with one dose of hydroxychloroquine

Chloroquine

- Highest concentrations of drug found in melanin-containing cells in the retina and skin – potential for eye toxicity
- Remains in the skin for 6–7 months after cessation of therapy

Hydroxychloroquine (Plaquenil)

- Max is 6.5 mg/kg/day *lean body weight* → www.halls.med/ideal-weight/body. htm
  ○ Commonly started at 200 mg PO BID
- 2/3 rd as effective as chloroquine, but ½ the toxicity
- Maximal efficacy may not be seen for 3–6 months
  ○ Dose leading, with administration of higher doses (up to 1,200 mg/day) for the first 6 weeks, has been shown to accelerate clinical response in rheumatoid arthritis, albeit with an increase in gastrointestinal intolerance
- If hydroxychloroquine not effective, can add quinacrine 100 mg/day (Atabrine)

Quinacrine (Atabrine)

- Skin deposition may occur as a yellow cast

Clinical Uses

- Lupus erythematosus
- Porphyria cutanea tarda
- Polymorphous light eruption
- Dermatomyositis
- Solar urticaria
- Sarcoidosis
- Granuloma annulare
- Oral lichen planus
- Panniculitis
- Chronic ulcerative stomatitis
- Some cases of – epidermolysis bullosa, atopic dermatitis, eosinophilic fasciitis, scleroderma, urticarial vasculitis, reticular erythematous mucinosis
- Patients with highest risk of side effects:
  ○ Increased body fat, >60 years of age, >5 years of use, high dose of medication

Side Effects

- Myopathy/cardiomyopathy
- Lower seizure threshold
- Aplastic anemia
- Blue-black pigmentation (in up to 30% of patients)

- Rare side effects
  - Iatrogenic phospholipids mimicking Fabry disease. Due to decrease in α-galactosidase activity due to chloroquine. (*Am J Kidney Dis 2006*) → investigate new-onset proteinuria
  - Hepatitis (<1%, but higher in PCT and chronic viral hepatitis). Adverse reaction to one does not preclude the use of another. (*Clin Rheum 2007*)

References:

Kalia, S and Dutz JP. New Concepts in antimalarials use and mode of action in dermatology. Dermatologic Therapy 2007; 20: 160–74.

Antimicrobials, Topical

Bacitracin

- Inhibits bacterial cell wall synthesis – inhibits peptidoglycan synthesis
- Gram (+): *S. aureus, S. pneumoniae, Neisseria, H. influenzae, T. pallidum* – [bactericidal against gram + and *Neisseria* species]
- Gram (–): minimal coverage
- SE: contact sensitization, rare anaphylaxis

Mupirocin (Bactroban)

- Inhibits bacterial RNA and protein synthesis (isoleucyl tDNA synthetase)
- Gram (+): Staphylococci (MRSA), Streptococci – [bactericidal against both MRSA and Strept]
- Gram (–): Some gram (–) cocci
- SE: local irritant
- Does not cross-react with other topical antimicrobials
- Renal toxicity when used on large denuded areas
- Uncommon contact sensitization

Neomycin

- Inhibits protein synthesis (binds 30s subunit)
- Gram (+): good coverage vs. *S. aureus* (weak for *Strep)* – [bactericidal against both gram + and gram–]
- Gram (–): yes
- SE: ototoxic and nephrotoxic; contact sensitization; virtually always used in combination
- Neosporin is – neomycin + bacitracin + polymyxin B

Polymyxin B

- Antibacterial via surface detergent-like mechanisms. Increases permeability of bacterial cell membrane by interacting with phospholipid components of cell membrane
- Gram (+): No activity
- Gram (–): *Proteus,Pseudomonas, Serratia* – [bactericidal]
- SE: rare contact sensitization

Retapamulin (AltaBax)

- Newest topical antimicrobial – FDA approved in 2007-06-25
- Useful for impetigo – BID treatment × 5 days
- Not approved for MRSA

Silvadene

- Binds to bacterial DNA and inhibits its replication
- Bactericidal against gram + and gram – organisms
- Reports of neutropenia and kernicterus; contact dermatitis in those with sulfa allergy; monitor for leukopenia if extensive use

Antiseptic Cleaners

Chlorhexidine (Hibiclens™)

- Disrupts cell membranes
- Excellent gram-positive and good gram-negative coverage
- Intermediate onset (~1 min scrub)
- Ototoxicity and keratitis
- Residual chemical activity on skin
- Antimicrobial activity not affected by blood
- Low skin absorption

Hexachlorophene (pHisoHex™)

- Good gram-positive coverage only
- Can be absorbed through skin → neurotoxic in infants
- Teratogenic

Iodine/Iodophores (Betadine)

- Iodine + surfactant → iodophore
- Oxidation/substitution by free iodide (active agent)
- Excellent gram-positive and good gram-negative coverage
- Intermediate onset
- Inactivated by blood and serum products
- May sensitize patient
- Must dry to be effective

Isopropyl alcohol (70%)

- Denatures proteins
- Good gram-positive/negative coverage (mainly gram-positive)
- Most rapid onset
- Caution with lasers (flammable)
- No killing of spores, antibacterial only

Triclosan

- Disrupts cell wall
- Good gram-positive/negative coverage
- Intermediate onset

Azathioprine

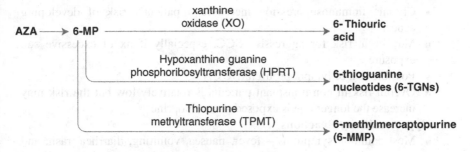

Fig. 4 Effect of Azathioprine on TPMT pathway

- Defect in TPMT – genetic predisposition
- Defect in HPRT – Lesch–Nyan disease
- Blockage of XO – from allopurinol
- **Pharmacokinetics**
  - Available as 50-mg scored tablets
  - $T_{1/2}$ is 5 h
  - Rapidly converted to 6-mercaptopurine (by liver and RBC)
  - Activate metabolites slowly accumulate – max clinical immunosuppression by 8–12 weeks
  - Pregnancy category D
  - Therapeutic response usually occurs between 6 and 8 weeks but may take up to 12 weeks
- TPMT activity
  - TPMT < 6.3 U (**low**): No treatment with azathioprine
  - TPMT 6.5–15 U/ml (**intermediate**): 1 mg/kg/day
  - TPMT 15.1–26.4 U/ml (**normal**): 2 mg/kg/day
  - TPMT > 26.4 U/ml (**high**): may require more aggressive dosing to see any effect
    - In last scenario – still start at 2 mg/kg/day then increase the dose every 4–6 weeks by 0.5 mg/kg/day to a max of 3 mg/kg/day
- **Side Effects**
  - **Hematologic (dose related)**
    - Occurs weeks to years after starting med
    - Leukopenia – not necessarily related to TPMT level
    - Bone marrow toxicity
  - **Gastrointestinal** – symptoms may resolve over time
    - Usually between first and fourteenth day of treatment (not subtle)
    - Nausea, diarrhea
    - Patient can take med in divided doses or with food to try to relieve these symptoms

- ○ **Hepatotoxicity**
  - ■ Increase in LFTs/hepatotoxicity – may be delayed in onset
- ○ **Carcinogenesis**
  - ■ Chronic immunosuppression increases a patient's risk of developing cancer
  - ■ May be at risk for aggressive SCC, especially if hx of excessive sun exposure
  - ■ Possible risk of lymphoproliferative CA
  - ■ Overall risk in non-transplant patients is relatively low but the risk may increase the longer one is exposed to azathioprine
- ○ **Hypersensitivity Reactions**
  - ■ Most common symptoms – fever, nausea, vomiting, diarrhea, rash, and occasionally shock
  - ■ Usually occurs within 4 weeks of initiating therapy and only a few cases reported to occur within hours of ingestion of the first dose or after years of therapy
- ○ **Infection risk**
- • Contraindications– hypersens to drug, preg females (cat D), veno-occlusive dz
- • **Drug Interactions**
  - ○ Allopurinol (increased risk of toxicity)
  - ○ Sulfasalazine, ACE-inhibitors, and Bactrim → have been reported to increase the risk of azathioprine-induced myelotoxicity. Avoid these drugs or use with caution
  - ○ Warfarin → effects of warfarin are reduced. Patients on this med may require 3–4x the dose of warfarin and should be monitored closely
- • **Dermatologic Uses**
  - ○ Immunobullous diseases – pemphigus vulgaris, pemphigus foliaceus, para-neoplastic pemphigus, bullous pemphigoid, cicatricial pemphigoid
  - ○ Eczematous disorders – atopic dermatitis (AZA not recommended as a first-line agent for this), pompholyx, contact dermatitis
  - ○ Photodermatoses – chronic actinic dermatitis, actinic reticuloid, PMLE
  - ○ Other – cutaneous lupus erythematosus, psoriasis, pyoderm gangrenosum (mixed reports of efficacy), cutaneous vasculitis, erythema multiforme, lichen planus, GVHD

Biologics – TNF-α Inhibitors

Overview

- Drugs (all are pregnancy category B)
- Etanercept (Enbrel) – oldest drug in this class
- Infliximab (Remicade)
- Adalimumab (Humira)

Side Effects

- Malignancy and Lymphoma
  - Unclear association
  - Some patient populations receiving drug have inherent increased risk of lymphoma. Psoriasis patients and RA patients have inherent risk of Non-Hodgkin's Lymphoma. Not clearly linked to TNF-α inhibitors
- Tuberculosis – get baseline and annual PPD
- CHF – soft contraindication; stop if symptoms. Consider consulting cardiology if unclear what the patient's status is
- Demyelinating diseases
  - Reported with all TNF-α inhibitors. Stop if symptoms and avoid rechallenge
  - Avoid in first-degree relatives with history of demyelinating disease
  - Symptoms – numbness, tingling, weakness, incoordination, diplopia
  - Unilateral symptoms more worrisome than bilateral symptoms
- Lupus-like syndrome
- TNF and hepatotoxicity → Rare reports of hepatotoxicity. However, TNF-alpha inhibitors may be helpful for some times of liver hepatitis
  - Increased TNF levels in NASH (nonalcoholic steatohepatitis) and alcoholic hepatitis
  - TNF <u>does</u> cause liver damage *(Cancer 1992)* – a major mediator of hepatotoxicity
  - Fat (LPS and free fatty acids) also activates TLR4 to increase TNF

Comorbidities

- Hepatitis
  - Anti-TNF meds are generally **good** in hepatitis C *(J Hep 2005)* – patient should be followed by hepatology
  - Anti-TNF and hepatitis B (use caution → get hepatology's input)
    - No good guidelines in literature
    - Goal is to maintain high surface Ab level – can give vaccination to boost this
    - If surface Ag positive and have viral replication → send to hepatologist
    - Reactivation of hepatitis B can occur if going on Anti-TNF

Table 42 Biologics used in psoriasis

	Alefacept (Amevive®)	Etanercept (Enbrel®)	Infliximab (Remicade®)	Adalimumab (Humira®)	Ustekinumab (Stelara®)
Description	Fusion protein of human LFA-3 and the Fc portion of IgG1	Fusion protein of the Fc of human IgG1 and the extracellular TNF receptor	Chimeric antibody against TNFα composed of a human IgG1 constant domain and murine variable regions	Recombinant human IgG1 monoclonal antibody against TNFα	Monoclonal antibody (fully human)
Mechanism	Inhibits T-cell activation and proliferation by blocking LFA-3/CD2 interaction, resulting in selective apoptosis of T-cells	Binds soluble TNF and blocks its interaction with cell surface receptors	Binds soluble and bound TNFα	Binds TNF and blocks its interaction with cell surface TNF receptors	Target the p40 subunit of interleukin (IL)-12 and IL-23 which are related to the differentiation of naïve T-cells into Th1 and Th17 cells
FDA indication	Moderate-to-severe plaque psoriasis in adults	Moderate-to-severe plaque psoriasis in adults; psoriatic, rheumatoid, and juvenile RA; ankylosing spondylitis	Severe recalcitrant psoriasis, Crohn's disease, RA	Moderate-to-severe RA in adults	Moderate-to-severe plaque psoriasis in adults
Dosing	15 mg IM q week × 12 weeks, wait 12 weeks, then consider a second course × 12 weeks	50 mg SC BIW × 12 weeks, then 50 mg SC q week	3 mg/kg IV over 2 h at weeks 0, 2, 6, then 5 mg/kg q 8 weeks (preferred psoriasis dose)	40 mg SC over 3–5 min q2 weeks × 12 weeks; can ↑ to q week doses if not on methotrexate	<100 kg 45 mg SC at week 0, week 4, q 12 weeks >100 kg 90 mg SC at week 0, week 4, q 12 weeks
FDA monitoring	CD4 at baseline and weekly (hold dose if <250 cells/µL)	Screen for latent TB (PPD and/or CXR) at baseline	Screen for latent TB (PPD and/or CXR) at baseline	Screen for latent TB (PPD and/or CXR), routine CBC/ chemistries at baseline; anti-dsDNA Ab if lupus-like sx present	Screen for latent TB (PPD and/or CXR) at baseline

Pregnancy and nursing	Preg Cat B, lactation safety unknown	Preg Cat B, lactation safety ? (secreted in breast milk)	Preg Cat B, lactation safety unknown	Preg Cat B, lactation safety unknown	Preg Cat B, lactation safety unknown
Optional monitoring	PPD and/or CXR, and β-HCG at baseline	PPD and/or CXR, BUN, Cr, SGOT, SGPT, Hep C serology and/or β-HCG at baseline Consider periodic CBC, ESR, and clinical follow-up q 3 months	BUN, Cr, SGOT, SGPT, Hep C serology and/or β-HCG at baseline. Consider periodic CBC and clinical follow-up q 3 months	PPD and/or CXR and β-HCG at baseline	PPD and/or CXR, and β-HCG at baseline
Side effects, common	Cough, dizziness, nausea, pharyngitis, pruritus, myalgias, chills, injection site reaction, transaminitis	Injection site reactions (37%), cough and resp sx (45%), headaches (35%), infections (17%), positive ANA (11%)	Nausea, abdominal pain, back pain, arthralgia, fatigue, headache	Injection site reaction (8%), positive ANA (12%)	Nasopharyngitis, URI, headache, fatigue, diarrhea, back pain, dizziness, pruritus, injection site reaction
Side effects, serious	Lymphopenia, malignancies, serious infections, hypersensitivity, transaminase elevations (rare), cardiovascular events	Allergic rxns (<2%), leukopenia, pancytopenia, new onset or exacerbation of CNS demyelinating d/o(rare). ↑ incidence of lymphoma, infections	Hypersensitivity rxn, infusion rxn, exacerb of CHF, infections (same as placebo), TB, invasive fungal infections, lupus-like syndrome	Hypersensitivity rxn, confusion, MS, paresthesia, subdural hematoma, tremor, infections, sepsis, malignancy, TB	Infection, malignancy, reversible posterior leukoencephalopathy syndrome
Contraindications	Hypersensitivity to alefacept, dc if CD4 <250 × 1 month	Hypersens to etanercept or components, active infections or sepsis. No live vaccines. CHF, poorly controlled diabetes, or immunosupp	Hypersens to infliximab or murine products, CHF (NYHA Class III/IV)	Hypersens to adalimumab, chronic or recurrent infections, latent TB, immunosupp. Avoid concomitant tx with anakinra and TNF-blocking agents	Hypersensitivity to ustekinumab
					Acute infection, caution if latent tuberculosis, caution if chronic/recurrent infections

(continued)

Table 42 (continued)

	Alefacept (Amevive®)	Etanercept (Enbrel®)	Infliximab (Remicade®)	Adalimumab (Humira®)	Ustekinumab (Stelara®)
Precautions	Infection, history of malignancy, live vaccines	Concurrent tx with anakinra, natalizumab, TNF-blockers or use in patients with preg, renal dz, asthma, CNS demyelin dz or blood dyscrasias	High risk of infection, those with preexisting or recent onset of CNS demyelin dz or seizure d/o, or who have received live vaccines	Mild CHF (NYHA Class I/II) – close cardiac monitoring. DC if lupus-like rash develops. Caution in elderly, patients with preexisting or recent onset of CNS demyelin dz	Infection, history of malignancy
Manufacturer	Astellas	Amgen, Wyeth Pharmaceuticals	Centocor	Abbott	Centocor
Other	* Can use with phototherapy * Max reduction in psoriasis at 8 weeks after last dose * 16-week cycles are under investigation	* Can use with methotrexate	* Can use with MTX * Improvement after first few weeks	* Can use with MTX, steroids, salicylates, NSAIDs	
Relative efficacy	PASI 75: 21% at week 14 (2 weeks post dosing) PASI 50: 42% at week 14 PASI 50 began 60 days after start Most maintain PASI 50 through 3 months observation period	PASI 75: 47% at 3 months, 54% at 6 months PASI 50: 71% at 3 months Median time to PASI 50 and 75 was 1 and 2 months, respectively, after start	PASI 75: 82% at week 10 and 33% at week 26 (5 mg/kg) PASI 50: 40% at week 26 (on 5 mg/kg) Statistically significant reduction in PASI w/respect to placebo 2 weeks after start	PASI 75: achieved by week 20 in one out of two patients (maintained though week 40) PASI 50: achieved by week 12 and week 16 in 2 out of 2 patients	PASI 75 (week 12): 67% with 45 mg dose, 78% with 90 mg

Off-label Uses

- Used in many skin conditions including sarcoidosis, hidradenitis suppurativa, Wegener's granulomatosis, neutrophilic, immunobullous disorders, vasculitis, etc. Infliximab may be more beneficial than others

TNF-α Inhibitors and Vaccinations

- Get any live vaccinations *prior to* going on Anti-TNF
- Should a patient need a live vaccination while on therapy such as the inhaled flu vaccine or the pneumonia vaccine, it would be prudent to stop therapy for at least 2 weeks prior to and after therapy

Tuberculosis Screening – Positive PPD

- If patient has a positive PPD and has never been treated as a converter, many recommend therapy with isoniazid or other appropriate therapy for at least 1 month prior to initiating therapy with a TNF-α inhibitor
- Some patients with a positive PPD have been treated in the past – check a baseline CXR with follow-up CXRs at 6 months, then at 1 year, then annually
- If patient is from outside the US, they may have received vaccination with the BCG vaccine which creates a positive PPD in many patients
  - ○ In cases where BCG vaccination is documented, then a baseline CXR should suffice. Do not repeat PPD – will usually be positive
  - ○ If BCG vaccination cannot be documented, treat these patients like a positive PPD patient prior to initiating anti-TNF therapy
  - ○ **QuantiFERON-TB-Gold test, an IFN-Y release assay, is the screening method of choice in patients who have had prior BCG vaccination**
    - ■ Not recommended in young children (not enough data)
    - ■ Data in immunocompromised patients (such as HIV) is somewhat conflicting. Recommend screening for TB with more than one method. These meds, however, are rarely used in this population

TNF-α Inhibitors and Methotrexate

- Low-dose MTX (7.5–12.5 mg) can help to blunt decreased efficacy with TNF-α Inhibitors and can help prevent formation of antibodies to the medications

Reference:

Patel R, Cafardi JM, Patel N, Sami N, Cafardi JA. Tumor necrosis factor biologics beyond psoriasis in dermatology. Expert Opin Biol Ther. 2011; 11(10): 1341–59.

Corticosteroids (CS)

- Dermatologists are some of the few physicians who prescribe high-dose corticosteroids, but do not always routinely screen for adverse side effects. We use some of the highest doses!
- No clear guidelines for dosing
- **Side Effects**
  - Acute SE → weight gain, headache, increased TG, peptic ulcers, increased appetite, sleep disturbances, aggravate mood disorders/depression, psychosis is rare
  - HPA axis – major concern is reduction of cortisol production due to exogenous CS
  - Avascular necrosis (acute and chronic SE)
    - Risks: lupus, ESRD, increased alcohol consumption, low BMI??, increased dosage and duration
    - MRI best for diagnosis
  - Ocular disease
    - Posterior subcapsular cataracts (usually on CS for at least 1 year on dose equivalent to 10 mg/day), glaucoma
  - Cushingoid appearance – moon facies, buffalo hump
  - Myopathy
    - Muscle weakness → falls → hip fracture → poor healing
      - Mortality of 11% in first year
      - Risk is higher in ages 65–84
      - 20% bedridden, 20–25% wheelchair bound
  - Infections
    - Mycobacterial (CXR, PPD at baseline)
    - Activation of Hepatitis C
  - Avoid live vaccinations like PO polio vaccine, yellow fever, intranasal flu,
  - Osteoporosis
    - **Bisphosphonates** – Only 20% of derm patients are on them *(Arch Derm 2006)*Begin bisphosphonate therapy with CS (if planning>5 mg for>3 months); Also begin calcium and vitamin D
      - Drug of choice for glucocorticoid-induced osteoporosis
      - Stop smoking, no alcohol; weight-bearing exercise recommended
      - SE: teratogenic, avascular necrosis of jaw (low incidence, associated with tooth extraction)
      - Fosamax 70 mg q week, Actonel, Boniva q month, Zoledronic (Reclast) 5 mg IV q year – afib in 5%
      - Teriparatide – recombinant form of PTH that is self-administered injection. NEJM 2007 *(Saag)* → Fewer vertebral fractures but not fewer hip fractures
    - SE after ceasing medication
      - HA, muscle weakness, arthralgias, depression → stops after couple of weeks

Prednisone – Directions for Oral Prednisone Taper

2 Week Taper	100 Tablets (5 mg tabs)
1st Day	12 tablets
2nd Day	12 tablets
3 rd Day	11 tablets
4th Day	10 tablets
5th Day	10 tablets
6th Day	9 tablets
7th Day	8 tablets
8th Day	7 tablets
9th Day	6 tablets
10th Day	5 tablets
11th Day	4 tablets
12th Day	3 tablets
13th Day	2 tablets
14th Day	1 tablet

Courtesy of Dr. Boni Elewski

Prednisone – Directions for Oral Prednisone Taper

3 Week Taper	150 Tablets (5 mg tabs)
1st Day	12 tablets
2nd Day	12 tablets
3 rd Day	11 tablets
4th Day	11 tablets
5th Day	10 tablets
6th Day	10 tablets
7th Day	9 tablets
8th Day	9 tablets
9th Day	8 tablets
10th Day	8 tablets
11th Day	7 tablets
12th Day	7 tablets
13th Day	6 tablets
14th Day	6 tablets
15th Day	5 tablets
16th Day	5 tablets
17th Day	4 tablets
18th Day	4 tablets
19th Day	3 tablets
20th Day	2 tablets
21st Day	1 tablet

Courtesy of Dr. Boni Elewski

Dapsone

- **Pharmacokinetics** – Crosses placenta, excreted in breast milk, Elimination $t_{1/2}$ is 24–30 h
- **Metabolism**
  - N-hydroxylation occurs in the liver and this metabolic product responsible for the hematologic adverse effects associated with dapsone including methemoglobinemia, hemolytic anemia
    - N-hydroxylation of dapsone can be inhibited by the use of **cimetidine 1.6 g daily (divided 400 mg TID-QID)**
    - **Vitamin E 800 IU daily**may also help prevent against hemolysis
- **Side Effects**
  - Pharmacologic – hemolytic anemia, methemoglobinemia, sulfhemoglobinemia
    - Note – oral methylene blue (100–300 mg/day) can be used to acute decrease methemoglobin levels, although this drug is not effective if patient is G6PD deficient
  - Idiosyncratic
    - Hematologic – leukopenia, agranulocytosis
    - Hepatic – hepatitis, infectious mononucleosis-like syndrome, cholestatic jaundice, hypoalbuminemia
    - Cutaneous hypersensitivity reactions – morbilliform eruption (including dapsone hypersensitivity syndrome), exfoliative erythroderma, TEN (rare)
    - Gastrointestinal – gastric irritation, anorexia
    - Neurologic – psychosis, peripheral neuropathy (motor predominantly)
- **Drug Interactions**
  - Drugs that increase Dapsone levels → Trimethoprim, Probenicid, Folic acid antagonists (such as pyrimethamine)
  - Drugs that decrease Dapsone levels → Activated charcoal, para-aminobenzoic acid, Rifampin
  - Drugs (oxidants) that ↑oxidative stress to RBCs → Sulfonamides, Hydroxychloroquine
- **Monitoring Guidelines**
  - Baseline
  - History and Exam, Labs – **CBC+diff, LFTs, Renal (BUN/Cr, GFR), UA, G6PD**
    - G6PD deficiency most common in African-Americans, Middle Eastern, and Far Eastern ancestry
  - Follow-Up and Labs
  - Assess for peripheral motor neurologic dysfunction
  - Assess for signs, symptoms methemoglobinemia
  - CBC+diff q week × 4 weeks, then q 2 weeks × 8 weeks, then q 3–4 months
  - Reticulocyte count prn to assess response to dapsone hemolysis
  - LFTs q month at least, then q 3–4 months
  - Renal function test q month at least, then q 3–4 months
  - Methemoglobin levels as clinically indicated

Drug Monitoring

Table 43 Drug monitoring – Baseline laboratory assessment

Drug	CBC with diff, plts	Serum chemistries, LFTs	Renal	Special tests
Azathioprine	✓	✓	✓	TB skin test, βHcG, TPMT, CXR, hepatitis panel, consider HIV testing
Cyclophosphamide	✓	✓	✓	UA, βHcG
Cyclosporine	✓	✓	✓	Cr clearance, Mg, uric acid, BP × 2, UA, βHcG
Dapsone		✓		G6PD, βHcG
Hydroxyurea	✓	✓	✓	βHcG
IVig	✓	✓	✓	Urinalysis, IgA levels, HIV, hepatitis A/B/C, serum immunoglobulins, RF, cryoglobulins
Methotrexate	✓	✓	✓	Liver bx, HIV in high-risk patients, CR clearance in DM and elderly, CXR, folate, B12, βHcG
Mycophenolate mofetil	✓	✓	✓	Baseline hepatitis panel, PPD
Plaquenil	✓	✓	✓	Ophtho exam, G6PD, βHcG
Prednisone	✓	✓	✓	BP, PPD, spinal bone density in post-menopausal women. Fasting glucose and lipids in high-risk patients
Retinoids	✓	✓	✓	Fasting triglycerides and cholesterol, βHcG

Table 44 Drug monitoring – Follow-up laboratory assessment

Drug (Major or serious side effects)	CBC with Diff, Plts	LFTs	Renal	Special tests
Azathioprine • Myelosuppression • Hepatotoxic (<1%) • GI disturbance – N/D • Oncogenic potential	Q 2 weeks × 2 Q month × 2, if stable Q 2–4 months	Q month × 2, if stable then Q 2–4 months .	Q month × 2, if stable Q 2 months	– βHcG (preg Cat D) – If GFR < 10, decrease AZA by 50% – If GFR < 50, decrease AZA by 25%
Cyclophosphamide • Leukopenia • Hemorrhagic cystitis	Q week × 3 months, if stable then Q 2 weeks	Q month	Q month	– βHcG – Serum chem. Q 2 months – UA Q week × 3 months, if stable then Q 2 weeks
Cyclosporine • Nephrotoxic • HTN • Hypertrichosis • Gingival. Hyperplasia	Q 2 weeks	Q 2 weeks	Q week × 4 weeks then Q 2 weeks if stable; CrCl Q 2–3 months; if Cr ↑ by >30%, stop	– βHcG Q month during and until 3 months after tx – BP Q week initially then Q 2 weeks if stable – Cycl. Level Q week initially, then Q 2 weeks – K, uric acid and Mg Q 2 weeks – Chol, TG
Dapsone • Hemolysis • Agranulocytosis • Methemoglobinemia • Peripheral neuropathy	Q week × 1 months then Q 2 weeks × 2 months; if stable then Q 2–3 months	Q month until stable, then Q 3–4 months	Q month until stable, then Q 3–4 months; Urinalysis also recommended	– Neuro exam Q 6–12 months (rare peripheral *motor* neuropathy) – Methemoglobin levels as indicated – Pregnancy Category C
Hydroxyurea • Myelosuppression • Flu-like symptoms • Rare leg ulcers	Q week × 3 months, if stable Q 2 weeks, then Q month	Q month initially, then Q 3–6 months if stable		– βHcG – Serum chem. Q month, then if stable Q 3–6 months

IVig • Nephropathy (sucrose-cont soln) • Thrombotic events • Constitutional sx • Anaphylaxis if IgA deficient • Infectious transmission • Serum sickness • DIC	Prior to each infusion	Prior to each infusion	Prior to each infusion	– Baseline IgA level – Screen for hepatitis A, B, C and annual – HIV testing and annual – RF, cryoglobulins – Serum immunoglobulins
Methotrexate Myelosuppression Hepatotoxic Rare pneumonitis	1–2 days prior to each dose	Q week till dose stable then Q 3–4 months	Q 6 months	– Liver bx after 1–1.5 g cumulative dose – βHcG
Mycophenolate mofetil • N/V, cramping, diarrhea • Neutrophil dysplasia – Pseudo-Pelger–Huet anomaly • Urinary – urgency, frequency, dysuria, sterile pyuria • No nephrotoxicity from MMF • Fever, myalgias, headache, insomnia • Peripheral edema • HTN • Rash • Increase in infections	Q 2 weeks after dose escalation and then q 2–3 months once dosage is stable	Q 2 weeks after dose escalation and then q 2–3 months once dosage is stable	Q 2 weeks after dose escalation and then q 2–3 months once dosage is stable	– βHcG (preg cat D) – Patients with GFR < 25 ml/min should not receive doses greater than 2 g/day – Relatively contraindicated in peptic ulcer dz, hepatic or cardiopulmonary dz

(continued)

Table 44 (continued)

Drug (Major or serious side effects)	CBC with Diff, Plts	LFTs	Renal	Special tests
Plaquenil • Retinopathy • Weak hemolytic • Phospholipids mimicking Fabry's • Hepatitis < 1%	Q month × 3, then Q 3–6 months	Q month × 3, then Q 3–6 months	Q month × 3, then Q 3–6 months	– Ophtho exam Q 6–12 months – βHcG
Prednisone • Osteoporosis • Avascular necrosis • Glaucoma/cataract • HTN, ↑ Chol, ↑ TG • PUD			Q 3–6 months	– BP Q month then Q 2–3 months – Inquire about joint ROM/pain, psychological dist and sx of PUD – Ophtho exam Q 6–12 months – Fasting glucose/TG Q 1 months, then Q 3–6 months – AM cortisol near time of cessation – Repeat bone density Q 1 year
Retinoids • Teratogen – iPLEDGE for isotretinoin • ↑ TG, Chol	Q month	@ 2 weeks then Q month	Q month until stable, then Q 3 months	– Fasting TG and cholesterol q month – βHcG q month during and 1 month after Rx – Yearly x-ray of ankle, thoracic and cervical spine – Bexarotene – add FT4, TSH, fasting blood glucose (will likely need cholesterol med and Synthroid). Gemfibrozil contraindicated
Thalidomide • Teratogen – STEPS program • Neuropathy • Sedation, constipation, dizziness • Rash, weight gain • Tachycardia, bradycardia, hypotension • Thrombosis • Ovarian failure, amenorrhea	No guidelines	No guidelines	No guidelines	– βHcG; men and women both need birth control – Baseline nerve conduction studies in all patients and q 6 months – Assess routinely for thrombotic events

Drug Reactions

Table 45 Medications and their associated cutaneous eruptions

Cutaneous eruption	Associated medications
Acneiform and pustular	Azathioprine, beta-lactam ABX, bromides, chloral hydrate, cyclosporine, disulfiram, epidermal growth factor receptor inhibitors (erlotinib, cituximab, panitumumab, gefitinib), hormones (ACTH, steroids, OCPs, androgens), haldol, iodides, INH, lithium, phenobarbital, phenytoin, quinadine, scopolamine, SSRIs, thiouracil, trazodone, vitamin B12
Acral erythema	Ara-C (cytarabine, cytosine arabinoside), doxorubicin, 5-FU, MTX, hydroxyurea, mercaptopurine, mitotane
Acute generalized exanthematous pustulosis (AGEP)	Beta-lactam antibiotics, cephalosporins, macrolides, mercury
Bullous pemphigoid	Lasix, neuroleptics, PUVA, sulfa drugs, thiol drugs
Erythema multiforme	Allopurinol, bactrim, barbiturates, cimetidine, codeine, dilantin, griseofulvin, ketoconazole, lasix, NSAIDs, penicillin, phenothiazines, sulfonamides, tetracyclines (including minocycline)
Erythema nodosum	Accutane, halogens, OCPs, penicillin, sulfonamides, tetracycline
Erythroderma	Alefacept (high doses), allopurinol, antibiotics, aspirin, barbiturates, carbamazepine, codeine, dilantin, iodine, isoniazid, omeprazole, penicillin, quinidine, sulfa drugs, vancomycin
Exanthem	Amoxicillin, ampicillin, bactrim, cephalosporins, ipodate sodium, whole blood
Exfoliative dermatitis	Antimalarials, arsenic, aspirin, barbiturates, captopril, cepha-losporins, codeine, gold, iodine, isoniazid, mercury, NSAIDs, penicillin, phenytoin, quinidine, sulfonamides, terbinafine
Fixed drug	**Barbituates**, **carbamazepine**, ciprofloxacin, erythromycin, gold, hydrochlorothiazide, metronidazole, **NSAIDs** (including diclofenac, ibuprofen, naproxen, piroxicam), nystatin, OCPs, phenacetin, **phenolphthalein**, phenylbutazone, pseudoephedrine, quinidine, salicylates, sulfa drugs, tetracyclines (including doxycycline and minocycline)
Gingival hyperplasia	Calcium channel blockers, cyclosporine, dilantin
Hypersensitivity syndrome	Allopurinol, anticonvulsants, azathioprine, dapsone, erythromycin, imatinib (rare), minocycline, rifampin, retinoids, sulfa meds
Lichenoid	**ACE-inhibitors**, allopurinol, **antimalarials,** beta-blockers (including timolol ophthalmic solution), **bismuth**, calcium channel blockers, carbamazepine, dapsone, furosemide, **gold**, **HCTZ**, hydroxyurea, interferon-α, lithium, lorazepam, metformin, methyldopa, NSAIDs, **penicillamine,** phenytoin, proton pump inhibitors (omeprazole, lansoprazole, pantoprazole), **quinine, quinidine,** simvastatin (and other statins), spironolactone, sulfonylureas (including chlorprop-amide, tolbutamide), tetracyclines (including doxy and minocycline) , TNF-alpha inhibitors
Linear IgA	Amiodarone, captopril > other ACE-inhibitors, cephalosporins, diclofenac, glyburide, lithium, PCN, phenytoin, PUVA, sulfa, **vancomycin**
P450 inducers	Carbamazepine, dilantin, ETOH, griseofulvin, INH, omeprazole, phenobarbital, propranolol, retinoids, rifampin, tobacco

(continued)

Table 45 (continued)

Cutaneous eruption	Associated medications
P450 inhibitors	Allopurinol, bactrim, cimetidine, clarithromycin, coumadin, cyclosporine, danazol, diltiazem, diuretics (furosemide, thiazides), erythromycin, ETOH (acute), flagyl, fluoroquinolones, grapefruit juice, ketoconazole and azoles, methylprednisolone, OCPs, protease inhibitors, St. John's Wort, verapamil
Pemphigus	Aspirin, **Captopril (or other ACE-inhibitor)**, Furosemide, **NSAIDs** (including indomethacin), penicillamine, penicillin, phenacetin, phenylbutazone, piroxicam, propranolol, rifampin, sulfa drugs, thiazides
Photoallergic	Sunscreens (PABA, benzophenones, digalloyl trioleate), antibacterial cleansers (chlorhexidine, hexachlorophene, bithionol), antifungal agents, antimalarials, carbonilide, fragrances (musk ambrette, sandalwood oil, 6-methylcoumarin), gold, griseofulvin, quinidine, quinine, tricyclic antidepressants, NSAIDs, phenothiazines (chlorpro-mazine, promethazine), silver, sulfa drugs, thiazide diuretics
Phototoxic	Amiodarone, artificial sweeteners (saccharin), coal tars (acridine, anthracene, pyridine), dyes (anthraquinone, eosin, rose bengal), furocoumarins (psoralens, 8-MOP, TMP), furosemide, NSAIDs (especially naproxen, piroxicam), phenothiazines, sulfonamides, sulfonylureas (orinase, diabenase), tetracyclines (especially demeclocycline, doxycycline), thiazides (especially HCTZ), quinolones (ciprofloxacin)
Pigmentary changes	**Slate Gray:** Chloroquine, hydroxychloroquine, minocycline, phenothiazines **Slate Blue:** Amiodarone **Blue-Gray:** Gold **Yellow:** Beta-Carotene, quinacrine **Red:** Clofazimine **Brown:** ACTH, AZT, Bleomycin, OCPs
Pityriasis rosea	ACE-inhibitors, flagyl, gold, NSAIDs, metronidazole, isotretinoin, arsenic, beta-blockers, barbiturates, sulfasalazine, bismuth, clonidine, imatinib, organic mecurials, methoxypromazine, D-penicillamine, tripelennamine, ketotifen, salvarsan
Porphyria cutanea tarda	(Drugs that unmask or aggravate PCT): **Alcohol**, barbiturates, chlorinated hydrocarbons (including hexachlorobenzene), estrogens (including **OCPs**), griseofulvin, **iron**, nalidixic acid, NSAIDs, phenytoin, rifampin, sulfa drugs, tetracyclines
Pseudoporphyria	Amiodarone, barbiturates, dapsone, **diuretics** (especially furosemide, bumetanide, and thiazides), **estrogens** (including OCPs), griseoful-vin, nalidixic acid, **NSAIDs** (especially naproxen), pyridoxine, sulfonamides and sulfonylureas, tetracycline, voriconazole
Psoriasis-aggravating meds	Corticosteroid withdrawal, inderal (beta-blockers), interferons, interleukin2, Lithium
Purpuric drug reaction	Aspirin, chloroquine, indomethacin, iodide, penicillin, phenothiaz-ines, phenylbutazone, quinidine, sulfa drugs, thiazides
Radiation recall	Dactinomycin, MTX, bleomycin, etoposide, suramin, cyclophosphamide
SCLE-like eruption	ACE-inhibitors, aldactone, antihistamines, azathioprine, CCB (Diltiazem), glyburide, griseofulvin, HCTZ, NSAIDs, PCN, penicillamine, piroxicam, sulfonylureas, terbinafine, TNF-alpha inhibitors

(continued)

Table 45 (continued)

Cutaneous eruption	Associated medications
Serum sickness-like syndrome	**Cefaclor**, streptokinase, IVIG, PCN, minocin, rifampin
SLE	Acebutolol, alpha-ethyldopa, 5-aminosalicylic acid (pentasa, mesalamine, asacol), **chlorpromazine**, chlorprothixene, chlorthalidone, estrogens (including OCPs), furosemide, griseofulvin, **hydralazine, HCTZ, INH, methyldopa**, methylthiouracil, NSAIDs (including ibuprofen, naproxen), **penicillamine**, PCN, phenytoin, phenothiazines, **procainamide, PTU, psoralens**, quinidine, streptomycin, sulfa drugs, **TCN** (including doxycycline and minocycline), **thiazides** –*Positive antihistone antibodies often, antibodies to ssDNA in many cases, ds-DNA negative, ± Ro Ab
Sweet's	All-trans retinoic acid, anticonvulsants, GCSF, lithium, lasix, minocycline, hydralazine, Sulfa
Telogen effluvium	ACE-inhibitors, allopurinol, amphetamines, anticoagulants, azathioprine, beta-blockers (especially propranolol), boric acid, mouthwashes, chloroquine, iodides, lithium, methysergide, OCPs, oral retinoids
TEN	Allopurinol, ampicillin, aminothiozone (thioacetazone), barbiturates, carbamazepine, chlormezanone, dilantin, lamotrigine, NSAIDs, penicillin, phenylbutazone, piroxicam, sulfadiazone, sulfadoxine, sulfasalazine, thiabendazole, trimethoprim–sulfamethoxazole
Urticaria and angioedema	ACE-inhibitors, blood products, NSAIDs, penicillin, sulfonamides
Vasculitis	ACE-inhibitors, allopurinol, AZT, cimetidine, dilantin, gold, hydralazine, ketoconazole, NSAIDs, penicillin, phenothiazines, propylthiouracil, quinidine, quinolones (ciprofloxacin, levofloxacin, etc), retinoids, sulfonamides, tetracycline, thiazides, vancomycin

Intravenous Immunoglobulin (IVig)

- Human plasma derived from pools of 1,000–15,000 donors
  - Risk of transmitting infectious diseases, although screened carefully
- Contains >90% IgG and low amounts of IgM and IgA
- $T_{1/2}$ – 35–40 days, though much variance between individuals
- For most derm diseases, we use "high-dose" IVig
  - 2 g/kg over 3–5 days – can be given over 2 days in younger patients with normal renal and cardiovascular function. Rate of infusion varies between products
- Multiple commercial preparations available in US. Distributed as either lipophilized powders or liquid concentrates. Lipophilized powders require reconstitution; concentrates do not
  - Sugars are often added to IVig preparations to stabilize the product and prevent reaggregation
  - Differences in production methodologies impact the product's pharmacologic and physiologic profile – these, in turn, impact tolerability and efficacy
    - Differences in volume load, osmolality, sodium content, sugar content, pH and IgA content, clinical tolerability
    - Decision to use one product over the others is NOT trivial; small differences affect the outcome
- **Mechanism of Action**
  - Not clearly understood
  - Probably works via a number of pathways:
    - (1) Neutralizing and/or reducing tiers of circulating pathogenic Ab by anti-idiotype Ab in IVig
    - (2) Accelerating the catabolism of pathogenic IgG autoantibodies by saturating FcRn receptors
    - (3) Inhibiting the pathogenic activation of T-lymphocytes by antibodies to CD4, αβT-cell receptor, CCR5, and other T-cell receptors
    - (4) Inhibiting complement-mediated damage
    - (5) Modulating cytokines
    - (6) Blocking the fxn of Fc-γ receptors on phagocytes by saturating, altering, or downregulating their affinity of the Fc receptors
    - (7) Interfering with effector fxns of T-cells, B cells, and monocytes (including Fas-Fas ligand interaction)
    - (8) Inhibiting differentiation and maturation of dendritic cells
    - (9) Increasing disease sensitivity to corticosteroids
    - (10) Modulating endothelial cell fxn (including inhibiting thromboxane A2)
- **Clinical Uses in Dermatology**
  - Autoimmune collagen–vascular diseases
    - Dermatomyositis and Polymyositis – May be better for muscle than for skin, but probably more helpful than Rituximab
    - Cutaneous and systemic lupus erythematosus
    - Systemic sclerosis, Mixed CT disease, Hyper-IgE syndrome

- ○ Autoimmune blistering diseases (no FDA-approved therapies for these!)
  - Bullous pemphigoid – 2 g/kg q 4 weeks. Clear within 3 months
  - Pemphigus vulgaris – 2 g/kg q 3–4 weeks until clear. Then taper off steroids and other immunosuppressants, then start to decrease IVig. Average time to clearing is 4.5 months. More helpful in milder disease; can be combined w/ Rituximab
  - Pemphigus foliaceus – 2 g/kg q 4 weeks. Clear in 3–5 months. Minimal help
  - Cicatricial pemphigoid – give cycle of IVig q 2 weeks if aggressive dz
  - Epidermolysis bullosa acquisita, linear IgA bullous disease, pemphigoid gestationis
- ○ Drug-induced disorders
  - TEN – *Prins* et al. recommend 3 g/kg given over 3 days (Arch Derm 2003; 139: 26–32)
  - DRESS syndrome
- ○ Vasculitis
- ○ Urticaria – often used first-line by allergy/immunology, especially those with angioedema
- ○ Infectious
  - Streptococcal toxic shock syndrome
  - Necrotizing fasciitis
- ○ Atopic dermatitis
- ○ Psoriasis and psoriatic arthritis – 1 report
- ○ Scleromyxedema
- ○ Kaposi's Sarcoma
- ○ PMLE
- ○ NFD – difficult to infuse that much fluid in patients with poor renal fxn
- **Lab Monitoring** – See *Drug Monitoring*
- **Side Effects**
  - ○ Constitutional – **headache** (may be from elevated blood pressure), low-grade fever, flushing, chills, rhinitis, myalgias, wheezing, tachycardia, back pain, abdominal pain, nausea, vomiting
  - ○ Hx of migraines may predispose patient to higher risk of aseptic meningitis
  - ○ Skin – eczematous rxn, **urticaria**, lichenoid reactions, pruritus of palms, petechiae
  - ○ May interfere with live vaccines – defer these until 6 months after tx
  - ○ Maltose-containing IVig
  - ○ Can cause a falsely high reading on glucometer –> Beware
  - ○ Sucrose-containing IVig (stabilizer)
    - Can cause renal dysfunction → sucrose is a disaccharide that cannot be enzymatically broken down when administered intravenously and is known to cause renal dysfunction as a result of osmotic nephrosis
    - Greater than 90% of causes of renal dysfunction reported in association with IVig are from sucrose-containing products

○ Thrombotic events → stroke, MI, DVT, pulmonary embolism
  ▪ Many reported cases have had risk factors for stroke → hx of stroke or TIA, CAD, chronic HTN, arrhythmias, hypercoagulable states
○ Anaphylactic reactions can occur in IgA-deficient recipients who have anti-IgA antibodies of the IgE subclass in their serum (approximately 30–40% of IgA-deficient individuals have anti-IgA antibodies in their serum)
  ▪ IgA deficiency common – about 1 in 300
  ▪ Recommend screening for IgA deficiency beforehand
○ Rare side effects → hypotension, serum sickness, disseminated intravascular coagulation, aseptic meningitis, alopecia, acute renal failure, acute tubular necrosis, proximal tubular nephropathy, osmotic nephrosis, stroke, MI, DVT, anaphylaxis, SJS, hemolysis, seizure, syncope, acute respiratory distress, pulmonary edema, pulmonary embolism, acute bronchospasm, transfusion-associated lung injury (TRALI)

Pearls and Pitfalls

– Initial frequency of dosing is generally one cycle of IVig q 3–4 weeks
– Control of immunobullous diseases generally seen in 5–8 months; can slowly taper
  ○ Some sequentially add Dapsone 100–200 mg QD if no response
  ○ If still no response in 3–4 months, can add MTX 25 mg q week
  ○ If still no response, rituximab 375 mg/m² is added
  ○ These meds are slowly discontinued once patient has clearing for a number of months
  ○ Once control, maintain same dose of IVig, but increase time between infusions gradually to 6, 8, 10, 12, 14, 16 weeks. Proposed endpoint is two infusions 16 weeks apart. (Arch Derm 2003; 139: 1051–59)
– Premedicate
  ○ Acetaminophen 650 mg
  ○ Diphenhydramine 50 mg

Reference:

Fernandez AP and Kerdel FA. The use of i.v. IG therapy in dermatology. Derm Therapy 2007; 20: 288–305.

Methotrexate

Table 46 Start-up algorithm: Screening and H & P

PMH	*Consider alternative therapy if "yes" to the following …*
	Hepatotoxicity risk factors:
	1. Significant lifetime alcohol consumption. Past or current use of > 1–2 drinks per day; may be less in some patients
	2. Persistently abnormal liver function tests
	3. Inherited or acquired liver disease
	4. Chronic hepatitis B or C
	5. Obesity
	6. Diabetes mellitus
	7. Exposure to hepatotoxic drugs or chemicals
	MTX contraindicated in the following …
	Childbearing Female
	1. Desiring to get pregnant
	2. Pregnant
	3. Nursing
	4. (NOTE – adequate contraception and patient reliability must be ensured)
	Renal Insufficiency
	1. Severe renal insufficiency – calculate CrCl or GFR in all patients (especially elderly)
	2. Dialysis
	Estimated CrCl by Cockcroft–Gault equation:
	$\text{Est CrCl} = \dfrac{(140 - \text{age}) \times (\text{weight in kg}) (0.85 \text{ if female})}{Cr \times 72}$
Medications	Sulfonamides – don't use with MTX!
	Diuretics – intermittent use can alter GFR → less excretion of MTX → ↑ levels
	NSAIDS – impair MTX clearance; may require lower dose
	Other interactions – Trimethoprim, dapsone, triamterene, salicylates, dipyridamole, probenacid, chloramphenicol, phenothiazines, phenytoin, tetracyclines, systemic retinoids, alcohol, caffeine?
Physical Exam	Signs of cirrhosis
	Signs of renal insufficiency
	Pregnancy
Labs	LFTs, hepatitis serologies, CBC, pregnancy test, renal function

Methotrexate Hepatotoxicity Monitoring in Psoriasis Patients: Two Alternative Approaches

1. **AAD Guidelines**
   (Roenigk HH Jr, Auerback R, Maibach H, Weinstein G, Lebwohl M. Methotrexate in psoriasis: consensus conference. J Am Acad Dermatol 1998; 38: 478 – 485.)
   a. Low-risk patients:
      i. Liver biopsy every 1–1.5 g of therapy in low-risk patients
      ii. After a cumulative dose of 4 g, biopsy after each 1 g of therapy
   b. High-risk patients:
      i. Consider delayed baseline liver biopsy (after 2–6 months of therapy, to establish medication's efficacy and tolerability) in at-risk patients
      ii. Repeat liver biopsy after every 0.5–1 g of therapy
   c. After abnormal biopsy results
      i. For histologic grades IIIA (fibrosis, mild), repeat every 6 months; consider alternative therapy
      ii. For histologic grades IIIB (fibrosis, moderate to severe) and IV (cirrhosis), discontinue therapy

2. **Manchester Guidelines**
   (Chalmers RJG, Kirby B, Smith A, et al. Replacement of routine liver biopsy by procollagen III aminopeptide for monitoring patients with psoriasis receiving long-term methotrexate therapy: a multi-center audit and routine health economic analysis. Br J Dermatol 2005; 152: 444 – 450.)
   a. Baseline PIIINP (procollagen III aminopeptide) level (if possible)
   b. Repeat PIIINP levels every 2–3 months while on therapy
   c. Indications for considering liver biopsy:
      i. Pretreatment PIIINP > 0.8 µg/L
      ii. At least three abnormal PIIINP levels (>4.2 µg/L) over a 12-month period
      iii. Elevated PIIINP level above 8.0 µg/L in two consecutive samples
   d. Indications for considering withdrawal of therapy:
   i. Elevated PIIINP level > 10.0 µg/L in three consecutive sample in a 12-month period
   e. "The decision whether to perform liver biopsy, withdraw treatment, or continue treatment despite elevated PIIINP levels must take into account other factors such as disease severity, patient age, and the ease with which alternative therapies may be used in place of methotrexate"

Table 47 Side effects of methotrexate

Most common	Nausea, anorexia, fatigue, malaise – usually occur around time medication is taken; are dose dependent
Hepatic	Elevated transaminases, steatotic hepatitis, cirrhosis (can be silent)
Hematologic	Leucopenia, thrombocytopenia, megaloblastic anemia, pancytopenia (rare, but 25% mortality, mucositis is precursor)
Pulmonary	Acute pneumonitis, slowly progressive pulmonary fibrosis. (Pulm SE are extremely rare, but may be increased in patients with preexisting disease)
Malignancy	Risk of lymphoma is probably increased in patients with rheumatic and psoriatic disease, BUT unclear whether this risk is related to underlying disease, their therapy, or both
Infection	May be safe to use in HIV patients if more conservative therapy has failed or is contraindicated
Mucocutaneous	Mucositis (more common in patients without adequate folic acid supplementation and may herald bone marrow toxicity), photosensitivity, alopecia, drug hypersensitivity rxns, radiation-recall reactions
Cardiovascular	Elevates homocysteine levels (folic acid helps counteract this)
Reproductive	Teratogenic (category X) – D/C med 4 months prior to attempting conception. Reversible oligospermia in males

Pearls and Pitfalls

- Leucovorin (**folinic acid**)=rescue drug if MTX toxicity; Give 25 mg PO q 6 h until stable. Check MTX level
- Folic acid – administered in doses ranging from 1 to 5 mg QD. Usually start at 1 mg PO QD and escalate the amount if doses greater than 15 mg weekly or side effects (particularly, if early signs of bone marrow toxicity – $\uparrow$ MCV)
- BUN and creatinine are not sufficient in assessing for normal renal function. Elderly patients, especially women with little muscle mass, can often have a serum BUN/Cr in normal range but nevertheless have significantly reduced glomerular filtration rate

Mycophenolate Mofetil (MMF)

- Average retail cost of MMF therapy is $600–$900 per month ($6 per 500 mg tablet), roughly five times that of azathioprine
- **Mechanism of Action**
  - Selective inhibition of the purine biosynthesis enzyme inosine monophosphate dehydrogenase (IMPDH). Two isoforms of IMPDH exist …
    - Type I – seen in most cell types, including resting lymphocytes
    - Type II – detected in multiple leukemia-derived cell lines; expression dramatically increases in lymphocytes when they are stimulated
      - This type is 5x more sensitive to MMF, thus conferring a specificity of MMF to activated lymphocytes
  - Other cells that may be affected by MMF – smooth muscle cells, fibroblasts, dendritic cells involved in antigen presentation and activation of naïve T-lymphocytes
- **Side Effects**
  - (Extremely well tolerated in general)
  - Gastrointestinal – Sx generally abate with continued use
    - Diarrhea (most common), nausea, vomiting, and abdominal cramps – occur in 12–36% of patients
      - Tend to occur early
      - Can limit maximum plasma concentration by BID and TID dosing and administering with food
      - An enteric form does exist and may be associated with less SE
      - If persistent or severe symptoms – consider opportunistic infection, GI ulceration and/or bleeding
    - Can elevate LFTs, although MMF is not thought to have significant hepatotoxicity
  - Hematologic (11–34%) – typically rapidly reverse with dose reduction or discontinuation
    - Leukopenia – most common, but still infrequent
    - Anemia
    - Thrombocytopenia
    - Neutrophil dysplasia (pseudo-Pelger-Huet anomaly) characterized by a left shift on CBC and nuclear hypolobulation on cytologic examination. This, in many cases, portends the subsequent development of neutropenia
  - Genitourinary – Sx generally abate with continued use
    - Urgency, frequency, dysuria, sterile pyuria
    - MMF does not exhibit nephrotoxicity
    - Decreased libido – rare
  - Pregnancy category D
    - MMF reduces estrogen/progestin blood levels and could reduce efficacy of oral contraceptives

- Two methods of contraception for 4 weeks before. Continue contraception for 6 weeks after discontinuing med
- Linked to ear/facial abnormalities
  o Constitutional
    - Fever, myalgias, headache, insomnia
  o Cardiovascular – Peripheral edema, HTN
  o Derm – nonspecific rash, acne, urticaria, dyshidrotic eczema – all reported
  o Infection and malignancy
    - Unclear how applicable the data is to derm patients → most of the data from organ transplant patients who generally have a higher burden of systemic illness and comorbidities
    - Increase in infections – viral (CMV risk when MMF > 3 g/day), bacterial, mycobacterial (similar to azathioprine)
- **Labs** – similar to azathioprine; see *Drug Monitoring*
- **Drug Interactions**
  o Any med reducing renal clearance may increase serum levels of MMF
  o Should be taken 1–2 h away from divalent cations (Ca, Fe, Mg, Na, etc) to improve absorption
  o Concomitant use with antiviral agents may increase levels of both
  o ABX may decrease MMF plasma levels – cephalosporins, fluoroquinolones, macrolides, penems, PCN, sulfonamides
- **Clinical Uses of MMF in Dermatology**
  o Psoriasis – better alternatives out there
  o Immunobullous diseases
    - PV/PF – an excellent adjuvant to corticosteroids
    - BP, Linear IgA
    - CP – might not respond as well. Imuran has better anti-inflammatory properties
  o Atopic dermatitis
  o Connective tissue diseases
    - Lupus – has helped lupus-associated glomerulonephritis
    - Dermatomyositis, vasculitis, systemic sclerosis
  o Neutrophilic Diseases: Pyoderma gangrenosum, Sweet's → May not be super effective
  o Sarcoidosis
  o Lichen planus, Lichenoid dermatoses → respond well

Pearls and Pitfalls

– Start 1.5–2 g/day and increase by 500 mg q month until reach benefit or 3 g/day max
  o Some start 500 mg QD and then increase to 500 mg BID after 1 week to decrease GI side effects
  o Can increase dosage every 2–4 weeks until a dose of 1.5 g BID (3 g total) is reached

- Once stable, may decrease dose by 500 mg/day per month
- Most patients require 2–3 g/day
- Use in conjunction with another agent (cyclosporine, prednisone) – works best this way
- Once control of disease is attained, begin tapering the more potent agent slowly
- Relatively safe – lack of hepatonephrotoxicity
- Although MMF's safety in patients with hepatitis B and C is well documented, reports have linked the med to rising hep C viral titers and hepatitis C-induced acute hepatitis
  o Obtain baseline hepatitis panel
- PPD before starting immunosuppressives

Reference:

(1) 2008 AAD lecture by Dr. J. Mark Jackson (Univ of Louisville).
(2) Zwerner J and Fiorentino D. Mycophenolate mofetil. Derm Therapy 2007; 20: 229–38.

Photodynamic Therapy (PDT)

Table 48 PDT protocols

	Incubation	Light source	Time of light source
Actinic keratoses	60 min - face, chest 90 min - arms 120 min - legs	Blue - face IPL, PDL - lips, chest, arms, legs	16:40 min (usual)
Acne vulgaris	30 min	IPL, PDL	Usual
Photorejuvenation	30 min	IPL	Usual
Hidradenitis suppurativa	60 min	IPL/Blue	Usual
Basal cell carcinoma	60–120 min	IPL, PDL	Usual
Bowen's disease	60–120 min	PDL, IPL	Usual

Courtesy of Dr. Amy Taub, Chicago, IL

Protocol and Information

1. Make sure patient can practice complete sun avoidance for 2 days prior to proceeding!!
2. Patient may be premedicated with Tylenol
3. Acetone scrub → 2 × 2 inch gauze. Scrub vigorously for 2 min, then clean with alcohol
4. Application of levulan
   (a) Apply in small circles over the entire area
   (b) Double pass areas of obvious disease
5. After applying the medication, escort patient to dark area or an area that is away from windows and skylights for the prescribed incubation time. (Touma et al.)
6. Set a timer and leave at the nurses' station
7. Put a note in the chart re: time that the Levulan was placed on the patient (and when it was removed). Person applying and removing the Levulan should initial the chart
8. Taub recommends washing off Levulan (to make it standard) prior to using the light source
9. Position patient within 4 inches of the light source. Best to have them lie down
10. Can use a room air fan during treatment, but avoid the Zimmer

After the Treatment (Post-Op)

1. Apply Avene Thermal Spring Water Gel immediately after
2. Prescription for Biafine cream in the AM
3. If in serious pain, give PO steroids. Usually helps in an hour
4. Hat/Sunglasses – for drive home

5. Sunscreen – Apply thick zinc oxide-based sunblock
   a. Prescribed soln – "Up the Anti" – made especially for PDT
   b. Zinc/Titanium based
6. Complete light avoidance is essential for 48 h!! Patient must avoid windows, skylights, outdoors. Patient may go out when it is completely dark outside
7. Skinceuticals – antioxidant C & E, ferrulic – may be helpful
8. Side Effects → Will get erythema and swelling. H1 Blockers can be helpful for the edema (appears to be from mast cell degranulation)

Other Notes

1. Patients prefer PDT to cryotherapy (in all studies) by a large margin!
2. For acne, IPL/PDL > Blue light. Best for severe acne and nodules, but off-label
3. Red light more painful
4. Take patients off tretinoin cream 1 week prior to minimize exuberant results
5. Levulan kerastick 2% → 5-ALA
6. Metvixia → methylester of 5% (MAL)

Coding

96567 – can use if > 15 AK's and this is documented

J7308 – for Levulan

Know what your main carriers require or need (some require a prior authorization)

Photodynamic Therapy (PDT) Dictation Form

Procedure
Photodynamic therapy with 20% 5-ALA (Levulan) to _____(the Scalp, etc)

Preprocedure Diagnosis
Actinic keratoses > 15

Postprocedure Diagnosis
(same)

Attending –

Resident –

Procedure:

- The benefits and risks were discussed with the patient prior to the procedure and informed consent was obtained
- The patient was prepped for PDT. The patient washed his/her face with a cleanser. The skin was then degreased with vigorous scrubbing of acetone on a 2×2 gauze for 2 min. The skin was secondarily degreased with alcohol swabs Cryotherapy and Curettage was used for the thick lesions prior to applying the medication
- The incubation time of the ALA for PDT was _____ *(1 h)*
  - The Levulan was applied at _____ PM/AM (time) by _____
  - The Levulan was removed at _____ PM/AM (time) by _____
  - 1 (or 2) stick was used
- The patient was premedicated with _____ (NSAID, acetaminophen) 1 h prior to the treatment
- The Levulan was activated by the Blu light (*or IPL vs. PDL*) for _____ minutes *(Blu light – 16 min, 40 sec)*
- The patient tolerated the procedure _____ *(Well, Not so well – had to be stopped and started several times, etc.)*
- No complications were observed

Postprocedure Care:

- Avene Thermal Spring Water Gel was applied to the skin. The patient may apply this to the skin 4–6x/day. (Alternative – Rx for Biafine cream)
- An opaque sunscreen was applied to the treated skin and patient was advised to avoid complete sun exposure for 48 h, including windows, doors, skylights, etc. The patient was advised that noncompliance may lead to a severe phototoxic reaction
- Side effects including burning, stinging, pruritus, and swelling were reviewed with the patient. Should *he/she* experience intense pain and swelling, would recommend starting an antihistamine such as Benedryl
- Patient was advised to contact our office if any blistering occurs

Patients with history of recurring cold sores should start oral Valtrex 500 mg or Famvir 250 mg tablets, one tablet BID for 3 days. Start prescription the morning of the PDT therapy

Retinoids

This medication may initially cause worsening of your acne in the first few weeks of treatment. This means the medication is working

Side Effects

- Scaling – the medication acts as a chemical exfoliant, and it is common to see some peeling in the morning and in the evening. You may *gently* massage the dead skin off with your hands or a washcloth when you clean your face. It is important NOT to scrub your face, as this can make acne worse
- Redness
- Burning
- Stinging
- Dryness

Instructions

Place a pea-sized amount of the medication on the finger and dot to 4–5 areas on the face. Rub these dots into the surrounding skin. Too much medication is only more irritating, not more effective

Tips

- Retinoids should be avoided during pregnancy and nursing
- It is important to stop your topical retinoid 2 weeks on the *entire face* prior to waxing (eyebrows, upper lip, etc.). By not doing so, it is very likely that you will get scab formation at the areas that are waxed. You may resume treatment the day of the waxing
- Concomitant therapy with abrasive soaps, astringents, toners, scrubs, buff puffs may cause increased irritation
- If significant irritation occurs, use the medication EVERY OTHER NIGHT for the first 2 weeks of use. It also sometimes helps to wait 30 min after washing your face before applying the medication (if time permits)
- If irritation continues or worsens, stop the medication and alert your dermatologist
- Applying more than the recommended pea-sized amount does NOT make the medication more effective or work faster; it does cause more irritation!
- Retinoids may cause a greater sensitivity to the sun. We recommend an oil-free, noncomedogenic moisturizer with sunscreen. The moisturizer will help with dryness and protect you from sunburn

Rituximab

- Murine–human chimeric Ab to CD20 → reduces B cells
  - CD20 expressed on B cells. Not expressed on T-cells, monocytes, or stem cells
  - Since plasma cells are mostly CD20-, immunoglobulin levels are not greatly affected immediately
- May also inhibit B cell-dependent activation of T-cells
- **Side Effects**
  - Mostly infusion-related events (fever, chills, headache, etc.)
  - Rash – including SJS/TEN
  - Slight increase in infection rate over placebo
  - Progressive multifocal leukoencephalopathy (may be more common in lymphoma patients)
  - Hepatitis B reactivation
  - Hypogammaglobulinemia – rare (may be related to repeated courses)
  - Hypotension, cardiogenic shock
  - Anti-chimeric Ab in 1–4% → can have hypersensitivity reaction
- Initial approved dosing regimen → Four weekly infusions of 375 mg/m^2
  - 50 mg/h and increase by 50 mg/h every 30 min to a max of 400 mg/h
- **Off-Label Uses**
  - Pemphigus vulgaris
    - Ab levels correlate with disease activity. IgG4 pathogenic (not IgG1). IgG4 produced by memory B cells while IgG1 produced by plasma cells
    - NEJM 2006 (Ahmed) – 2 cycles of Rituximab for 3 weeks, then IVig 2 g/kg for 4 months. 9 out of 11 had remission
  - Paraneoplastic pemphigus
  - Bullous pemphigoid
  - Epidermolysis bullosa acquisita
  - Cutaneous B-cell lymphoma
  - Dermatomyositis
    - Cutaneous findings tend to be very resistant to treatment in general
    - Standard dosing 375 mg/m^2 q week × 4 weeks
    - Get myositis improvement in some; skin may or may not improve
    - NIH study at Univ of Pitt
  - GVHD
  - Wegener's granulomatosis
  - Microscopic polyangiitis
  - Cryoglobulinemic vasculitis
  - Churg–Strauss syndrome

Thalidomide

- Costs approximately $3600 for two tablets
- FDA-approved for erythema nodosum leprosum (ENL), myeloma
- **Mechanism of Action**
  - Inhibition of production of TNF-α *in vitro* and *in vivo* but NOT helpful in rheumatoid arthritis. (Likely works via other MOA that we don't know about)
  - Accelerates the degradation of TNF-α ribonucleic acid transcripts
  - Decreases IgM production
  - Inhibits angiogenesis
  - Inhibits chemotaxis
- **Off-Label Derm Uses**
  - Aphthous stomatitis, aphthous ulcers in association with HIV, Behçet's syndrome, Kaposi's sarcoma, prurigo nodularis, actinic prurigo, Langerhans cell histiocytoses, uremic pruritus, lichen planus, pyoderma gangrenosum, Jessner's lymphocytic infiltrate, sarcoidosis, erythema multiforme, GVHD, metastatic melanoma, cutaneous lupus, scleroderma, scleromyxedema
- Contraindicated in TEN – one study showed an increase in mortality
- **Precautions**
  - Teratogenic – STEPS program; sexually active males need to practice contraception
  - Common – constipation, rash, drowsiness
  - Other – edema, bradycardia, dryness, pruritus, headache, hypotension, increased appetite, mood changes, male sexual dysfunction, nausea, tachycardia, weight gain
  - Caution with neutropenic patients – can cause neutropenia
  - Peripheral neuropathy – primarily affects sensory fibers in lower extremities
    - Nerve conduction velocity may be done, but careful questioning preferred b/c symptoms can occur despite normal NCV, and NCVs can be abnormal in asymptomatic patients
    - May be dose related and can be irreversible side effect
    - Numbness, pins and needles, sensation of tightness, cold intolerance, and burning
  - Amenorrhea – in most cases, menses resume within 3 months of discontinuing thalidomide. Long-term effects in terms of fertility are unknown
  - Ovarian failure
  - Procoagulation and thromboembolism – ? If related to oral contraceptives

Note – antimalarials have known antithrombotic properties, and care should be taken when withdrawing these agents from patients on thalidomide

General Derm

Acanthosis Nigricans

Etiology

Depends on type (see below)

Classification

- Acanthosis Nigricans (AN) is divided into two broad categories: **benign and malignant**
  - **Benign** – Few, if any, complications of their skin lesions
    - Many of these patients have underlying insulin-resistant state. Severity of the insulin resistance is highly variable
    - Severity of skin findings may parallel the degree of insulin resistance, and a partial resolution may occur with tx of the insulin-resistant state. Insulin resistance is the most common association of AN in the younger age population
  - **Malignant** – underlying malignancy is often an aggressive tumor. Average survival time of patients with signs of malignant AN is 2 years, although cases in which patients have survived for up to 12 years have been reported. In older patients with new onset AN, most have an associated internal malignancy

Clinical Presentation and Types

- **Obesity-associated AN** – is the most common type
  - Lesions may appear at any age but are more common in adulthood
  - Weight dependent; lesions may completely regress with weight reduction
  - Insulin resistance is often present in these patients; however, it is not universal

- **Syndromic AN** is the name given to AN that is associated with a syndrome
  - *Type A syndrome* – [hyperandrogenemia, insulin resistance, and AN syndrome (HAIR-AN syndrome)]. Often familial, affecting primarily young women (especially black women). Associated with polycystic ovaries or signs of virilization (e.g., hirsutism, clitoral hypertrophy). High plasma testosterone levels common. Lesions of AN may arise during infancy and progress rapidly during puberty
  - *Type B syndrome* – generally occurs in women with uncontrolled diabetes mellitus, ovarian hyperandrogenism, or an autoimmune disease such as SLE, scleroderma, Sjögren syndrome, or Hashimoto thyroiditis. Circulating antibodies to insulin receptor may be present. Lesions of AN vary in severity
- **Acral AN** occurs in patients who are in otherwise good health.
  - Most common in dark-skinned individuals, especially African Americans
  - Hyperkeratotic velvety lesions are most prominent over the dorsal aspects of the hands and feet
- **Unilateral AN**, aka **nevoid AN**, is believed to be inherited AD
  - May become evident during infancy, childhood, or adulthood
  - Lesions tend to enlarge gradually before stabilizing or regressing
- **Familial AN** – rare genodermatoses; seems to be transmitted in AD fashion with variable phenotypic penetrance
  - Typically begin during early childhood but may manifest at any age
  - Often progresses until puberty, at which time it stabilizes or regresses
- **Drug-induced AN** – uncommon
  - May be induced by several meds – including nicotinic acid, insulin, pituitary extract, systemic corticosteroids, and diethylstilbestrol
  - Rarely, triazinate, oral contraceptives, fusidic acid, and methyltestosterone
  - May regress following the discontinuation of the offending medication
- **Mixed-type AN** – situations in which patient with one of AN develops new lesions of a different etiology
  - An example of this would be an overweight patient with obesity-associated AN who subsequently develops malignant AN

Labs

- For patients with adult onset of AN, perform a basic workup for underlying malignancy
- Screen for diabetes with a glycosylated hemoglobin level or glucose tolerance test
- Screen for insulin resistance; a good screening test for insulin resistance is a plasma insulin level, which will be high in those with insulin resistance. This is the most sensitive test to detect a metabolic abnormality of this kind because many younger patients do not yet have overt diabetes mellitus and an abnormal glycosylated hemoglobin level, but they do have a high plasma insulin level

Differential Diagnosis

- Addison Disease, hemochromatosis, pellagra, Becker nevus, confluent and reticulated papillomatosis of Gougerot and Carteaud syndrome (CARP), Dowling–Degos disease, hypertrophic SK, ichthyosis hystrix, linear epidermal nevus, parapsoriasis en plaque, pemphigus vegetans

Treatment

- Correct the underlying disease process
  - Correction of hyperinsulinemia often reduces the burden of hyperkeratotic lesions
  - Weight reduction in obesity-associated AN may result in resolution of the dermatosis
- Treatment of the lesions of AN is for cosmetic reasons only
  - Keratolytics
    - Topical tretinoin
    - Salicylic acid (Salex cream)
    - Urea cream – (Carmol cream)
- Oral agents – some benefit include etretinate, isotretinoin, metformin, and dietary fish oils
  - Dermabrasion and long-pulsed alexandrite laser therapy may also be used to reduce the bulk of the lesion
- Cyproheptadine has been used in cases of malignant AN because it may inhibit the release of tumor products

Prevention

- Weight management

Pearls and Pitfalls

- Do not apply salicylic acid to large body surface area, as there is a risk of salicylicism
- Tretinoin cream can be irritating. Start by using 3x/week
- Generic tretinoin must be applied at bedtime as sun exposure will inactivate the product

Acne Vulgaris

Etiology and Pathogenesis

- Four key contributing components
  1. Follicular epidermal hyperproliferation with subsequent plugging of follicle
  2. Excess sebum
  3. Presence and activity of *Propionibacterium acnes*
  4. Inflammation
- Consider hormonal role, especially in setting of hirsutism or dysmenorrhea
- Genetics may play role
  - Family history of cystic acne
  - Severe acne may be associated with XYY syndrome (Klinefelter's)
- Toll-like receptor 2 (TLR-2) recently implicated in pathogenesis of acne. TLR-2 is a receptor recognized by *P. acnes*. When bound, TLR-2 upregulates production and the release of proinflammatory cytokines such as interleukin-12 and interleukin-8 from monocytes. TLR-2 is expressed on infiltrating inflammatory cells around the pilosebaceous follicle in those with acne
- 5a-reductase type 1 – is present in the sebaceous gland and converts testosterone dihydrotestosterone (DHT). It has been hypothesized that those with acne might have more active 5a-reductase type 1, but studies haven't been significant

Clinical Presentation and Types

- **Acne conglobata** – Severe cystic acne presenting as nodules, cysts, abscesses, sinus tracts, and ulcerations
- **Acne cosmetica** – due to comedogenic cosmetics
- **Acne excoriee** – Mild acne that has been extensively picked at, often leading to scarring. Often due to emotional and psychological issues such as depression, obsessive-compulsive disorder, etc.
- **Acne fulminans** – Acute onset of severe cystic acne with concomitant suppuration and ulceration. Patients have malaise, fatigue, fever, arthralgias, leukocytosis, increased erythrocyte sedimentation rate (ESR)
- **Acne in adult women** – Common issue. May be associated with irregular menses, hormonal irregularities
- **Acne mechanica** – flares of preexisting acne because of pressure from sports helmets/gear, facial masks, leaning on the hands, etc.
- **Acne with facial edema** – Acne associated with disfiguring facial edema. Woody induration may be present with or without erythema
- **Chloracne** – some overlap with occupational acne. This is due to exposure to chlorinated hydrocarbons in electrical conductors, insecticides, herbicides. Often involves face and postauricular areas

- **Comedonal acne** – Keratin plugs are called *comedones,* which may be open or closed. When acne is primarily composed of this type, may be called comedonal acne
- **Cystic acne** – Prominence of cystic lesions
- **Infantile acne** – comedones, superficial inflammatory papules and pustules, and, in some cases, nodulocystic lesions on the face, particularly the cheeks. Not associated with underlying endocrinopathies. DDx includes neonatal cephalic pustulosis and neonatal sebaceous gland hyperplasia. Scarring possible if cystic lesions present and not treated aggressively
- **Inflammatory acne** – Prominence of inflammatory acne papules. Person also typically has comedones
- **Neonatal acne** – Typically on nose and cheeks. Acne related to *Malessezia spp.* Treat with topical antifungals
- **Occupational acne** – Often due to exposure to tar derivatives, cutting oils, chlorinated hydrocarbons. Not restricted to sites where acne typically occurs
- **Pomade acne** – Acne on the face in areas where hair (with oil-based products) typically sits such as forehead and lateral cheeks
- **Recalcitrant acne** – Consider hormonal evaluation, congenital adrenal hyperplasia (11B- or 21B-hydroxylase deficiencies)
- **Tropical acne** – flare of acne lesions in tropical climates. Often have a folliculitis overlap. Present with folliculitis, inflammatory nodules, and sometimes cysts

Labs

- Consider checking these if hirsutism present, relcitrant to therapy
  - Total testosterone, free testosterone, DHEA-S, LH, FSH, prolactin

Differential Diagnosis

- Comedones are required for diagnosis of any type of acne. Comedones are not a feature of:
  - Folliculitis
  - Rosacea
  - Perioral dermatitis
  - Steroid acne – monomorphous folliculitis with small erythematous papules and pustules. No comedones present
  - Drug-induced acne – monomorphous acne-like eruption due to medications such as corticosteroids, isoniazid, lithium, phenytoin, EGFR blockers. No comedones present
  - Acne aestivalis – papular eruption after sun exposure. May be a form of polymorphous light eruption. No comedones. Usually on arms, neck, and chest

Treatment

- Typically consists of a combination of: Topical retinoids, topical antibiotics, oral antibiotics, benzoyl peroxide, and/or salicylic acid
  - Always try to use a topical retinoid as this is the backbone of acne therapy
  - Systemic retinoids (isotretinoin) reserved for severe and/or recalcitrant disease

Details:
- **Topical retinoids** = backbone of acne therapy → targets microcomedo

Table 49 Topical retinoids used in the treatment of acne vulgaris

Trade name	Generic	Formulations	Comments
Retin-A	tretinoin	0.01, 0.025% cream or gel	Sunlight, benzoyl peroxide inactivates this form
Retin-A Micro	tretinoin	0.04, 0.1% gel	0.04%=gray tube 0.01%=purple
Atralin	tretinoin	0.05% gel	Pkg insert says to avoid in patients with fish allergy
Avita	tretinoin	0.025% cream or gel: 20 and 45 g tubes	
Renova	tretinoin	0.02% cream	Used primarily for wrinkles, mottled hyperpigmentation in older individuals
Refissa	tretinoin	0.05% cream	Used primarily for wrinkles, mottled hyperpigmentation in older individuals
Tazorac	tarazotene	0.1% cream: 30 g, 60 g 0.1% gel: 30 g, 100 g	Gel formulation may cause pruritus in some individuals
Tretin-X	tretinoin	0.01% or 0.025% gel: 35 g 0.025%, 0.05%, or 0.1% cream: 35 g	Packaged with complimentary foaming cleanser and soothing moisturizer
Tretinoin emollient cream	Tretinoin	0.05%	Similar to Renova cream 0.05%
Ziana	Clindamycin 1.2%+tretinoin 0.025% – 30 g, 60 g		Recommend using benzoyl peroxide products in conjunction to avoid resistance to clindamycin
Veltin	Clindamycin 1.2%+tretinoin 0.025% – 30 g, 60 g		

Summary of retinoids (weak to strong): Differin and Avita cream/gel<tretinoin cream 0.025% (gray)<tretinoin cream 0.05% (blue)<tretinoin cream 0.1% (red)<tretinoin gel 0.01% (green)<tretinoin gel 0.025% (orange)<retin-A micro gel 0.04% (gray)<retin-A micro gel 0.1% (purple)<tretinoin liquid

- **Benzoyl peroxide and topical antibiotics**
  - Benzoyl peroxide is antimicrobial and has weak comedolytic properties

Table 50 **Topical benzoyl peroxide and topical antibiotics used in the treatment of acne vulgaris**

Trade name	Formulations	Comments
Acanya	1.2% clindamycin + 2.5% benzoyl peroxide – 50 g, pump	May be slightly better tolerated by patients with sensitive skin
Benzac	5, 10% gel (alcohol) or wash	
Benzac AC (emollient base)	2.5, 5, 10% gel (water): 60 and 80 g tube	
Benzac W	5% and 10% – 8 oz	Wash
BenzaClin	1% clindamycin + 5% benzoyl peroxide – 25 g, 35 g, 50 g	
Benzamycin	3% erythromycin + 5% benzoyl peroxide	Needs refrigerated. Not used as much b/c of resistance to erythromycin.
BenzaShave	5%, 10% shaving cream	Good for pseudofolliculitis barbae, acne
BenzEFoam	5.3% foam – 60 g, 100 g	
Benziq LS gel	2.75% – 50 g tube	
Benziq Gel	5.25% – 50 g tube	
Benziq Wash	5.25% – 175 g tube	
Brevoxyl	4% and 8% creamy wash – 170 g 4% and 8% gel – 42.5 g 5% bar – 113 g	
Clindamycin	Cleocin-T 1% gel, lotion, soln ClindaReach 1% kit with applicator arm and head with pledgets Clindets – 1% pledgets/50% alcohol Evoclin – 1% foam in 50 and 100 g cans Ziana – 1.2% clindamycin + 0.025% tretinoin gel	
Desquam-E (emollient base)	5, 10% gel (water)	
Desquam-X	5, 10% gel (water)	
Duac	1% clindamycin + 5% benzoyl peroxide	Also supplied as "Duac Care System" which contains SFC lotion
Inova Easy Pad	4% and 8% 4% BPO + 1% salicylic acid = Inova 4/1 acne control therapy 8% BPO + 2% salicylic acid = Inova 8/2	
Pacnex MX	4.25% wash – 16 oz 4.25% LP cleansing pads – 6 g, 60 pads 7% HP cleansing pads – 6 g, 60 pads	
PanOxyl Bar	5, 10% bar soap	OTC
Sulfoxyl Lotion Regular	5% BPO + sulfur 2% → 59 mL	
Sulfoxyl Lotion Strong	10% BPO + sulfur 5% → 59 mL	
Triaz	3, 6, 9% cream, gel (water), cleanser, pads	
ZoDerm	4.5, 8.5% cream, gel or wash	

Table 51 Other topical medications used in the treatment of acne vulgaris

Generic name	Dosing	Comments
Azelaic acid	Azelex 20% cream – 30 g, 50 g Finacea 15% gel: 50 g	May cause hypopigmentation of skin
Dapsone 5% gel	Aczone gel 5% – 30 g, 60 g	Pkg insert does NOT require checking G6PD prior to starting treatment Not recommended in those on oral dapsone, TMP/SMX, antimalarials – increased risk of hemolysis
Salicylic acid	**Rx:** 2% Salicylic acid in 70% ethanol; apply to chest and back BID. Disp: 240 mL	The Clinique 3-Step system's exfoliator has salicylic acid in it. Strength depends on the Clinique number (1, 2, 3, 4) Many over-the-counter products contain salicylic acid. Not recommended during pregnancy
Sodium sulfacetamide	Clarifoam EF Clenia Klaron 10% lotion: 59, 118 mL Ovace 10% foam, wash Plexion cleanser, cleansing cloths, topical suspension Rosac 5, 10% cream Rosanil 5, 10% wash Rosula cleanser, gel, medicated pads (urea base) Sulfacet-R 5, 10% lotion Zetacet 10% ss + 5% sulfur lotion; also in wash	Sulfur meds may potentially cause hypersensitivity rxn

Table 52 Oral antibiotics used in the treatment of acne vulgaris

Generic name	Trade names	Dosing	Side effects and adverse events	Comments
Tetracycline	Sumycin	500 mg PO BID 125 mg/ 5 mL 250 mg tabs	Nausea, vomiting, vaginitis, esophagitis	Take on empty stomach (2 h after a meal and 1 h prior) with water Avoid dairy or iron-containing products for 1 h Class of Tetracyclines – Do not use with PO retinoids (risk of pseudotumor cerebri increases) – Don't use in kids < age 8 (staining of teeth) – Do not use in pregnant, lactating women

(continued)

Table 52 (continued)

Generic name	Trade names	Dosing	Side effects and adverse events	Comments
Doxycycline	Adoxa 150 mg Doryx 75, 100 ER Monodox 50, 75, 100 Periostat – low dose Vibramycin – 50, 100 Oracea – low dose	50 – 100 mg PO QD-BID for generic	Photosensitivity, especially in summer. Nausea if taken on empty stomach, esophagitis	Safe in renal insufficiency
Minocycline	Minocin 50, 100 Solodyn 45, 90, 135 ER Dynacin 50, 75, 100	100 mg PO QD-BID for generic	Pigmentary changes, vertigo, hepatitis, DRESS syndrome	Minocin Kit – contains complimentary T3 calming wipes
Erythromycin (EES)		400 mg 200 mg/5 mL 400 mg/5 mL	Nausea, GI upset, QT prolongation	Not commonly given b/c of resistance. Can be used in lactation Many drug interactions (CYP450 3A4) – discuss with patients

Table 53 Systemic retinoids used in the treatment of severe acne vulgaris

Generic	Brand	Dosing	Side Effects	Comments
Isotretinoin	Accutane (dc'd in US) Amnesteem Claravis Sotret	0.5–1.5 mg/kg for total dose of 120– 150 mg/kg	Teratogenic, elevated TG/ cholesterol, dryness, myalgias, arthralgias, depression, pseudotumor cerebri	iPLEDGE program – patient comes every 30 days; must fill prescription within 7 days – Need two negative pregnancy tests prior to starting – Patient needs two forms of birth control – Baseline labs: CBC, LFTs, fasting cholesterol panel, HcG, BUN, Cr – Repeat labs monthly prior to renewing prescription – **pseudotumor cerebri** (persistent headache, N/V, stiff neck, visual changes, papilledema)

- **Oral contraceptives**
  - All combination oral contraceptive pills have a net effect of increasing sex hormone binding globulin and decreasing circulating free testosterone and thus have the potential to improve acne
  - Drospirenone = a component of some contraceptives. Drospirenone is an analog of spironolactone which has antiandrogenic and anti-mineralocorticoid properties
    - Yasmin – The drospirenone component in Yasmin is equivalent to 25 mg of spironolactone
    - Yaz

- **Procedures** – (few studies, insurance typically does not cover these)
  - ○ Blue light (405–420 nm) – reacts with porphyrins produced by *P. acnes*, creating reactive oxygen species that damage the bacterial cell wall leading to bacterial death
  - ○ Red light (660 nm) – anti-inflammatory
  - ○ Photodynamic therapy – utilizes blue light reacting with a porphyrin in the sebaceous gland. Possible mechanism of PDT is destruction of sebaceous glands

Pearls and Pitfalls

- **Topical Retinoids:** Apply pea-sized amount of the medication sparingly to dry skin. To decrease side effects, apply 30 minutes after washing the area. Consider mixing with a non-comedogenic moisturizer if irritation persists.
- Expect flare of acne in first month (indication that it is working)
- Expect exfoliation of skin – *gently* massage off when washing face
- Some need to be applied at night b/c are inactivated by sunlight – generic tretinoin, atralin gel
- Need to stop topical retinoids 2 weeks prior to facial waxing
- Warn patient to hold topicals for a couple of days if skin becoming too irritated, red
  - ○ **Benzoyl peroxide**
    - Will bleach fabrics and possibly hair
    - Allergic contact dermatitis can occur
  - ○ **Oral antibiotics**
    - Tetracycline (TCN, doxycycline, minocycline) are Preg Category D and can rarely cause pseudotumor cerebri. Minocycline can cause hepatitis, DRESS syndrome

Acne Keloidalis Nuchae (AKN)

Etiology and Pathogenesis

- Injury produced by short haircuts (especially when the posterior hairline is shaved with a razor, a practice common in African-American men) and curved hair follicles (analogous to pseudofolliculitis of the beard in African Americans) may be the precipitating factors
- Other suggested etiologic possibilities – constant irritation from shirt collars, chronic low-grade bacterial infections, and an autoimmune process (AKN usually responds to systemic steroid therapy)

Clinical Presentation

- A scarring form of chronic folliculitis that manifests as follicular-based papules and pustules, which eventuates in keloid-like lesions. Does not look keloidal histologically
- Small, smooth, firm papules with occasional pustules on posterior scalp and neck
- Often coalesce to form one or several large plaques, which gradually enlarge for years
- 10x more common in African Americans than in whites

Differential Diagnosis – bacterial folliculitis, tinea capitis, sarcoid, acne, follicular occlusion triad

Medical Treatment and Management

- Bacterial culture and sensitivities if pustules present
- BID application of topical corticosteroid (class 2 or 3) with topical retinoid → seems to be more effective than class 1 or 2 topical corticosteroid alone
- Potent topical corticosteroid + long acting tetracycline such as doxycycline
- Topical clindamycin BID if pustules present; PO ABX based on culture results
- In the rare cases where large abscesses or draining sinuses are present, give patients a 7- to 10-day course of prednisone after starting appropriate systemic antibiotics
- Intralesional steroid injections (10–40 mg/mL) are another method
- Laser therapy (carbon dioxide or Nd:YAG) has been successful for some patients. Postoperative intralesional triamcinolone injections (10 mg/mL q 2–3 week) help prevent recurrence
- Cryotherapy has also proven to be successful in some cases. The area is frozen for 20 s, allowed to thaw and is then frozen again a minute later. (Will cause hypo- or depigmentation → warn patient)

Surgical Treatment

- Removing each papule with a hair transplant punch is the next therapeutic option if combined retinoic acid/corticosteroid treatment is not successful. The punch should extend deep (past the deepest level of the hair follicle) into the subcutaneous tissue, as superficial removal seems to have a much higher incidence of recurrence
  - After removal, inject the wound edges with a bolus of Kenalog 40 mg, and, then, it should be closed with 4-0 sutures. Or, use an equal amount of 2% lidocaine with epinephrine and triamcinolone acetonide at 40 mg/mL to anesthetize the surgical site
  - The ends of the nylon sutures often irritate the skin if patients sleep on their back or have a short neck. Use silk sutures to prevent this problem. Instruct patients to clean the postoperative area three times a day with alcohol or sodium chloride solution followed by the application of a topical antibiotic ointment
  - Remove the sutures in 6–14 days, and start patients on a twice-daily topical retinoid/corticosteroid regimen for 4–6 weeks
  - Kenalog (10–40 mg/mL) is also injected into the postoperative site or sites every 2–3 weeks for four sessions, starting 1 week after suture removal
- The preferred method of removal for larger linear lesions (1 cm or less in diameter) is a horizontal ellipse for excision with primary closure. The base of the excision should extend below the hair follicles. Close the postoperative site with 4–0 silk sutures
  - The postoperative site often splays to the diameter of the initial excision. Always remember when closing primarily not to close when the posterior part of the neck is flexed or patients will spend a week or more having to look upward. Under this amount of tension, the resultant scar splays and will be the same size as the amount of area removed, often creating an area of alopecia as large as the initial defect
  - For large lesions that cannot be excised and closed primarily, the area of AKN is excised to the fascia or to the deep subcutaneous tissue and left to heal secondarily
    - Complete wound healing takes 8–12 weeks. Give patients explicit verbal and written postoperative care instructions
    - If possible, show patients and postoperative caregivers a set of photographs showing the before; immediate postoperative, 1-week postoperative, and monthly postoperative healing progression; and final healing
    - Initiate a broad-spectrum antibiotic (e.g., erythromycin) on the day of surgery and continue for 10 days because sterilizing the scalp is impossible
    - Tie off or coagulate all bleeders after excision. Then, apply pressure to the postoperative site for 10 min, and check for bleeding again. If most of the oozing has stopped, apply an antibiotic ointment to minimize bacterial colonization, and place a nonadherent dressing (e.g., Telfa, vaseline gauze, adaptic) over the defect. Wrap gauze over the dressing to help secure it and absorb the exudate. Use paper tape to secure the gauze

- Pain medication may be necessary for the first 48 h
- Dressing changes BID
○ Do not give corticosteroid injections prior to complete wound closure because they prevent wound contraction

Prevention

- Do not shave occipital scalp with a razor
- Avoid tight-fitting clothes and other sources of mechanical irritation
- Instruct males who play football to make sure their helmets fit properly and do not cause irritation on the posterior part of the scalp

Actinic Keratoses

Etiology and Pathogenesis

- Prolonged exposure to the sun in susceptible individuals leads to cumulative damage to keratinocytes (especially in Fitzpatrick Types I, II, and III)
- Can progress to squamous cell carcinoma

Clinical Presentation

- Scaly patches and/or papules which are distributed on sun-exposed areas – especially the head, neck, arms, hands, chest and sometimes the shoulders and legs
  - Often red, but may be flesh-colored or brown
  - Easier to feel than to see
- May be seen as a rare, single lesion or in confluent patches
- Usual onset begins around age 40, but occasionally seen in individuals < age 30
- Almost never seen in dark-skinned individuals
- Outdoor occupation puts person at risk, as does outdoor sports
- Common on the scalps of men with androgenetic alopecia
- Usually not painful. Can come and go.
- Variants
  - **Actinic cheilitis (lips)**
  - **Hypertrophic actinic keratosis**

DDx – seborrheic keratosis, superficial SCC in situ, superficial BCC, guttate psoriasis (occasionally), discoid lupus (occasionally)

Histology – mild to moderate pleomorphism in the basal layer of the epidermis, extending into follicles. Atypical keratinocytes and parakeratosis is present

Treatment

- Hypertrophic AK's often need biopsy to rule out SCC (in situ or invasive)

Table 54 Common treatments for actinic keratoses

Generic name	Trade name	Treatment regimen	Comments
Liquid nitrogen	–	Apply to lesion with 1–2 mm border with two freeze/thaw cycles. 10–20 s thaw time Hypertrophic AK – 30–40 s thaw time	SE – pain, blistering, scar, pigment changes
5-Fluorouracil (5-FU)	**Efudex** 5% cream or soln, 2% soln, 1% cream or soln, 0.5% micronized cream (Carac)	Apply BID for 2–4 weeks (2 weeks for actinic cheilitis and 4 weeks to arms)	Avoid sun; Redness, erythema Carac tolerated better Some recommend Retin A 0.025% cream to arms BID × 2 weeks before 5-FU
	Carac 0.5% cream	Apply QD for 1–4 weeks	**Rx**: 5-FU; Mix 1 vial (500 mg) in 40 cc of 40% propylene glycol; Apply BID × 3 weeks (2 weeks for actinic cheilitis and 4 weeks to arms)
Imiquimod	Aldara 5% cream Zyclara 3.75% cream	Aldara: 2–3x per week for 16 weeks Zyclara: once daily (QHS) × 2 weeks, off × 2 weeks, once daily (QHS) × 2 weeks	Apply QHS × 8 h, Wash off in AM
Diclofenac	Solaraze 3% gel	BID for 8–12 weeks	
Jessners/TCA 35% peel			Jessner's peel – combination of salicylic acid 14%, lactic acid 14%, and resorcinol 14% in alcohol. No timing necessary. Apply the agent, wait for a light frost, and then *neutralize* with water

(continued)

Table 54   (continued)

Generic name	Trade name	Treatment regimen	Comments
Photodynamic Therapy (PDT) – *see PDT section*	5-Aminolevulinic acid (ALA), Methyl aminolevulinate (MAL)	1) ALA PDT → Apply ALA, incubate for 1–18 h later, apply blue light. Can retreat at 8 weeks. Most allow ALA to incubate for 1–2 h	**ALA** – Levulan Kerasticks available in boxes of six. The topical solution (final ALA concentration of 20%) must be prepared just prior to application by breaking the glass ampules with gentle pressure and subsequently mixing the contents by shaking the applicator
		2) MAL PDT → MAL on skin lesions for 3 h with occlusion, then exposure to 75 J/cm² of red light using the Curelight device. Repeat in 7 days	**MAL** – final conc is 16.8% (Metvixia); contains peanut and almond oils

Pearls and Pitfalls

- It can be difficult to distinguish between AK's and psoriasis on the arms of patients with psoriasis. Try to get the psoriasis under control with topical steroids and have them return to re-assess. Biopsy if unclear. These pts often do have a combination of both because many have had light treatments which can contribute to actinic damage
- Prevention – highly effective UVB/UVA sunscreens can slow the rate at which these develop
- PDT (also see section on PDT)
  - ○ After PDT, patients must avoid complete sun exposure for 48 hrs (the half-life of the medication). Failure to do so may result in a blistering phototoxic reaction
  - ○ Many pts prefer PDT over creams and cryotherapy (better to lerated). PDT, however, can be very painful if the ALA is left to incubate overnight
- Topical 5-FU can be very irritating! Consider having pts return in 2-3 weeks for assessment
- Imiquimod can be very irritating on the face and an irritant dermatitis common. Review in detail with patient and follow closely

Acute Generalized Exanthematous Pustulosis (AGEP)

Etiology and Pathogenesis

- Acute febrile drug eruption characterized by numerous, small pustules
- Over 90% of cases are drug-induced → usually due to antibiotics
  - Beta-lactams – penicillins, aminopenicillins, cephalosporins
  - Calcium-channel blockers – especially diltiazem
  - Other – antimalarials, carbamezapine, acetaminophen, terbinafine, nystatin, isoniazid, metronidazole, vancomycin, doxycycline, icodextrin during peritoneal dialysis
- Occasionally due to hypersensitivity reaction to mercury or in association with an enterovirus
- Genetic predisposition → HLA-B5, –DR11, and –DQ3

Clinical Presentation

- High fever, which generally begins on the same day as the pustular rash, or less often, a few days before or after the eruption
  - Distribution – lesions begin either on the face or in the major intertriginous areas (axillae, groin, inguinal folds). Dissemination occurs over a few hours
  - Morphology – numerous tiny, primarily non-follicular, sterile pustules which arise in large areas of erythema and edema
  - May be associated burning and/or pruritus
  - May see – Edema of the face and hands, purpura, vesicles, bullae, EM-like lesions, mucous membrane involvement
- Time between the drug administration and the skin eruption is relatively short, usually < 2 days
- Lesions last 1–2 weeks and are followed by superficial desquamation

Labs

- CBC + diff → leukocytosis, eosinophilia
- CMP → transient renal dysfunction
- Ca → hypocalcemia
- LFTs and culture of pustules → normal

DDx – acute pustular psoriasis (von Zumbusch type), skin infection

Histology

- Spongiform pustules seen in the superficial layers of the epidermis, beneath the stratum corneum
- Edema of the papillary dermis and a perivascular infiltrate of neutrophils and eosinophils usually present
- In a minority of patients, may see foci of necrotic keratinocytes or small vessel vasculitis

Treatment

- Withdraw drug
- Topical steroids
- Antipyretics

Pearls and Pitfalls

- Patients have usually been started on antibiotics by other physicians because of the fever and pustules. Stop antibiotics unless there is a definitive reason to continue them

Amyloidosis

Table 55 Forms of Amyloidosis

Types	Fibril protein	Other features
Systemic		
Primary	AL (lambda λ chain)	• Involves tongue, heart, GI tract, and skin • Petechiae, purpura, waxy skin-colored papules, alopecia, carpal tunnel syndrome, neuropathy
Secondary	AA	• Result of chronic disease: TB, leprosy, Hodgkin's, RA, Reiters, syphilis • **No skin involvement** • Amyloid in the adrenals, liver, spleen and kidney
Localized cutaneous		
Macular	Altered keratin	Rippled brown macules in interscapular region on back, nostalgia paresthetica
Lichen	Altered keratin	Brown, scaly papules on bilateral shins
Nodular	AL chains	Single or multiple nodules on extremities, genitals, trunk, or face
Hereditary		
Familial mediter-ranean fever	AA	• AR, intermittent fevers, renal amyloidosis, peritonitis, pleurisy • Defect: pyrin
Muckle wells	AA	• AD, periodic attacks of urticaria, fever, deafness, renal amyloidosis
Other		
Hemodialysis association	B2 microglobulin	
Senile	B amyloid protein	Senile or neuritic plaques, Alzheimer's disease

Angioedema

Etiology and Pathogenesis

- Most cases are idiopathic, but medications, allergens, and physical agents have been implicated
- **Drugs** → ACE inhibitors, aspirin, NSAIDs, dextran, opiates, radiocontrast agents
- **Common** → hymenoptera envenomations, food allergies (fresh berries, shellfish, fish, nuts, tomatoes, eggs, milk, chocolate, food additives, preservatives), local trauma (dental procedure, tonsillectomy), exposure to elements (sunlight, water, cold, heat), animal dander, emotional stress, postinfection or illness
- **Other** → lymphoproliferative disease (low-grade lymphoma, CLL, MGUS, systemic amyloidosis) or rheumatologic illness where immune complexes consume C1q and functionally and quantitatively lower the amounts of C1 esterase inhibitor
- Can also occur in setting of **autoimmunity** directed against the C1 esterase protein
- Inherited form – Quincke's edema

Clinical Presentation

- Angioedema involves vessels in the layers of the skin below the dermis, while urticaria is localized superficial to the dermis. This results in varying clinical presentations
- Commonly see edematous face, lips, and tongue – associated with breathing difficulties in some cases (anaphylaxis). Urticarial lesions typically present
- **Inherited (Quincke's edema) – Normal C1q levels**
  - Detected in first to second decade of life, AD
  - Serum **C1q normal** in inherited form
  - Defect in synthesis and/or function of C1 esterase inhibitor
  - **Type I: low amounts of normal C1 esterase inhibitor**
  - **Type II: Normal amounts of dysfunctional C1 esterase inhibitor**
- **Acquired – Low C1q**
  - Affects adults or elderly with no family history
  - Serum C1q decreased in this form

Labs

- Screen with C3, C4 levels → C4 low, C3 normal in angioedema
  - Best screening – **C4** (but won't tell you difference between inherited or acquired). **C2 and C4** will be decreased in both forms

- C1q level low in acquired, but normal in hereditary (see above)
- C1 inhibitor
- C1 inhibitor function

DDx – urticaria, drug-hypersensitivity reaction

Treatment

- Airway management key; patient should have EpiPen on them at all times
  - Epinephrine → No signs of circulatory compromise: 0.3–0.5 mg of 1:1000 SC
    Signs of shock: 0.3–0.5 mg of 1:10,000 IV or via ET
  - Terbutaline 2 puffs MDI q 4–6 h prn OR 0.25 mg SC OR 5 mg PO tid (β2
    agonist)
- Severe reactions – steroids, H1 and H2 blockers, and epinephrine
  - Methylprednisolone 40–125 mg IV, depending on severity of symptoms; may
    be repeated q 4–6 h
  - H2 blocker – Tagamet 300 mg IV may be repeated q 6–8 h (IM also
    available)
  - H1 blocker – Benedryl, Atarax, Claritin, Zyrtec, Xyzal, etc.
- Hereditary angioedema – more refractory to epinephrine, antihistamines,
  steroids
  - Stanozolol and danazol may be used for acute attacks (Preg Cat X)
    - Stanozolol 2 mg PO tid; reduce to maintenance dose of 2 mg/day or 2 mg
      QOD after 1–3 months
    - Danazol 200 mg PO bid/tid initially; if efficacious, taper dosage by 50%
      over following 2–3 months
- Acute – fresh frozen plasma (FFP) or C1 inhibitor

Antibodies in Connective Tissue Diseases

Helpful website: www.rdlinc.com

Table 56 Antinuclear antibody patterns

Pattern	Nuclear antigen	Clinical associations
Homogenous	Double-stranded DNA	Systemic lupus erythematosus
Diffuse	Histone Topoisomerase I	Drug reaction Systemic lupus erythematosus Systemic sclerosis (scleroderma)
Speckled	Extractable nuclear antigens (Sm, RNP) Ro-SSA/La-SSB Other	Mixed connective tissue disease Systemic lupus erythematosus Sjögren's syndrome Poly/dermatomyositis Various autoimmune diseases Infection Neoplasia
Nucleolar	RNA-associated antigens	Systemic sclerosis (scleroderma)
Peripheral	Double-stranded DNA	Systemic lupus erythematosus
Centromere	Centromere	Limited systemic sclerosis

Table 57 Autoantibodies in rheumatic disease

Type	Description	Clinical association
Anti-dsDNA	Autoantibodies to double-stranded DNA	• High specificity for SLE • Often correlated with more active, severe disease • ELISA test is very sensitive and can be positive in other diseases, normal people
Anti-histone	Five major types exist	• SLE, drug-induced SLE, other autoimmune disease • SLE patients will likely be positive for other autoantibodies as well
Anti-ENA	Sm (Smith) ⟶ RNP (ribonucleoprotein) ⟶ RNA-protein complexes ⟶	High specificity for SLE High specificity for SLE Higher prevalence in African-American and Asian patients
Anti-SSA (Ro)	Ribonucleoproteins	• SLE (especially subacute cutaneous lupus) • Neonatal lupus • Sjögren's syndrome
Anti-SSB (La)	Ribonucleoproteins	• Sjögren's syndrome • SLE • Neonatal lupus
Anti-centromere	Antibody to centromere/kinetochore region of chromosome	• Limited scleroderma • High rate of pulmonary hypertension • Primary biliary sclerosis

Table 57   (continued)

Type	Description	Clinical association
Anti-Scl 70	Antibodies to DNA topoi-somerase 1	• Diffuse scleroderma • Risk of pulmonary fibrosis
Anti-Jo-1	Antibody to histidyl tRNA synthetase	• Poly/dermatomyositis • Patients tend to have interstitial lung disease, Raynaud's phenomenon, **mechanic's hands**, arthritis • Typically resistant to treatment
Anti-SRP	Antibody to Signal Recognition Protein (SRP)	• Cardiomyopathy • Poor prognosis
Anti-PM-Scl	Antibody to nucleolar granular component	• Polymyositis/scleroderma overlap syndrome
Anti-Mi-2	Antibodies to a nucleolar antigen of unknown function	• Dermatomyositis • **Favorable prognosis**

Aphthous Stomatitis, Recurrent (RAS)

Etiology and Pathogenesis

- Unclear etiology, but appears to be multifactorial – stress, trauma, hormonal changes, drugs, infection, acidic foods, etc.
  - EBV and CMV infections hypothesized to be potential causes

Clinical Presentation and Classification

- Clinical Classifications
  - Minor aphthous ulcers (80–85% of RAS) are 1–10 mm in diameter and heal spontaneously in 7–10 days
  - Major aphthous ulcers (also called Sutton disease) constitute 10–15% of RAS. These lesions are greater than 10 mm in diameter, take 10–30 days or more to heal, and may leave scars
  - Herpetiform ulcers (5–10% of RAS) are multiple, clustered, 1- to 3-mm lesions that may coalesce into plaques. These usually heal in 7–10 days
- Predisposing factors
  - Hematinic deficiency
  - Malabsorption (Crohn's, Celiac disease, DH, pernicious anemia)
  - Cessation of smoking
  - Stress
  - Trauma
  - Endocrine in some women – RAS is clearly related to the progesterone level fall in the luteal phase of the menstrual cycle
  - Allergies to food – Food allergies occasionally underlie RAS; the prevalence of atopy is high
  - Acidic foods
  - Sodium lauryl sulfate (SLS) – This is a detergent in some oral health care products (many toothpastes) that may produce oral ulceration
  - Immune deficiencies – Ulcers similar to RAS may be seen in patients with HIV and some other immune defects
  - Drugs – especially NSAIDs, alendronate, nicorandil, methotrexate

Labs – consider checking for vitamin deficiencies, Celiac disease

DDx – iron/thiamine/folate or B12 deficiency, Celiac disease, Crohn's disease, Neumann bipolar aphthosis, Behçet's syndrome, Sweet syndrome, HIV infection, neutropenia, other immunodeficiencies, Periodic fever + aphthous stomatitis + pharyngitis + and cervical adenitis syndrome (PFAPA) in children, SCC, burn, trench mouth, lichen planus, histoplasmosis, syphilis, coxsackievirus infection, MAGIC syndrome, pemphigus vulgaris, herpesvirus 6 infection

Histology – looks like an ulceration

Treatment

- Ensure that patients brush atraumatically (e.g., with a small-headed, soft toothbrush) and avoid eating particularly hard or sharp foods (e.g., toast, potato crisps), and avoid other trauma to the oral mucosa. Avoid acidic foods
- Topical corticosteroids are mainstay of treatment
  - Hydrocortisone hemisuccinate pellets (Corlan), 2.5 mg
  - Triamcinolone dental paste, administered QID
  - Betamethasone sodium phosphate as a 0.5-mg tablet dissolved in 15 mL of water to make a mouth rinse, used QID
    - *Note*: Betamethasone, fluocinonide, fluocinolone, fluticasone, and clobetasol are more potent and effective than hydrocortisone and triamcinolone, but they carry the possibility of oral candidiasis
- Topical tetracyclines may reduce the severity of ulceration, but they do not alter the recurrence rate
  - A doxycycline capsule of 100 mg in 10 mL of water administered as a mouth rinse for 3 min
  - *Or* tetracycline 500 mg plus nicotinamide 500 mg administered four times daily may provide relief and reduce ulcer duration
  - Avoid tetracyclines in children younger than age 9 who might ingest them and develop tooth staining
- Chlorhexidine gluconate mouth rinses reduce the severity and pain of ulceration but not the frequency
- B complex vitamins can be very helpful for some patients
  - Anti-inflammatory agents can help; a spectrum of topical agents such as benzydamine and amlexanox may help. Benzydamine hydrochloride mouthwash, though no more beneficial than a placebo, can produce transient pain relief
    - Other – sodium cromoglycate lozenges, dapsone, colchicine, pentoxifylline, thalidomide (especially in Behçet's), levamisole, colchicine, azathioprine, prednisolone, azelastine, alpha 2-interferon, cyclosporin, deglycerinated licorice, 5-aminosalicylic acid (5-ASA), prostaglandin E2 (PGE2), sucralfate, diclofenac, and aspirin
    - See *lichen planus (oral)* for other treatment options – such as mouthwashes

Pearls and Pitfalls

– Acute necrotizing gingivitis (trench mouth) is a painful disorder which is on the differential of apthous ulcers
  ○ Typically affects adolescents and young adults and occurs mainly in setting of poor oral hygiene, malnutrition, and/or immunosuppression
  ○ Cause is a mix of bacterial pathogens – *Fusobacterium, Prevotella*, and spirochetes. Ulcers are covered by grayish pseudomembrane. Associated lymphadenopathy, foul breath. Send to dentist or periodontist. Chlorhexidine or saltwater rinses may be helpful. Need broad-spectrum antibiotics
– **Clotrimazole lozenges have a lot of sugar in them**. Do not use if patient has history of many dental caries

Atypical Fibroxanthoma (AFX)

Etiology and Pathogenesis

- Superficial fibrohistiocytic tumor with intermediate malignant potential because of its occasional ability to metastasize and even cause death
- Histiocytes and fibroblastic cells thought to play a role in its etiology
- Risk factors – UV radiation exposure, x-ray radiation exposure, transplant patients, elderly male, xeroderma pigmentosa

Clinical Presentation

- Usually on head/neck of elderly patient
- Presents as a pink or red, solitary, firm, asymptomatic papule or nodule. Ulceration and bleeding may develop and lesion usually < 2 cm in diameter. Tends to be larger on trunk or extremities
- May occur at unusual locations – ethmoid sinus, the eyelid, the cornea, and the ocular surface

DDx – basal cell carcinoma, squamous cell carcinoma, merkel cell carcinoma, pyogenic granuloma, melanoma, trichilemmal cysts, syringocystadenoma papilliferum, nevus sebaceous, adnexal tumors

Histology

- Poorly differentiated spindle cell malignancy with pleomorphism, hyperchromatism, atypical mitotic figures. Epidermis is thin and often ulcerated. May contain hemorrhagic areas, pseudoangiomatous areas, granular cell changes, keloidal areas, myxoid areas, osteoclast-like giant cells, prominent sclerosis, fibrosis, clear cell changes and perifollicular location. Histologic features that suggest a more aggressive tumor include – vascular invasion, invasion into the subcutaneous fat, and necrosis
- Immunohistochemical stains:
  - Vimentin + (but nonspecific stain that is also positive in spindle cell SCC, desmoplastic melanomas)
  - Alpha-1-antitrypsin and alpha-1-chymotrypsin are positive in majority of AFX cases
  - *Usually* negative for muscle markers such as desmin

Treatment

- Mohs surgery recommended – has better cure rate than wide local excision

Pearls and Pitfalls

- Patients should be examined at least every 6 months, because there is a risk of recurrence, metastasis, and the development of additional skin cancers

Reference:

Iorizzo LJ and Brown MD. Atypical Fibroxanthoma: A review of the literature. Dermatol Surg. 2011; 37: 146–57.

Axillary Granular Parakeratosis

Etiology and Pathogenesis

- Acquired keratotic dermatosis initially linked to the use of personal hygiene products including deodorants, antiperspirants, creams, and soaps that were used in excess. However, patients without known irritant also develop this
- Possible defect in processing of profilaggrin to filaggrin

Clinical Presentation

- Keratotic brown-red papules coalescing into plaques – usually in axillae, but other intertriginous areas can be involved
- Varying degrees of maceration secondary to local occlusion
- Usually seen in adult women, although an infantile form has been reported (thought to be from occlusion from diaper – under pressure points)

DDx – intertrigo, seborrheic dermatitis, candidiasis, inverse psoriasis, tinea, erythrasma, Hailey–Hailey disease, Darier disease, pemphigus vegetans, confluent and reticulated papillomatosis (CARP), acanthosis nigricans, irritant dermatitis, allergic contact dermatitis

Histology

- Stratum corneum is thickened and compacted with increased eosinophilic staining
- Parakeratosis
- Visible retention of basophilic keratohyalin granules within areas of parakeratosis

Treatment

- Many treatments reported:
  - Calcipotriene, topical steroids, cryotherapy, oral retinoids, behavioral modifications, emollients, oral antibiotics, topical keratolytics, oral antifungals, topical antifungals, triamcinolone mixed with silvadene

Pearls and Pitfalls

- Biopsy confirms the diagnosis
- Treatment may be trial and error as no standard treatment regimen has emerged as most successful

Reference:

Wallace CA, et al. Granular parakeratosis: a case report and literature review. J Cutan Pathol. 2003; 30: 332–5.

Basal Cell Carcinoma

Etiology and Pathogenesis

- Sun exposure and anatomic site appear to be important in development
- Most common gene alteration = **PTCH gene**
  - When Sonic Hedgehog (SHH) protein is present, it binds to Patched (PTCH), which then releases and activates smoothened (SMO). SMO signaling is transduced to the nucleus via Gli. When SHH is absent, PTCH binds to and inhibits SMO. Mutations in the *PTCH* gene prevent it from binding to SMO, simulating the presence of SHH. The unbound SMO and downstream Gli are constitutively activated, thereby allowing hedgehog signaling to proceed unimpeded
  - The same pathway may also be activated via mutations in the **SMO gene**, which also allows unregulated signaling of tumor growth
- Second most common gene alteration = **p53** mutation
- Mutations in **CDKN2A** (INK4A) locus which encodes p16 and p14 are detected in smaller number
- **Ras** mutation in some
- Activated **BCL2** (an antiapoptosis proto-oncogene) also is commonly found in BCCs

Clinical Presentation and Types

- Most common malignancy in humans. It typically occurs in areas of chronic sun exposure
- BCC is usually slow growing and rarely metastasizes, but it can cause clinically significant local destruction and disfigurement if neglected or inadequately treated
- Prognosis is excellent with proper therapy
- **Variants**
  - **Nodular** – most common
    - Papule or nodule, translucent or "pearly". Skin-colored or reddish, smooth surface with telangiectasias. Well-defined
  - **Pigmented** – most common in individuals with dark pigment
    - May be brown to blue-black. Smooth, glistening surface. Can mimic melanoma or blue nevus
  - **Cystic**
    - Round, oval shape with depressed/umbilicated center
  - **Superficial**
    - Pink or red, scaly, eczematous patch
  - **Micronodular** – aggressive
  - **Morpheaform and Infiltrating** – aggressive BCC subtypes; sclerotic plaques or papules
    - May appear as a scar, clinically

- Syndromes
  - Xeroderma pigmentosum
    - AR; starts with pigmentary changes and progresses to BCC, squamous cell carcinoma, and malignant melanoma. The effects are due to an inability to repair UV-induced DNA damage. Other features include corneal opacities, eventual blindness, and neurologic deficits
  - Nevoid BCC syndrome (basal cell nevus syndrome, Gorlin syndrome)
    - Multiple BCCs occur in this autosomal dominant condition, often starting at an early age. Odontogenic keratocysts, palmoplantar pitting, intracranial calcification, and rib anomalies may be seen. Various tumors, such as medulloblastomas, meningioma, fetal rhabdomyoma, and ameloblastoma can also occur
  - Bazex syndrome (Bazex–Dupre–Christol syndrome)
    - X-linked dominant condition with features of follicular atrophoderma (ice-pick marks, especially on dorsum of the hands), multiple BCCs, local anhidrosis (decreased or absent sweating), and congenital hypotrichosis
  - Rombo syndrome
    - AD, BCC and atrophoderma vermiculatum, trichoepitheliomas, hypotrichosis milia, and peripheral vasodilation with cyanosis

DDx – AKs, SCCis, fibrous papule, keratoacanthomas, nevus, sebaceous hyperplasia, SK, SCC, trichoepithelioma, merkel cell carcinoma, melanoma (pigmented lesions)

Histology – There are various histologic patterns of BCC. More aggressive tumors include the micronodular form, morpheaform/sclerosing/infiltrative form.
- Basaloid tumor cells budding from epidermis or follicles, or within the dermis, with variable atypia
- Retraction artifact (clefting) – stroma separates from tumor lobules
- Peripheral palisading of nuclei
- Mucin in stroma
- Solar elastosis
- Perineural invasion in some aggressive forms (not commonly)

Treatment

- Electrodessication & Curettage (ED&C)
  - Vigorous scraping in different directions followed by curettage; repeat three times
  - Overall cure rate is 80–90%
  - Not recommended on the face and ears – high-risk areas
  - Not a good option for – aggressive subtypes of BCC, such as morpheaform, infiltrating, micronodular, and recurrent tumors, are usually not friable and therefore unlikely to be removed by using the curette

- Surgical Excision
  - Margins: at least 4 mm to achieve 95% cure rates (even for least aggress tumors)
- Mohs surgery
  - Recommended for face, ears, and for aggressive histologic subtypes
  - With the Mohs technique, almost 100% of the tissue margins are examined, compared with standard vertical (bread-loaf) sectioning, in which less than 1% of the outer margins are examined
  - Cure rates for 1° BCC are 98–99% with Mohs excision; 94–96% for recurrent BCC
- Radiation therapy
  - For most BCCs, cure rate over 90%; if tumor recurs, tends to be more aggressive. Limit to those patients who cannot undergo surgery
- Cryotherapy – operator dependent, not for aggressive tumors
- Imiquimod 5% cream – for superficial BCCs
  - Apply 5x/week for 6 weeks
  - Frequency and duration should be tailored to patient's response
  - Cure rates 70–100%; immune stimulant – caution in transplant patients, autoimmune disorders
- 5-Fluorouracil – small, superficial BCCs
  - Apply BID for at least 6 weeks; may need 10–12 weeks
  - Penetrates only 1 mm into the skin
- Photodynamic therapy – off-label, superficial BCCs, various protocols
- Interferon alfa-2b – some success in treating small (<1 cm), nodular, and superficial BCCs. Not typically utilized
  - Intralesional injection 3x/week for 3 weeks
  - 1.5 million units per injection (total of 13.5 million U)
  - Cure rates up to 80% in the appropriate tumor
  - Immune stimulant – flu-like symptoms, not for transplant patients or those with autoimmune diseases

Pearls and Pitfalls

- BCCs rarely metastasize

Behçet's Syndrome

Etiology and Pathogenesis

- Genetic and environmental factors contribute to the development of this disease
  - HLA-B5 and HLA-B51 confer an increased risk of developing the syndrome; Patients with sacroiliitis have an increased frequency of HLA-B27
- Circulating immune complexes and neutrophils appear to be responsible for the mucocutaneous lesions. The neutrophils of Behçet's produced an increased amount of superoxides and lysosomal enzymes → tissue injury

Clinical Presentation

- Characterized by recurrent aphthous ulcers, genital ulcers, and uveitis or retinal vasculitis. Other manifestations of the disease include skin lesions, arthritis, GI lesions, CNS involvement, and vascular lesions, including aneurysms and thrombosis. Primary process = vasculitis
  - Skin – sterile pustules, oral ulcers, genital ulcers, erythema nodosum-like lesions
- Pathergy present; usual age of onset → 30–40 but childhood cases reported
- Diagnostic Criteria (Defined by International Study Group)
  - At least three episodes of oral ulceration must occur in a 12-month period
  - Must be observed by a physician or the patient
  - May be herpetiform or aphthous in nature
  - At least two of the following must occur
  - (1) recurrent, painful genital ulcers that heal with scarring
  - (2) ophthalmic lesions, including anterior or posterior uveitis, hypopyon, or retinal vasculitis
  - (3) skin lesions, including erythema nodosum, superficial thrombophlebitis, pseudofolliculitis, or papulopustular lesions (may also include atypical acne)
  - (4) pathergy, which is defined as a sterile erythematous papule larger than 2 mm in size appearing 48 h after skin pricks with a sharp, sterile needle (a dull needle may be used as a control)

Labs

- CRP, ESR, leukocyte count, complement and acute-phase reactants all may be elevated during an acute attack
- Elevations are occasionally found in IgA, immunoglobulin G (IgG), alpha-2 globulin, immunoglobulin M (IgM) levels, and immune complexes
  - (None of these findings is specific for the diagnosis of Behçet disease, but they can corroborate active disease)

- Up to 1/3 of patients with thrombosis have Factor V Leiden mutation; r/o other causes
- Viral culture/PCR – to rule out HSV

DDx – erosive lichen planus, herpes simplex infection, cicatricial pemphigoid, pemphigus vulgaris, linear IgA, Stevens-Johnson syndrome

Histology – Epidermis has ulceration or pustule formation. Diffuse dermal neutrophils, lymphocytes, and/or histiocytes sometimes with vasculitis

Treatment and Management

- Eye exam
  - Eye involvement is the leading cause of morbidity in this disease and occurs in 90% of patients
  - Posterior uveitis is most common, but can get anterior uveitis, hypopyon, secondary glaucoma, and cataracts
- Erythema nodosum – may be treated with colchicine or dapsone
- Colchicine or azathioprine can be used for systemic manifestations, such as severe ulcers or skin disease
  - Alternatives – cyclophosphamide, cyclosporine, chlorambucil, thalidomide, sulfasalazine
- Joint involvement → prednisone, local corticosteroid injections, and NSAIDs. Colchicine, sulfasalazine, IFN-alpha, levamisole, and azathioprine may be alternatives
- Tumor necrosis factor (TNF) antagonists, such as etanercept or infliximab may be effective. Thalidomide also helpful
- Oral lesions – see *Lichen Planus for treatment options*

Pearls and Pitfalls

- Patients with oral and genital ulcers are often inappropriately labeled as "Behçet's". A thorough exam of skin, oral mucosa, and nails can help sort this out. A biopsy may be helpful to rule out other diseases
- It is helpful to test for pathergy

Reference:

Yazici H, Fresko I, Yardakul S. Behçet's syndrome: disease manifestations, management and advances in treatment. Nat Clin Pract Rheumatol. 2007; 3(3): 148–55.

Bullous Lupus

Etiology and Pathogenesis

- Autoantibody-mediated blistering disease which occurs in patients with SLE

Clinical Presentation

- Rapid development of a widespread bullous eruption
  - The blistering activity does not necessarily correlate with the underlying SLE, but parallel exacerbations (often involving lupus nephritis) have been described
  - Bullous systemic lupus erythematosus occasionally represents the initial clinical manifestation of systemic lupus erythematosus
  - Mucosal lesions may be present and are painful
- The diagnosis of BSLE requires the following elements
  - Fulfillment of the American College of Rheumatology criteria for SLE
  - An acquired vesiculobullous eruption
  - Histologic evidence of a subepidermal blister and predom neutrophilic dermal infiltrate
  - DIF microscopy demonstrating IgG (with or without IgA and IgM) deposits at BMZ
  - Evidence of antibodies to type VII collagen via DIF or indirect immunofluorescence (IIF) on salt-split skin, immunoblotting, immunoprecipitation, enzyme-linked immunosorbent assay (ELISA), or immunoelectron microscopy
- Presence of immunoglobulin G (IgG) autoantibodies specific for the hemidesmosomal BP antigens BP230 (BPAg1) and BP180 (BPAg2). Autoantibodies against alpha 6 integrin and laminin-5 may occur

Labs

- Bullous lupus may occur in the setting of SLE; thus, ANA test results generally positive. Anti-dsDNA, anti-Sm, anti-Ro/SS-A, anti-La/SS-B, and anticardiolipin antibodies may also be positive
- Other laboratory abnormalities related to SLE can include ↓ complement (i.e., C3, C4, CH50), anemia, ↓ WBC, ↓ plts, proteinuria or cellular casts on urinalysis, and an ↑ ESR

DDx – Bullous pemphigoid, dermatitis herpetiformis, drug-induced bullous disorders, EB, EBA, erythema multiforme, GVHD, hydroa vacciniforme, Linear IgA dermatosis, porphyria cutanea tarda, Pseudoporphyria, Rowell syndrome (lupus that looks like TEN)

Histology

- Subepidermal blister containing many neutrophils instead of lymphocytes. Often more mucin in dermis
- **Type 1 BSLE** → DIF of salt-split perilesional skin and/or IIF microscopy following incubation of the patient's serum with salt-split normal human skin reveals immunoglobulin deposits localized to the dermal floor of the split
- **Type 2 BSLE** → Cases with negative IIF and an undetermined sublocalization of anti-BMZ antibodies (or Ab recognizing a dermal antigen other than collagen VII)
- **Type 3 BSLE** → characterized by immunoglobulin binding the epidermal roof or both the roof and the dermal floor of salt-split skin. Antigens in such patients have included bullous pemphigoid antigen 1, laminin-5, and laminin-6

Treatment

- **Dapsone** – 25–200 mg/day PO QD – usually quite effective
  - Interestingly, although type 1 BSLE and EBA both have antibodies targeting type VII collagen, EBA differs considerably in its marked resistance to treatment
  - Response usually dramatic, with cessation of new blister formation within 1–2 days and rapid healing of existing lesions
  - Low doses (**25–50 mg/day**) often effective; higher dose sometimes required
  - Rapid recurrences may occur w/withdrawal of dapsone, with prompt remission after reinstitution of therapy. However, may be able to d/c med within year
- **Prednisone** – for those who cannot tolerate dapsone (G6PD deficiency) or who are not controlled on dapsone alone
- **Methotrexate** (MTX), **azathioprine**, and **mycophenolate mofetil** represent additional therapeutic options

Pearls and Pitfalls

- Not all blistering eruptions in patients with SLE are BSLE

Bullous Pemphigoid

Etiology and Pathogenesis

- Interaction of autoantibody with bullous pemphigoid antigen (BPAG1 and BPAG2) in hemidesmosome of basal keratinocytes is followed by complement activation and attraction of neutrophils and eosinophils. Autoantibodies against α-6-integrin and laminin-5 may occur
- Certain drugs have been implicated in some cases → furosemide, ibuprofen and other NSAIDs, captopril, penicillamine, and antibiotics

Clinical Presentation

- Erythematous, papular or urticarial-type lesions that evolve into bullae
  - Bullae → large, tense, firm-topped, oval or round. Bullae rupture less easily than in pemphigus
  - Eruption may be localized or generalized
  - Distribution → axillae, medial thighs, groin, abdomen, flexural arms, lower legs (often first manifestation). Blistering on palms/soles can interfere with patients' daily activities
  - Mucous membranes → practically only in the mouth (10–35%), but less severe than pemphigus, but pain may limit oral intake
- Primarily affects elderly age 50–70
- **Variants** – generalized bullous, vesicular, vegetative, generalized erythroderma, urticarial, nodular, acral

DDx – cicatricial pemphigoid, dermatitis herpetiformis, drug-induced bullous disorders, epidermolysis bullosa, EBA, erythema multiforme, Linear IgA dermatosis, chronic bullous dermatosis of childhood, dyshidrosis, bullous lupus, pemphigus vegetans, urticaria, urticarial vasculitis, herpes gestationis

Labs and Histology

- Histopathologic analysis from the edge of a blister
- DIF studies on normal-appearing perilesional skin – usually demonstrate IgG (70–90% of patients) and complement C3 deposition (90–100% of patients) in a linear band at the dermal–epidermal junction. This pattern of immunoreactants is not specific for BP and may be seen in CP and EBA
  - BP can be differentiated from EBA and CP by incubating the patient's skin biopsy sample in 1 mol/L salt prior to performing the DIF technique. This process induces cleavage through the lamina lucida

- o DIF on salt-split skin reveals IgG on the blister roof (epidermal side of split skin) in patients with BP, while, in CP and EBA, the IgG localizes to the blister floor (dermal side of split skin)
- If the DIF result is positive, indirect immunofluorescence (IDIF) is performed using the patient's serum. The preferred substrate for IDIF is salt-split normal human skin substrate
  - o Document the presence of IgG circulating autoantibodies in the patient's serum that target the skin basement membrane component
  - o The titer of circulating antibody is not correlated with the disease course

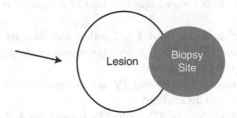

Fig. 5 Where to biopsy SKIN lesions of bullous pemphigoid for DIF

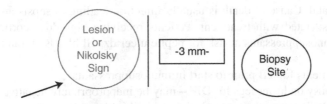

Fig. 6 Where to biopsy MOUTH lesion of bullous pemphigoid for DIF

Treatment and Management

- Lesions may flare in patients with oral disease after eating hard and crunchy foods, such as chips, raw fruits, and vegetables
- Oral lesions – see section on *Lichen planus*
- Those on steroids for longer than 1 month (or who you anticipate will be) need to be on calcium and vitamin D. Consider a bisphosphonate as well
  - o See *Corticosteroids*
- Anti-inflammatory agents
  - o PO corticosteroids – 1 mg/kg/day not to exceed 80 mg/day; taper as symptoms resolve
  - o Topical corticosteroids

- ○ Tetracyclines – 500 mg qid; may combine with niacinamide (2 g/day)
- ○ Dapsone 50–200 mg PO qd (check G6PD prior)
- • Steroid-sparing Immunosuppressants
  - ○ Azathioprine – 1 mg/kg qd/bid (empiric) or by TPMT level; increase by 0.5 mg/kg q 4 week until response, not to exceed 2.5 mg/kg/day
    - ■ TPMT < 6.3 U (low): No treatment with azathioprine
    - ■ TPMT 6.5–15 U/ml (intermediate): 1 mg/kg/day
    - ■ TPMT 15.1–26.4 U/ml (normal): 2 mg/kg/day
    - ■ TPMT > 26.4 U/ml (high): may require more aggressive dosing to see any effect
      - □ *In last scenario – still start at 2 mg/kg/day then increase the dose every 4–6 weeks by 0.5 mg/kg/day to a max of 3 mg/kg/day*
  - ○ Methotrexate
  - ○ Mycophenolate mofetil → Start 1.5–2 g/day and increase by 500 mg every month until reach benefit or 3 g/day maximum. Once stable, may decrease dose by 500 mg/day every month
  - ○ Cyclophosphamide → 50–100 mg IV qd in combination with prednisone; 2.5–3 mg/kg/day PO divided qid
  - ○ Rituximab → Initial dose of 375 mg/m^2 IV q week for 4–8 week

Pearls and Pitfalls

- – May be fatal. Cause of death is usually infection leading to sepsis and adverse events associated with treatment. Patients receiving high-dose corticosteroids and immunosuppressants at risk for peptic ulcer dz, GI bleeds, agranulocytosis, diabetes
- – Screen patients for TB prior to start immunosuppressants
- – Avoid biopsy on lower legs for DIF – may be inappropriately negative
- – Consider PCP prophylaxis when using cyclophosphamide

Calciphylaxis

Etiology and Pathogenesis

- Etiology not well-understood
  - **Risk factors** include – renal disease (94%), females (5:1), obesity, oral corticosteroids, calcium-phosphate product > 70, liver disease, serum aluminum > 25 ng/mol, ESR > 30.

  Note: Many nephrologist say that Calcium-Phos product should be ≤ 55. If greater, there is an increased risk of calcific uremic arterialopathy

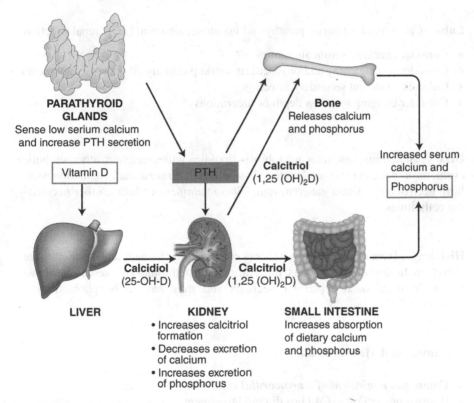

Fig. 7 Calcium-phosphorus homeostatic pathways

  - **Possible risk factors** – hyper- or hypoparathyroidism, vitamin D excess or deficiency, bone disease, bone relevant malignancy, hypercoagulable state (Protein c/s, factor V Leiden, hyperhomocysteinemia), systemic inflammatory state

Clinical Presentation

- Initially have a livedo reticularis pattern which becomes progressively more dusky red to violaceous. Bullae may form over ischemic tissue, which becomes necrotic
- Violaceous reticulated plaques develop a black, adherent crust (infarcted sites)
- Lesions gradually enlarge over weeks to month and are very painful. Ulcers may become very deep and become secondarily infected
  - Infection can remain localized or become generalized
- Distribution → most common on lower extremities, abdomen, buttocks
- Disease typically seen in patients with end-stage renal disease, often with hyperparathyroidism

Labs – Calcium, phosphorus, parathyroid hormone, albumin, LFTs, renal function

- Consider checking serum aluminum
- Consider coagulopathy and/or vasculitis workup initially (if diagnosis not clear)
- Cultures – rule out secondary infection
- Consider imaging to assess depth of ulcerations

DDx – panniculitis, vasculitis, necrobiosis lipoidica with ulceration, atheroembolic event, thrombotic event/coagulopathy, disseminated intravascular coagulation, warfarin necrosis, pyoderma gangrenosum, *Vibrio vulnificus* cellulitis, other necrotizing cellulitides

Histology – Incisional deep biopsy shows calcification of small- and medium-sized vessels in the dermis and subcutis. Intraluminal fibrin thrombi are present. Ischemia results in intralobular septal fat necrosis and may have a lymphohistiocytic infiltrate.

Treatment and Management

- *Cutaneous equivalent of a myocardial infarction*
- Primary prevention → Ca-Phos directed treatment
- After it occurs
  - Restore skin perfusion/oxygen
    - Low-dose tPA [Sewell LD, et al. Low-dose tissue plasminogen activator for calciphylaxis. Arch Derm 2004; 104]
    - Hyperbaric oxygen
    - Follow w/ chronic anticoag to prevent rethrombosis (warfarin, LMWH)

- ○ Wound care
  - ▪ Maggot larvae (middle stomach kills MRSA)
  - ▪ Antiseptic whirlpool and Antiseptic wet dressings
  - ▪ Surgical debridement
- ○ Infection control → most die of sepsis
- ○ Pain control → opiates, pain specialists very helpful
- ○ Halt further calcium deposits
  - ▪ Dialysis
  - ▪ Calcimimetic agents (cinacalcet): reduces PTH secretion
  - ▪ **Sodium thiosulfate** [Cicone JS et al. Successful treatment of calciphylaxis with intravenous sodium thiosulfate. Am J Kid Dis 2004; 43(6): 1104–8] – chelating agent – *25 grams IV QOD or tiw × 3–34 weeks*
  - ▪ Bisphosphonate
- ○ Halt further calcium deposits
  - ▪ Phosphate binding gels – give TID with meals
    - ▫ Renagel – also lowers LDL, very expensive
      - • PhosLo – don't use in patients with high calcium, because contains calcium acetate. Inexpensive
    - ▫ Fosrenol
  - ▪ Parathyroidectomy – reserved for uncontrolled hyperparathyroidism

Pearls and Pitfalls

- – Associated with very poor outcome

Reference:

Weenig RH, et al. Calciphylaxis: Natural history, risk factor analysis, and outcome. J Amer Acad Dermatol 2007; 56(4).

Cholestasis of Pregnancy

Etiology and Pathogenesis

- Exact etiology unclear, but likely due to both hormonal and mechanical factors
  - Example – Conjugated estrogens can reduce uptake of bile acids into hepatocytes

Clinical Presentation

- Patients typically present in third trimester (pregnancy typically uneventful)
- Intense generalized pruritus in invariably the presenting symptoms
  - Worse at night
  - Worst on trunk, palms, soles
- There may be no progression beyond pruritus but 50% develop dark urine, lightly colored stools or jaundice within 2–4 weeks
  - Jaundice stabilizes shortly after presentation and resolves in 1–2 weeks after delivery
- Symptoms wax and wane but usually disappear within 48 h of delivery
- Recurrence in subsequent pregnancies is between 60% and 70%. Recurrence with oral/hormonal contraceptives is routine
- **Maternal morbidity** – potential for malabsorption. If severe or prolonged, see depletion of vitamin K which can lead to bleeding abnormalities. Tendency for women to later develop cholelithiasis or gallbladder disease. It is generally accepted that there is an undefined tendency for women to have premature labor, fetal stress, and fetal death, which may be reduced by treatment

Labs

- Increased serum bile acids (cholic acid, deoxycholic acid, chenodeoxycholic acid) – confirms diagnosis in the absence of alternative explanations
  - May range from 3–100 times the normal level
- Conjugated (direct) bilirubin is increased but rarely above 2–5 mg/dl
- Serum Alk Phos, γ-glutamyltransferase (GGT), cholesterol – erratic during pregnancy
- AST typically remains within 4x normal, even in those with cholestasis of pregnancy. Higher elevations usually require an alternative explanation
- Hepatic ultrasound generally normal
- Rule out hepatitis with serologies

DDx – viral hepatitis, primary biliary cirrhosis, drug-induced hepatitis

Histology

- Liver biopsy is not indicated in uncomplicated cases but if done, shows centri-lobular cholestasis, which may be patchy or mild. Cholestasis can be severe, with bile thrombi found within dilated canaliculi. Hepatocellular necrosis and portal inflammation are not seen

Treatment

- Cholestyramine or phenobarbital useful for relatively mild elevations of bile acids but benefit is disputed
- UVB phototherapy
- Rest, low-fat diet
- Ursodeoxycholic acid (UDCA) has gained favor – 15 mg/kg/day. Its use reported to both control symptoms and decrease adverse effects to the fetus
- If cholestasis lasts beyond a few weeks, vitamin K absorption may be impaired, potentially leading to a prolonged prothrombin time → can lead to intracranial hemorrhage in baby
- Need careful monitoring by obstetrics – repeated non-stress tests and biophysical profiles. The presence of fetal distress dictates prompt delivery

Pearls and Pitfalls

- Meconium staining and premature labor occur in as many as 45%
- Evidence that maternal bile salts above 40 µmol/l are correlated with an increased incidence of fetal (but not maternal) complications
- Failure of pruritus to stop within days of delivery or the persistence of elevated LFTs following delivery suggest underlying liver disease, especially primary biliary cirrhosis

Table 58 Pregnancy dermatoses

Condition	Risk to baby	Skin involvement in baby
Cholestasis of pregnancy	Increased risk of premature labor, meconium staining, fetal distress, fetal death vitamin K deficiency	None
Pemphigoid gestationis	Increased risk of prematurity. Tendency toward small-for-gestational-age births	Lesions of pemphigoid gestationis in up to 10%
Prurigo of pregnancy	None	None
PUPPP	None	1 report

Chondrodermatitis Nodularis Helices (CNH)

Etiology and Presentation

- Common, benign, painful condition of the helix or antihelix of the ear
- Exact cause unknown, but believe to be from prolonged and excessive pressure
  - Ear has relatively little subcutaneous tissue for insulation and padding, and only small dermal blood vessels supply the epidermis, dermis, perichondrium, and cartilage
  - Dermal inflammation, edema, and necrosis from trauma, cold, actinic damage, or pressure probably initiate the disease. Focal pressure on the stiff cartilage most likely produces damage to the cartilage and overlying skin in most cases
- Right ear more commonly involved; more common in men (elderly)

Clinical Presentation

- Firm, tender nodule which is round to oval with a raised, rolled edge and central ulcer or crust Size may range from 3 to 20 mm. Removal of the crust often reveals a small channel
- Color is similar to surrounding skin, although a thin rim of erythema may exist
- The right ear > left, and bilateral distribution occasionally occurs
- Lesions develop on the most prominent projection of the ear. The most common location is the apex of the helix. Distribution on antihelix is more common in women

DDx – gout tophus, amyloid deposit, SCC, elastosis nodularis

Histology

- Epidermis usually ulcerated
- At the periphery, intact epidermis is edematous and hyperplastic
- Dermis below the ulceration demonstrates homogeneous acellular collagen degeneration with fibrin deposition
- Granulation tissue flanks the zone of necrosis on both sides
- Focus of cartilaginous degeneration may be present, although it is usually minimal

Treatment

- Primary goal – relieve or eliminate pressure at the site of the lesion
  - Often difficult because of the patient's preference to sleep on the side of the lesion
  - Pressure-relieving prosthesis can be fashioned by cutting a hole from the center of a bath sponge – device can then be held in place with a headband
  - **CNH Pillow** – special prefabricated pillow is available that helps relieve pressure on the ear. For more information on this pillow: www.cnhpillow.com; **$60**
- Topical and IL steroids
- Cryotherapy – can make it worse in some cases
- Collagen injections may bring relief by providing cushioning between skin and cartilage
- Surgical removal – wedge excision, curettage, electrocauterization, carbon dioxide laser ablation, and excision of the involved skin and cartilage (must remove all damaged cartilage)

Pearls and Pitfalls

- CNH rare in children but can be associated with dermatomyositis

Cicatricial Pemphigoid (CP)

Etiology and Pathogenesis

- Autoantibodies to laminin 5 (laminin 332)
- Predominantly Ocular CP→ β4 subunit of α6β4 integrin
- IgG antibodies to same target antigens as for BP, especially BP180 (distal C-terminal)
  - BP180 = BPAG2 = Collagen XVII
- Heterogeneous group with various antibodies

Clinical Presentation

- Autoimmune blistering diseases that predominately affects the mucous membranes, including the conjunctiva, and occasionally the skin
- Scarring of the mucous membranes is common ("cicatricial"), which can lead to decreased vision, blindness, and supraglottic stenosis with hoarseness or airway obstruction
- Most patients with CP are elderly, with a mean age of 62–66 years
- **Ocular**
  - May present with pain or sensation of grittiness in the eye and conjunctivitis
  - Erosions may be seen on the conjunctival surface
  - Early changes include keratinization of conjunctiva and shortening of fornices
  - Later, patients develop entropion with subsequent trichiasis
  - Often present after ocular surgery, especially for cataracts, with severe inflammation of the eye or eyes and scar formation
  - Progressive scarring – symblepharon (fibrous tracts that tether bulbar and conjunctival epithelium), synechiae (adhesion of the iris to the cornea or the lens), and ankyloblepharon (a fixed globe)
  - End result of ocular involvement is opacification and blindness
  - Lacrimal gland and duct involvement leads to decreased tear production
    - Diminished tear formation leads to ocular dryness and further trauma
- **Mouth**
  - Gingivae are most commonly involved, followed by the palate and the buccal mucosa; however, any mucosal site in the mouth may blister
  - Involvement of the oropharynx may present with hoarseness or dysphagia
    - Progressive scarring disease may lead to esophageal stenosis requiring dilatation procedures
    - Supraglottic involvement may lead to airway compromise requiring tracheostomy
- **Nose** – epistaxis, bleeding after blowing the nose, nasal crusting, discomfort
- **Perianal** and **genital areas** may be involved

- **Skin lesions**
  - In approx 1/3 of patients, manifesting as tense vesicles/bullae – may be hemorrhagic
  - Blisters may heal with scarring or milia
  - Scalp involvement may lead to alopecia
  - **Brunsting–Perry variant of localized CP** – cutaneous CP involving the head and the neck without mucosal involvement
    - Elderly, male patients presenting with a chronic, recurrent vesiculobullous eruption on the head and the neck that heals with atrophic scarring
    - Patients with this disorder have histologic immunofluorescent and immunoelectron microscopic features similar to other patients with CP

DDx – BP, drug-induced bullous disorders, desquamative gingivitis, EB, EBA, erythema multiforme, Linear IgA bullous dermatosis, pemphigus vulgaris, paraneoplastic pemphigus

Histology and Labs

- Criteria for the diagnosis of CP include an appropriate clinical presentation, histology demonstrating a subepidermal blistering process
- **Histology**
  - Biopsy of the edge of an early blister
  - Typically reveals a noninflammatory, subepidermal blister. When present, the inflammatory infiltrate localizes to the dermal–epidermal junction and the perivascular areas
    - This histologic feature can also be seen in other autoimmune subepidermal blistering diseases, including cell-poor BP, EBA, and linear IgA bullous dermatosis
    - The histologic features of porphyria cutanea tarda and variegate porphyria may also resemble CP

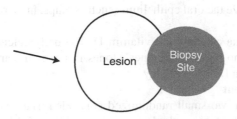

Fig. 8 Where to biopsy SKIN lesions of cicatricial pemphigoid for DIF

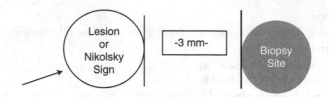

Fig. 9 Where to biopsy MOUTH lesions of cicatricial pemphigoid for DIF

DIF (perilesional skin) – continuous deposits of any one or the combination of the following along the epithelial basement membrane zone: IgG, IgA, and/or C3

- DIF study can be used to categorize the process as an autoimmune blistering disease, but it cannot be used to discriminate between CP, BP, or EBA
    - **IDIF** study of patients' sera depicts circulating antibasement membrane zone specific for IgG in 20% of patients, and, when present, it usually has a low titer (1:10–1:20)
    - **Salt-split skin** –
        - Healthy human skin preincubated in 1 mol/L sodium chloride is used as a substrate, autoantibodies in patients with CP associated with reactivity to *BPAG2* bind to the epidermal roof (similar to BP)
        - Patients with autoantibodies associated with <u>epiligrin</u> have circulating autoantibodies that bind to the blister floor, similar to that in patients with EBA

Treatment

- Goals – suppress extensive blister formation, promote healing, and prevent scarring
- Increased risk of malignancies has been documented in patients with antiepiligrin CP, especially in the first year of disease; hence, appropriate screening is warranted
- **Diet**
    - Patients with oral disease may benefit from avoiding foods high in acid (such as tomatoes and orange juice), and foods with hard surfaces that may mechanically traumatize the oral epithelium (such as chips, nuts, raw vegetables, and uncut fruit)
    - Ensure adequate calcium and vitamin D. The daily calcium requirement in patients with no history of kidney stones is 1.5 g/day, and daily minimum dose of vitamin D is 800 IU/day
- **Medical Treatment**
    - Evidence from two small randomized controlled trials indicates that ocular CP responds best to cyclophosphamide, while mild-to-moderate disease seems effectively suppressed by treatment with dapsone

- ○ **Cyclophosphamide** – 1–5 mg/kg/day IV; alternatively 2.5–3 mg/kg/day PO divided qid
  - ▪ Side Effects
    - □ Hematologic, regularly examine urine for RBCs, which may precede hemorrhagic cystitis
      - • Adverse effects – oligospermia or azoospermia, cardiomyopathy, infectious disease, interstitial pneumonia, increase risk of malignancy, possibility of increased toxicity in adrenalectomized patients
- ○ **Dapsone** – 50 mg PO qd initial; increase to 100 mg/day as tolerated; check G6PD prior to therapy
- ○ **Mycophenolate mofetil** – 1–1.5 g PO bid
- ○ **Azathioprine** – 1 mg/kg/day PO for 6–8 week; increase by 0.5 mg/kg q 4 week until response or dose reaches 2.5 mg/kg/day; check TPMT prior to therapy
- ○ **Cyclosporine** – 3–9 mg/kg/day PO QD
- ○ **High-dose IVig** has been used successfully in the treatment of CP in patients who were refractory to other therapies
- • **Surgical**
  - ○ Surgery to ablate ingrown eyelashes prevents further ocular damage
  - ○ Procedures to release entropion have been successful
  - ○ Patients with esophageal obstruction may require dilatation procedures
  - ○ Care should be taken to control the inflammatory component of the disease before and immediately after surgery because patients with CP frequently experience flare-ups after surgery
  - ○ Patients with upper airway disease may develop respiratory compromise requiring tracheostomy

Pearls and Pitfalls

- – With surgical management, be very careful! Can result in flares of the disease and patient should be clearly aware of this. Benefits of surgery should outweigh the risks
- – Patients with autoantibodies to laminin 5 (also known as antiepiligrin CP) have an increased risk for cancer

Condyloma Accuminata

Etiology and Pathogenesis

- Caused by human papillomavirus (HPV) usually types 6, 11

Table 59 Disease association of human papillomavirus (HPV) genotypes

Characteristic HPV lesion	Associated HPV type
Palmoplantar warts	1
Common warts	2 (less common – 4, 26, 27, 65, 78)
Flat warts	3, 10 (27, 28, 49)
Butcher's warts	7
Condylomata acuminata	6, 11 (70, 83)
Bowenoid papulomatosis	16
Cervical intraepithelial neoplasia and cancers, anogenital cancers	16 and 18 most common
Oral papillomas	6, 11
Oral focal epithelial hyperplasia (Heck's)	13, 32
Recurrent laryngeal papillomatosis	6, 11
Erythroplasia of Queyrat	16
Verrucous carcinoma	16, 6, 11
Epidermodysplasia verruciformis (EV)	5, 8
Myrmecia wart	63
Digital SCC	33, 51, 73, 16

Clinical Presentation and Types

- Warty growths in the genital area which vary in size
- May present as skin-colored, brown, pink or whitish (especially if macerated from moist location)
- May be sessile, pedunculated, large confluent plaques
- Distribution – genitals, perianal, inguinal folds. May extend into vagina, cervix in women. May extend into anal canal

DDx

- **Bowenoid papulosis** – multiple red-brown warty papules or confluent plaques on external genitalia. Resemble genital warts, but histologically are a high-grade squamous intraepithelial lesion (HSIL) or squamous cell carcinoma in situ. HPV-16
- **Erythroplasia of Queyrat** – presents as well-demarcated, velvety, erythematous plaque on glabrious skin of penis and vulva. Histologically is SCC in situ. Usually from HPV-16

- **Buschke–Löwenstein tumor** – Large tumor that is made up of a group of "semi-malignant" verrucous carcinomas that are locally invasive and destructive but rarely metastasize. HPV 6, 11. Histology resembles condyloma accuminata but may see focal malignant transformation
- **Focal epithelial hyperplasia (Heck's disease)** – multiple circumscribed papules found on gingival, buccal or labial mucosa and resemble flat warts or condylomata. HPV-13 or -32. Seen in Native Americans, Eskimos, Greenlander, South American Indians, South African communities
- **Oral florid papillomatosis (Ackerman tumor)** – multiple, confluent, verrucous lesions which coalesce. Usually in oral cavity or nasal sinuses. HPV-6 or -11. Thought to be promoted by smoking, irradiation, and chronic inflammation. May progress to verrucous carcinoma
- **Verrucous carcinoma**
- **Epidermodysplasia verruciformis (EDV)** – seen in either patients with familial cellular immunity defect or in HIV patients. Usually from HPV-5. Histologically, see bubbly bluish cytoplasm in keratinocytes, sometimes cytologic atypia. Transformation to SCC seen in familial EDV, but not typically in HIV patients. Clinically may resemble PR, verruca plana
- **Condyloma lata** – from syphilis
- **Pearly penile papules** – benign, common finding. Normal
- **Perianal pyramidal protrusion** – seen in infants and babies. Is a flesh-colored to pink soft tissue swelling that appears in the medial raphe of girls. Can be mistaken for condyloma accuminata. Benign finding and is often associated with constipation. May be a peculiar form of lichen striatus

Histology

- Epidermal hyperplasia, parakeratosis, koilocytosis, and papillomatosis → not all of these are found in all condyloma. Upper portions of the epithelia of mucosal surfaces normally have some degree of cytoplasmic vacuolization

Labs

- Consider ruling out syphilis with serologic tests
- Detection of subclinical genital HPV requires soaking with 5% acetic acid for 3–5 min. Leads to whitening of lesions. Used in gynecology. However – can get whitening with infectious and inflammatory conditions, so can be misleading

Treatment

- Important to treat as these are contagious to others and can transform into malignancy (SCC, verrucous carcinoma, vulvar carcinoma, cervical carcinoma)

- Infection control – most studies suggest that condom use will not prevent HPV infection. Limiting the number of sexual partners is mainstay of reducing transmission
- Local destructive therapy
  - **Cryotherapy** – most commonly used, although TCA may be more effective. Two freeze-thaw cycles recommended
  - **Trichloroacetic acid (TCA)** – 70–90%. Can be used during pregnancy. Apply carefully as can cause scarring
  - **Electrosurgery**
  - **Curettage**
  - **Scalpel or scissor removal**
  - **CO2 laser vaporization**
- Topical cytotoxic therapy
  - **Podophyllin** – microtubule perturbing agent. Applied in office. Contraindicated in pregnancy (teratogenicity reported). Falling out of favor because potential for systemic toxicity if used in large volumes
  - **Podophyllotoxin** – identified as the most active constituent of podophyllin. Can be prescribed so patient can apply at home. Apply 0.5% soln or 0.15% cream BID for 3 days each week
- Topical immunomodulators
  - **Imiquimod 3.75% or 5%** – interacts with TLR 7 and 8. Use 3x/week QHS. May increase frequency as tolerated

Pearls and Pitfalls

- Protective face mask should be worn if using cautery or laser to treat condyloma. Risk of inhalation of viral particles which could lead to lesions on vocal cords/ larynx
  - **Recurrent respiratory papillomatosis** is a rare disease of benign exophytic laryngeal papillomas caused by HPV-6 and -11. Triad of hoarseness, stridor, and respiratory distress which is often misdiagnosed as asthma, croup, vocal cord nodules. Malignant transformation may occur
- Mitotic figures can be seen histologically if recent treatment with podophyllotoxin (which is a microtubule perturbing agent and can thus cause abberant mitoses)
- Have a low threshold to biopsy periungual warts in HIV patients, as recent reports show that digital SCC can mimic benign conditions. These patients often have condyloma or history of condyloma. These lesions can often recur after therapy

– HPV vaccines not helpful in treating condyloma but can help in prevention. Encourage vaccination in young patients. Vaccine given (0.5 mL IM each) in a series @ 0, 2, 6 months. Stay with same brand during series. Cost is approximately $360 for series
  ○ Gardasil→HPV 6, 11, 16, 18
    ▪ Women ages 9–26
    ▪ Men ages 9–26
  ○ Cervarix→HPV 6, 11, 16, 18
    ▪ Women ages 10–25
– Condyloma accuminata in children
  ○ Should prompt consideration of possibility of sexual abuse. It should be remembered, however, that anogenital warts occur in large numbers of children as a result of innocent or vertical transmission. Take thorough history – age of onset, maternal history (known condyloma, abnormal pap smears, cervical biopsies), social environment, caregivers, etc. Much debate over approach and avoid reflexive reporting as this may cause unnecessary emotional devastation for the innocent. Refer, however, if any ambiguity or red flags. Consider nonsexual transmission if …
    ▪ Child < age 3
    ▪ If lesions developed within first year of life
    ▪ If patient has other nongenital warts
    ▪ If warts present in close contacts (especially genital warts)

Confluent and Reticulated Papillomatosis (CARP) of Gougerot and Carteaud

Etiology and Pathogenesis

- Unknown etiology. Many theories – insulin resistance, abnormal keratinization, abnormal host response to *Pityrosporum orbiculare (Malassezzia furfur)* or to a bacteria (Dietzia spp), genetic predisposition
- Reported worldwide and in all racial groups

Clinical Presentation

- Hyperkeratotic and verrucous papules coalescing into plaques in the center and reticulated at the peripheral border. Typically hyperpigmented
- Involves – intermammary region (most common), epigastric area, upper back. Less commonly involves neck, face, shoulders
- Seen primarily in adolescents and young adults
- May be more common in darker-skinned individuals, but new reports argue against this

Labs – Consider bacterial and fungal cultures. Rarely associated with hyperinsulinemia, obesity, and acanthosis nigricans. Consider checking fasting glucose if this is a concern.

DDx – acanthosis nigricans, tinea versicolor, seborrheic dermatitis, macular amyloidosis, prurigo pigmentosa, erythema dyschromican perstans, pigmented allergic contact dermatitis, epidermal nevus syndrome, Darier's disease, mycosis fungoides (if cigarette-paper appearance present), axillary granular parakeratosis, pityriasis rubra pilaris, syringomas (can rarely have reticulated appearance)

Histology

- No definitive histology. Looks like less pronounced acanthosis nigricans. Occasionally see decreased or absent granular layer. Mild lymphocytic infiltrate.
- Biopsy can help rule out other conditions

Treatment

- Oral minocycline 50–100 mg BID – can rarely cause drug-induced lupus, drug-hypersensitivity syndrome
- Oral azithromycin 250–500 mg 3x/week – more benign adverse effect profile compared to minocycline and is pregnancy category B
- Others – fusidic acid 1,000 mg QD, clarithromycin 500 mg QD, erythromycin 1,000 mg daily, tetracycline 500 mg BID, cefdinir 300 mg BID
- Isotretinoin, acitretin – effective, but disfavored for treatment because minocycline is better tolerated and very effective
- Mixed reports of topical treatments – rubbing alcohol, selenium sulfide, ketoconazole cream, tretinoin, tazarotene, calcipotriene, topical urea

Pearls and Pitfalls

- Minocycline in conjunction with a topical lactic acid-containing emollient is often very useful
- Usually no post-inflammatory pigment alteration with resolution (unlike tinea versicolor)
- Underdiagnosed, can relapse when treatment is discontinued

Cryoglobulinemia

Etiology and Pathogenesis

- Cryoglobulins are single or mixed immunoglobulins that undergo reversible precipitation at low temperatures. May be caused by ...
- **Infection**
  - Viral – Hep A, B, C; HIV; EBV, CMV; adenovirus
  - Fungal – Coccidioidomycosis
  - Bacterial – Endocarditis, strept. infections, syphilis, Lyme dz, leprosy, Q fever
  - Parasitic – Malaria, toxoplasmosis, others
- **Autoimmune**
  - SLE, rheumatoid arthritis, Sjögren syndrome
  - Vasculitis – Polyarteritis nodosa (especially, hepatitis B–associated), Henoch–Schönlein purpura
- **Lymphoproliferative**
  - Waldenström macroglobulinemia, multiple myeloma, lymphoma, leukemia (e.g., chronic lymphocytic leukemia, hairy cell leukemia)
- **Renal disease** – Proliferative glomerulonephritis
- **Liver disease**
  - Hepatitis A, B, and C (30–98% of patients with HCV infection have cryoglobulins, especially type II); cirrhosis
- **Post vaccination** – pneumococcal vaccine
- Disease associations variable based on type of cryoglobulinemia
  - Type I is observed in lymphoproliferative
  - Types II and III are observed in chronic inflammatory diseases such as chronic liver disease, infections (chronic HCV infection), and coexistent connective-tissue diseases (SLE, Sjögren syndrome). Mixed cryoglobulinemia is rarely associated with lymphoproliferative disorders

Clinical Presentation and Types– classified via Brouet classification

- **Type I cryoglobulinemia**, or simple cryoglobulinemia–
  - Result of a monoclonal immunoglobulin, usually IgM, or, less frequently, IgG, IgA, or light chains
  - This disorder is typically related to an underlying lymphoproliferative disease and, as such, may be clinically indistinguishable from Waldenström macroglobulinemia, multiple myeloma, or chronic lymphocytic leukemia.
  - May result in hyperviscosity due to high levels of circulating monoclonal cryoglobulin, leading to physical obstruction of vessels. Concentrations may reach up to 8 g/L
    - Hyperviscosity may manifest as acrocyanosis, retinal hemorrhage, severe Raynaud's phenomenon with digital ulceration, livedo reticularis, purpura, arterial thrombosis, etc.

- **Types II and III cryoglobulinemia** (mixed cryoglobulinemia)
  - ○ Contain rheumatoid factors (RFs), which are usually IgM and, rarely, IgG or IgA
  - ○ These RFs form complexes with the fragment, crystallizable (Fc) portion of polyclonal IgG
  - ○ The actual RF may be monoclonal (in type II cryoglobulinemia) or polyclonal (in type III cryoglobulinemia) immunoglobulin
  - ○ Types II and III cryoglobulinemia represent 80% of all cryoglobulins
  - ○ Associated with chronic inflammatory states such as systemic lupus erythematosus (SLE), Sjögren syndrome, and viral infections (particularly HCV)
  - ○ B-cell clonal expansion, particularly RF-secreting cells, is a distinctive feature in many of these disease states
  - ○ The resultant aggregates and immune complexes are thought to outstrip reticuloendothelial-clearing activity. Tissue damage results from immune complex deposition and complement activation
  - ○ In HCV-related disease, HCV-related proteins are thought to play a direct role in pathogenesis and are present in damaged skin, blood vessels, and kidneys
  - ○ Meltzer triad – purpura, arthralgia, and weakness (25–30%) of patients
  - ○ Specific clinical manifestations to Types II and III –
  - ○ Joint involvement (usually, arthralgias in the proximal interphalangeal [PIP] joints, metacarpophalangeal [MCP] joints, knees, and ankles), fatigue, myalgias, renal immune-complex disease, cutaneous vasculitis, and peripheral neuropathy

Table 60 Classification of cryoglobulins

Subtype	Molecular composition	Associations	Pathophysiology	Clinical
I	Monoclonal IgM or IgG	Plasma cell dyscrasias, lymphoproliferative disorders	Vascular occlusion	Raynaud's phenomenon, retiform purpura, gangrene, acrocyanosis
II	Monoclonal IgM* (>IgG*) against polyclonal IgG	HCV, HIV, autoimmune connective tissue diseases, lymphoproliferative disorders	Vasculitis	Palpable purpura, arthralgias, peripheral neuropathy, glomerulonephritis
III	Polyclonal IgM* against IgG			

*Typically have rheumatoid factor activity (i.e., are directed against the Fc portion of IgG)
Reference: Used with permission from Elsevier. Chung L, Kea B and Fiorentino DF. Cutaneous asculitis. In: Bolognia JL, Jorizzo JL, Rapini RP (eds). Dermatology, 2nd edn. London: Mosby, 2009: 357

- **Clinical Signs and Symptoms of Cryoglobulinemia** (Fever can occur)
  - ○ **Cutaneous and Mucosal**
    - ▪ Red-purple macules and papules (90–95%), ulcerations (10–25%)
    - ▪ Lesions in nondependent areas are more common in type I cryoglobuline-mia (head and mucosa), as are livedo reticularis, Raynaud's phenomenon, and ulcerations
    - ▪ Nail fold capillary abnormalities are common and include dilatation, altered orientation, capillary shortening, and neoangiogenesis
    - ▪ Acrocyanosis, cold urticaria, Sicca symptoms may occur
  - ○ **Musculoskeletal**
    - ▪ Arthralgias and myalgias are rare in type I cryoglobulinemia; common in II, III
    - ▪ Arthralgias common in PIP, MCP joints of hands, knees, ankles
  - ○ **Renal**
    - ▪ Renal disease may occur secondary to thrombosis (type I cryoglobuline-mia) or immune complex deposition (types II and III)
    - ▪ Membranoproliferative glomerulonephritis – seen in mixed cryoglobulinemia
    - ▪ Isolated proteinuria and hematuria more common than nephritic synd, nephrotic synd, or ARF
  - ○ **Pulmonary** – infiltrates may be present
  - ○ **Neuropathy**
    - ▪ Neuropathy is common in types II and III disease (as determined with electromyographic and nerve conduction studies), affecting 70–80% of patients
    - ▪ Sensory fibers more commonly affected than motor fibers
  - ○ **GI** – abdominal pain if GI vessels involved; splenomegaly may occur

Labs

- Cryoglobulins
  - ○ Type I tends to precipitate within first 24 h (at concentrations >5 mg/mL)
  - ○ Type III cryoglobulins may require 7 days to precipitate small sample (<1 mg/mL)
- UA, CBC+diff, LFTs, electrolytes, ANA, ESR, RF (and consider anti-CCP)
- CH50, C3, C4 – may have low complement, especially C4
- SPEP/UPEP and/or serum and urine IFE
- Measure serum viscosity if symptoms warrant
- Hepatitis testing – especially HCV, but also A, B

Histology – Depends on presentation – may be vasculitis or thrombotic event

Treatment

- **NSAIDs** (600–800 mg PO tid/qid) – for arthralgias, myalgias
- Immunosuppressive medications are indicated upon evidence of organ involvement such as vasculitis, renal disease, progressive neurologic findings, or disabling skin manifestations
  - ○ **Prednisone** – 1 mg/kg/day PO in divided doses; up to 120 mg/day has been reported
  - ○ **Cyclophosphamide** – 1–5 mg/kg/day PO QD
  - ○ **Azathioprine** – 1 mg/kg/day initial; then 2–3 mg/kg/day PO single or divided dose
  - ○ **Chlorambucil** – 0.1–0.2 mg/kg/day PO
- Plasmapheresis
  - ○ Indicated for severe or life-threatening complications related to in vivo cryoprecipitation or serum hyperviscosity. Concomitant use of high-dose corticosteroids and cytotoxic agents is recommended for reduction of immunoglobulin production
  - ○ Some authors recommend using concomitant cytotoxic medications or corticosteroids to reduce a rebound phenomenon that may develop after plasmapheresis
- GI evaluation – for treatment of hepatitis C
- Rituximab
  - ○ Some evidence for controlling dz manifestations such as vasculitis, peripheral neuropathy, arthralgias, low-grade B-cell lymphomas, renal disease, and fever
  - ○ NIH has trial looking at rituximab in treating mixed cryoglobulinemias
  - ○ 60–75 mg/m^2 IV as a single dose; repeat q 21 days
  - ○ Alternatively, 20–30 mg/m^2/day for 2–3 days; repeat in 4 week

Pearls and Pitfalls

- Tests for cryoglobulins can be falsely negative and need to be checked during clinical flares on more than one occasion. Blood sample needs to be kept around 37 °C, especially for first 15 min while the clot forms

Cutaneous T-Cell Lymphoma (CTCL)

Table 61 Classification of CTCL by WHO and the European Organization for Research and Treatment of Cancer (EORTC)

Indolent clinical behavior
• Mycosis Fungoides
o   Variants of mycosis fungoides (MF)
■ Pagetoid reticulosis (localized disease)
■ Follicular, syringotropic, granulomatous variant
o   Subtype of MF – Granulomatous slack skin (GSS) syndrome
• CD30⁺ T-cell lymphoproliferative disorders of the skin
o   Lymphomatoid papulosis
o   Primary cutaneous anaplastic large-cell lymphoma
• Subcutaneous panniculitis-like T-cell lymphoma
• Primary cutaneous CD4+ small or medium pleomorphic T-cell lymphoma
Aggressive clinical behavior
• Sézary syndrome
• Primary cutaneous natural-killer/T-cell lymphoma, nasal-type
• Primary cutaneous aggressive CD8+ T-cell lymphoma (provisional)
• Primary cutaneous gamma/delta (γ/δ) T-cell lymphoma (provisional)
• Primary cutaneous peripheral T-cell lymphoma (PTL), unspecified

Table 62 Algorithm for diagnosis of early mycosis fungoides

Clinical Criteria → Scoring: Two points for basic criteria and two additional criteria
One point for basic criteria and one additional criteria
Basic
■ Persistent and/or progressive patches or thin plaques
Additional
■ Non-sun exposed location
■ Variation in size or shape
■ Poikiloderma
Histopathological Criteria → Scoring: Two points for basic criteria and two additional criteria
One point for basic criteria and one additional criteria
Basic
■ Superficial lymphoid infiltrate
Additional
■ Epidermotropism without spongiosis
■ Lymphoid atypia – cells with enlarged hyperchromatic nuclei and irregular or cerebri-form nuclear contours
Molecular Biological Criteria → Scoring: One point for clonality
Clonal TCR gene rearrangement
Immunopathological Criteria → Scoring: One point for one or more criteria
< 50% CD2+, CD3+ and/or CD5+ T cells
< 10% CD7+ T cells
Epidermal or dermal discordance of CD2, CD3, CD5, or CD7 (*T-cell antigen deficiency confined to the epidermis*)

Table 63 TNMB staging system for mycosis fungoides and sézary syndrome

Tumor Stage	Clinical Signs
T1	Limited patches, papules, and/or plaques† covering < 10% of the skin surface
	May further stratify into T1a (patch only) vs. T1b (plaque ± patch)
T2	Patches, papules, or plaques covering ≥ 10% of the skin surface
	May further stratify into T2a (patch only) vs. T2b (plaque ± patch)
T3	One or more tumors (≥ 1-cm diameter)
T4	Confluence of erythema covering ≥ 80% BSA
Nodal Stage	
No	No clinically abnormal peripheral lymph nodes; biopsy not required
N1	Clinically abnormal peripheral lymph nodes; histopathology Dutch grade 1
N1a	(dermatopathic lymphadenopathy) or NCI LN_{0-2}
N1b	Clone negative#
	Clone positive#
N2	Clinically abnormal peripheral lymph nodes; histopathology Dutch grade 2 [DL;
N2a	early involvement by MF (presence of cerebriform nuclei > 7.5 µm)] or NCI LN_3
N2b	Clone negative#
	Clone positive#
N3	Clinically abnormal peripheral lymph nodes; histopathology Dutch grades 3 (partial effacement of LN architecture; many atypical cerebriform mononuclear cells) or grade 4 (complete effacement) or NCI LN_4; clone positive or negative
Nx	Clinically abnormal peripheral lymph nodes; no histologic confirmation
Visceral Organs (M)	
M0	No visceral organ involvement
M1	Visceral involvement with pathological confirmation; organ should be specified
Peripheral Blood	
B0	Absence of significant blood involvement: ≤ 5% of peripheral blood lympho-
B0a	cytes are atypical (Sézary) cells
B0b	Clone negative#
	Clone positive#
B1	Low blood tumor burden: > 5% of peripheral blood lymphocytes are atypical
B1a	(Sézary) cells but does not meet the criteria of B2
B1b	Clone negative#
	Clone positive#
B2	High blood tumor burden: ≥ 1,000/µL Sézary cells with positive clone#

ISCL/EORTC revision to the staging of mycosis fungoides and Sézary syndrome

	T	N	M	B
IA	1	0	0	0, 1
IB	2	0	0	0, 1
II	1, 2	1, 2	0	0, 1
IIB	3	0–2	0	0, 1
III	4	0–2	0	0, 1
IIIA	4	0–2	0	0
IIIB	4	0–2	0	1
IVA_1	1–4	0-2	0	2
IVA_2	1–4	3	0	0–2
IVB	1–4	0–3	1	0–2

- Recommended evaluation and initial staging of patient with MF/CTCL
  - **Complete skin exam including**...
    - Determination of type(s) of skin lesions
      - If only patch/plaque disease or erythroderma, then estimate percentage of body surface area involved and note any ulceration of lesions
      - If tumors are present, determine total number of lesions, aggregate volume, largest size lesion, and regions of the body involved
    - Identification of any palpable lymph node, especially those ≥ 1.5 cm in largest diameter or firm, irregular, clustered, or fixed
    - Identification of any organomegaly
  - **Skin biopsy**
    - Most indurated area if only one biopsy
    - Immunophenotyping to include at least the following markers: CD2, CD3, CD4, CD5, CD7, CD8, and a B-cell marker such as CD20. CD30 may also be indicated in cases where lymphomatoid papulosis, anaplastic lymphoma, or large-cell transformation is considered
    - Evaluation for clonality of TCR gene rearrangement
  - **Blood tests**
    - CBC with manual differential, LFTs, LDH, comprehensive chemistries
    - TCR gene rearrangement and relatedness to any clone in skin
    - Analysis for abnormal lymphocytes by either Sézary cell count with determination of absolute number of Sézary cells and/or flow cytometry (including $CD4^+/CD7^-$ or $CD4^+/CD26^-$)
  - **Radiologic tests**
    - In patients with T1N0B0 stage disease who are otherwise healthy and without complaints directed to a specific organ system, and in selected patients with T2N0B0 disease with limited skin involvement, radiologic studies may be limited to a CXR or ultrasound of peripheral nodal groups to corroborate absence of adenopathy
    - In all patients with other than presumed stage IA disease, or selected patients with limited T2 disease and the absence of adenopathy or blood involvement, CT scans of chest, abdomen, and pelvis alone ± FDG-PET scan are recommended to further evaluate any potential lymphadenopathy, visceral involvement, or abnormal lab tests. In patients unable to safely undergo CT scans, MRI may be substituted
  - **Lymph node biopsy**
    - Excisional biopsy is indicated in those patients with a node that is either ≥ 1.5 cm in diameter and/or is firm, irregular, clustered, or fixed
    - Site of biopsy
      - Preference is given to the largest lymph node draining an involved area of the skin or if FDG-PET scan data are available, the node with highest standardized uptake value (SUV)
      - If there is no additional imaging information and multiple nodes are enlarged and otherwise equal in size or consistency, the order of preference is cervical, axillary, and inguinal areas
    - Analysis: pathologic assessment by light microscopy, flow cytometry, and TCR gene rearrangement

- **Treatment of CTCL**
  - ○ **Skin-directed Therapies**
    - ▪ Topical corticosteroids
    - ▪ Topical bexarotene (Targretin gel)
    - ▪ Topical nitrogen mustard
    - ▪ Light tx
      - □ PUVA – Oxsoralen ultra 10 mg tabs. Dose is 0.4–0.6 mg/kg to be taken 1.5 h prior to UVA light
      - □ nbUVB
    - ▪ Total skin electron beam therapy
    - ▪ Superficial X-irradiation – palliative
  - ○ **Systemic Therapy**
    - ▪ Chemotherapy
    - ▪ MTX
    - ▪ Gemcitabine
    - ▪ CHOP (cyclophosphamide, doxorubicin, vincristine, prednisone) combo
    - ▪ Chlorambucil
    - ▪ Liposome-encapsulated doxorubicin
    - ▪ Purine analog (deoxycoformycin, 2-chlorodeoxyadenosine, fludarabine)
    - ▪ **Biologic Response Modifiers**
      - □ Interferon-α
      - □ Retinoids – acitretin and isotretinoin; typical starting doses are 25–50 mg/day and 1 mg/kg/day, respectively
      - □ Retinoids – Bexarotene – usually 300 mg/m^2/day
        - • Refractory to at least one prior systemic therapy
        - • Causes marked central hypothyroidism in significant number of patients with marked reduction in serum TSH and thyroxine
        - • Causes hypertriglyceridemia – gemfibrozil contraindicated
      - □ Denileukin diftitox
        - • Recombinant fusion protein comprising diphtheria toxin fragments and interleukin (IL)-2 sequences
        - • Typically administered for 5 consecutive days at 9 or 18 μg/kg/day for up to eight 21-day cycles, but only in patients with neoplastic T cells expressing the high-affinity IL2R
    - ▪ **Vorinostat** (suberoylanilide hydroxamic acid) – Zolinza
      - □ 400 mg PO QD with food; If patient is intolerant to therapy, the dose may be reduced to 300 mg orally once daily with food. If necessary, the dose may be further reduced to 300 mg once daily with food for 5 consecutive days each week
      - □ Histone deacetylases inhibitor approved by the FDA for the treatment of progressive, persistent, or recurrent CTCL on or after two systemic therapies have failed
      - □ SE – thrombocytopenia, diarrhea, taste changes, nausea, diarrhea, hyperglycemia, increased protein in urine, transient increase in creatinine. DVTs and PE – rare. Drink 2–3 quarts of fluid every day

- Immunotherapy
  - Alemtuzumab (Campath)
    - Humanized recombinant IgG1κ monoclonal antibody with human Fc and V region framework sequences. Specific for CD52 glycoprotein on cells
    - Dose of 30 mg IV 3x/ week, following an initial dose-escalation phase, for up to 12 weeks
  - Zanolimumab (HuMax-CD4®)
    - Human monoclonal antibody that acts as a CD4 antagonist and has been granted orphan drug status in the US and Europe
- Extracorporeal photoimmunotherapy (ECP)
  - Peripheral blood leukocytes are harvested, mixed with 8MOP, exposed to UV radiation, and then returned to the patient

References:

(1) Hwang ST, Janik JE, Jaffe ES, et al. Mycosis fungoides and Sézary syndrome. Lancet 2008; 371: 945–57.
(2) Trautinger F, Knobler R, Willemze R, et al. EORTC consensus recommendations for the treatment of mycosis fungoides/Sézary syndrome. Eur J Cancer 2006; 42(8): 1014–30.
(3) Pimpinelli N, Olsen EA, Santucci M, et al. Defining early mycosis fungoides. J Am Acad Dermatol 2005; 53: 1053–63.
(4) Olsen E, Vonderheid E, Pimpinelli N. Revisions to the staging and classification of mycosis fungoides and Sezary syndrome: a proposal of the International Society for Cutaneous Lymphomas (ISCL) and the cutaneous lymphoma task force of the European Organization of Research and Treatment of Cancer (EORTC). Blood 2007; 110(6): 1713–22.

Delusions of Parasitosis

Etiology and Pathogenesis – unknown

Clinical Presentation

- Patient has firm, fixed, false belief that he or she has pruritus due to an infestation with parasites in the absence of any objective evidence of an infestation
- May present with clothing lint, pieces of skin, or other debris contained in plastic wrap, on adhesive tape, or in matchboxes
  - Matchbox sign, or what the authors term the "Saran-wrap sign"
- Savely et al. introduced the term **Morgellon disease** to describe a condition characterized by fibers attached to the skin – appears to be little more than a new designation for DP
  - CDC is currently investigating Morgellon's disease
- Male-to-female ratio is 1:1 in age < 50 years, and 3:1 in those > 50 years
- In approximately 12% of patients, the delusion of infestation is shared by a significant other
  - Phenomenon is known as folie à deux (e.g., craziness for two) or folie partagé (i.e., shared delusions)
  - Variations in this are the conviction that a child, a spouse, or a pet is infested

Labs

- Rule out true infestation – scabies prep (KOH)
- Evaluate for other causes of pruritus – CBC + diff, anemia, thyroid dysfunction, urinalysis, LFTs, determinations of levels of serum electrolytes and glucose, blood urea nitrogen, serum creatinine, serum vitamin B-12, folate, and iron
- Consider biopsy if dermatitis herpetiformis is suspected
- Consider drug screen – for cocaine, amphetamines, methylphenidate (Ritalin)

DDx – The diagnosis is one of exclusion, and other diseases that can also cause a sensation of itching (e.g., internal disease, actual infestation) must be considered, investigated, and treated if present

- Formication involves the cutaneous sensation of crawling, biting, and stinging
  - Formication does not involve the fixed conception that skin sensations are induced by parasites. Patients with this condition can accept proof that they do not have an infestation. Formication is distinct from DP
- True infestations (e.g., scabies), pediculosis, cocaine or drug use, and primary systemic causes of pruritus must be excluded. Examples include hepatitis, HIV infection, dermatitis herpetiformis, thyroid disease, anemia, renal dysfunction, neurologic dysfunction, and lymphoma

- Schizophrenia – afflicted patients may think they are being attacked by insects as a manifestation of their paranoia
- Psychotic depression may cause the patient to believe he or she is contaminated or "dirty" because of insect infestation
- Drug-induced delusions of parasitosis reported with tx for Parkinson's disease
- At least one report of DP caused by ciprofloxacin

Histology – see only secondary changes – erosions, ulcers, prurigo nodules

Treatment

- Psychotropic meds – to treat the delusion; disease may remit on its own
  - Treatment of choice – risperidone or olanzapine
    - **Risperidone** 1–2 mg qd initially – May cause extrapyramidal reactions, hypotension, tachycardia, and arrhythmias
    - **Olanzapine** 2.5 mg/day – Caution in narrow-angle glaucoma, cardiovascular disease, cerebrovascular disease, prostatic hypertrophy, seizure disorders, hypovolemia, and dehydration. Can cause hyperglycemia, metabolic syndrome if used long term
  - Older choice – Pimozide
    - **Pimozide** – start 1 mg/day; EKG recommended at initiation and regular intervals thereafter (watch for prolongation of the QT interval, T-wave changes, and the appearance of U waves); careful observation for extrapyramidal symptoms (10–15%), especially in geriatric patients
  - After medication has cleared the DP, it should be continued for several months and then discontinued
- Treat secondary infection, pruritus if these are big factors
- Do NOT reinforce the delusion
  - Do NOT give permethrin "just in case" – can strengthen the delusion and make it more difficult to treat later
    - While getting the patient to take a medication, such as risperidone, don't tell them that it is a medication that "kills the parasites"; this reinforces and validates the delusion
  - While one should not say anything to confirm the delusion, it is usually not helpful to forcefully confront patients with DP
    - Statements such as the following might be helpful: **"I know you feel strongly that there are parasites here, and I'm sure that you itch severely, but I cannot prove that parasites are or have been the cause of your problem"**
- Serotonergic antidepressants may have a role in the treatment of these patients

- A psychiatrist should be consulted if the dermatologist cannot or will not prescribe the necessary medications
  - Most patients with DP are reluctant to see a psychiatrist, and the dermatologist may be more successful in giving the referral if they have gained the patient's trust after several clinic visits instead of immediately after meeting the patient

Pearls and Pitfalls

- Always check out the samples that patients bring in. Sometimes the patients actually DO have bugs on them or in their environment

Dermatitis Herpetiformis (DH)

Etiology and Pathogenesis

- Autoimmune blistering disease characterized by gluten-sensitive enteropathy in which IgA antiendomysial antibodies are directed against tissue transglutaminase
  - Gluten is a protein present in grasses of the species *Triticeae,* which includes barley, rye, and wheat
  - Rice, oats, corn belong to different species and are generally well tolerated
  - Strict compliance with a gluten-free diet results in normalization of the small bowel mucosal changes and control of the cutaneous manifestations of DH in most patients
- Strong genetic component → over 90% have HLA class II DQ2 genotype composed of the DQA1*0501 and DQB1*02 alleles

Clinical Presentation

- Exquisitely pruritic papulovesicles or excoriated papules on extensor surfaces which are often excoriated by the time of presentation
- Risk of non-Hodgkin's lymphoma, Hodgkin's disease, B-cell lymphomas, GI lymphoma
- **DH and Celiac Disease**
  - DH and Celiac disease represent one disease with varying clinical presentations
  - 10–20% of patients with Celiac Disease have DH
  - 4–7% of patients with DH have family members with disease and even higher number of relatives with Celiac
- **Associated diseases**: vitiligo, alopecia areata, Sjögren's syndrome, rheumatoid arthritis, Type I diabetes, autoimmune thyroid disorders, pernicious anemia, myasthenia gravis

Labs

- Endomysial IgA antibodies – highly specific for the disease
  - Presence of IgA antiendomysial antibodies correlates with the extent of the gut disease; however, some DH patients do not have detectable IgA antiendomysial antibodies, even during episodes of active skin disease
  - Can be negative in 10–30% (sensitivity)
- Anti-Tissue transglutaminase antibodies (is the autoantigen for the development of endomysial antibodies) – ELISA
- The titers of both endomysial antibodies and anti-tissue transglutaminase Ab correlate with the degree of mucosal damage

- IgA deficiency
  - This occurs in 1 in 40 patients with Celiac disease (much more common than in general population). If high suspicion for Celiac, rule out this deficiency. In such cases, a test for IgG antibodies against tissue transglutaminase should be performed
  - This phenomenon of IgA deficiency evaluated in DH patients – reports of this in the medical literature
    - Unclear if IgG antibodies against tissue transglutaminase will be helpful?

DDx – linear IgA disease, bullous lupus, inflammatory EBA, and bullous pemphigoid

Histology

- Dermal papillary neutrophilic microabcesses – best observed in early red lesions
- Neutrophilic infiltrate and fibrin are associated with degenerative changes of the collagen and the development of edema
- Microvesiculation follows, leading to the formation of multilocular subepidermal blisters
- Dermal inflammatory infiltrate – lymphocytes, histiocytes, and abundant neutrophils
- Nuclear dust (leukocytoclasis) is also characteristic, but no evidence of vasculitis
- Occasional eosinophils may be present

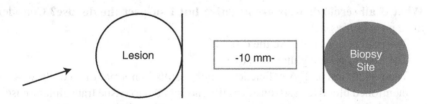

Fig. 10 Where to biopsy lesion of dermatitis herpetiformis for DIF

- **DIF** – should be performed for confirmation (**perilesional**)
  - Biopsy normal-appearing skin adjacent to an active lesion, as lesional skin often produces false-negative results
  - Granular deposits of IgA in the dermal papillae of perilesional skin – in papillae
  - Other immunoglobulins are not usually found, but C3 is often present
  - IgA deposition may disappear after a prolonged period on a gluten-free diet
  - Cutaneous IgA deposition is not seen in Celiac disease

- Biopsies of the jejunum show classic villous atrophy in >90% of patients with DH

Treatment

- Dapsone (or related drugs such as sulfapyridine)
  - Check G6PD prior
  - Most require 50–100 mg daily to control symptoms
  - Individuals on dapsone will have some degree of hemolysis
  - Most on 100 mg a day will have some degree of methemoglobinemia that may manifest as a headache
    - Cimetidine 1.6 g daily (Divided 400 mg QID) can reduce this SE – see *Dapsone*
    - Vitamin E 800 IU daily may protect against dapsone-induced hemolysis
  - Risk of agranulocytosis is multiplied 25–30 times that of normal individuals when there is severe inflammatory case of DH
- Gluten-free diet → Treatment of choice
  - Improves both the cutaneous symptoms and the GI pathology
  - Diet must be strictly gluten-free to be successful
  - Avoid what, barley and rye
    - Patients may eat rice, corn products
    - Oats are ok to eat
  - Cross-contamination of products is a challenge for patients
  - Only way to decrease the risk of GI lymphoma is to stay on gluten-free diet

Pearls and Pitfalls

- **What if all serologic tests are negative but I suspect the disease?** Consider three possibilities …
  - The patient does not have the disease
  - The patient is on a gluten-free diet
  - The patient has an IgA deficiency which results in normal titers of the above-mentioned blood tests. (Consider DIF and IgG Ab to tissue transglutaminase). IgA deficiency is more common in patients with Celiac disease/DH
- Reliable sources of information (Don't believe everything you read on the Internet):
  - Celiac Disease Foundation: www.celiac.org
  - The Gluten Intolerance Group of North America: www.gluten.net
  - National Foundation for Celiac Awareness: www.celiaccentral.org
  - The Canadian Celiac Association: www.celiac.ca

Dermatofibrosarcoma Protuberans (DFSP)

Etiology and Pathogenesis

- Not completely understood. Some have associated its development with trauma, vaccinations, and scarring
- Recently, chromosomal abnormalities have been discovered, which suggest a genetic basis for this tumor. Translocation between chromosomes 17 and 22 [t(17;22)] has been observed in more than 90% of cases, resulting in the activation of platelet-derived growth factor receptor

Clinical Presentation

- Locally aggressive sarcoma which favors young to middle-aged adults. Rarely seen in childhood or as a congenital presentation
- Location – trunk (50–60%), proximal extremities (20–30%), head and neck (10–15%)
  - Predilection for shoulder or pelvic area of trunk
- Slow-growing, asymptomatic, skin-colored indurated plaque that eventually develops violaceous to red-brown nodules

DDx – keloid, large dermatofibroma, dermatomyofibroma, morphea. Congenital and childhood-onset DFSP may have an atrophic appearance and/or hypopigmented to blue-red color which may be misdiagnosed as a vascular malformation or vascular tumor.

Histology

- Plaque lesions – proliferation of spindle-shaped cells arranged as long fascicles parallel to skin surface. Infiltrate thick collagen bundles which appear cellular and wavy. Adnexal structures are infiltrated and obliterated. Infiltration extends in subcutaneous tissue, often in a multilayered pattern
- Nodular lesions – histology more cellular → storiform pattern. Cells infiltrate subcutaneous tissue in honeycomb pattern. Cells have hyperchromatic nuclei, mitotic figures
- If pigment-containing cells (Schwannian differentiation) are present – "Bednar tumor"
- CD34+, Factor XIIIa –

Treatment

- Mohs surgery
- Imatinib mesylate (Gleevac®) may be useful because the translocation places the platelet-derived growth factor (PDGF) B-chain gene under the control of the collagen 1A1 promoter and imatinib targets the PDGF receptor

Pearls and Pitfalls

- Highly cellular dermatofibromas will be CD34-, Factor XIIIa +
- High rate of recurrence

Dermatomyositis (DM)

Etiology and Pathogenesis

- Immune-mediated process likely triggered by outside factors (e.g., malignancy, drugs, infections) in genetically predisposed individuals

Clinical Presentation

- Symmetric, proximal, extensor, inflammatory myopathy which is accompanied by a characteristic skin eruption
- Associated with malignancy in at least 30% of adults
- Children: peak ages 5–10 years old; Adults: peak age 50
- **Skin**
  - Diffuse erythematous rash of the trunk (often with poikiloderma), edematous, violaceous eyelids (heliotrope rash), periungual telangiectasias
  - Gottron's papules – papules on the knuckles of the hands
  - Gottron's sign – violaceous discoloration of the knuckles, elbows, and/or knees
  - Ragged cuticles common
  - Pruritus is a common sign of underlying dermatomyositis
- **Muscle**
  - Proximal muscle weakness with EMG abnormalities, myositis on muscle biopsy, and elevated muscle enzymes such as CPK and aldolase
  - Muscle dz may occur concurrently, precede skin dz, or follow skin dz by weeks to years
  - Amyopathic variant exists – Dermatomyositis sine myositis or Amyopathic Dermatomyositis (ADM)
- **Complications**
  - Calcinosis is a complication mostly observed in children or adolescents; rare in adults
  - Residual weakness and disability possible as a long-term complication
  - Contractures may develop in children with severe dz (immobility of joints and calcinosis)

Labs

- **Creatine kinase** (most sensitive/specific)
- **Aldolase**
- **Aspartate aminotransferase (AST)**
- **LDH** – ↑ LDH, AST, CK, aldolase precede myositis clinically

- **ANA** positivity is common
- **Anti-Mi-2** – Highly specific for DM but lacks sensitivity. Only 25% of patients have them. Associated with acute-onset classic DM and V-shaped and shawl rash and a relatively good prognosis
- **Anti-Jo-1**- More frequent in patients with polymyositis than in DM. Associated with pulmonary involvement, Raynaud's, arthritis, mechanic's hands
- **Anti-SRP** – Associated with severe polymyositis
- **Anti-PM-Scl, Anti-Ku** – Assoc w/ overlapping features of myositis, scleroderma

Imaging and Workup

- CT of the chest/abdomen/pelvis – to r/o malignancy
- Barium swallow to assess esophageal dysmotility
- CXR at time of diagnosis
- MRI – helpful in assessing for inflammation in patients without weakness. Useful in differentiating from a steroid myopathy
- EMG – (although MRIs more commonly used now)
- PFTs, EKG
- Muscle biopsy

DDx – GVHD, lupus, hypothyroidism, sarcoidosis, multicentric reticulohistiocytosis, CREST, parapsoriasis, pityriasis rubra pilaris, PMLE, psoriasis, morphea, lichen myxedematosus, rosacea, tinea capitis, urticaria (chronic), CTCL, photodrug eruption, airborne allergic contact dermatitis, atopic dermatitis, trichinosis

Histology

- Epidermis normal or atrophic with degeneration of the basal layer
- Thickening of the basement membrane is sometimes present
- Dermal edema and dermal mucin (latter seen with Alcian blue or colloidal iron stains)
- Sparse perivascular lymphocytic infiltrate – may be interface
- Dermal or subcutaneous calcification may be seen
- DIF negative
- Muscle – classic path findings include a combination of type II muscle fiber atrophy, necrosis, regeneration, and hypertrophy with centralized sarcolemmal nuclei, plus lymphocytes in both a perifascicular and a perivascular distribution

Treatment

- **Calcinosis** (mostly children and adolescents)
  - o Early aggressive treatment of myositis may aid in preventing this complication. Once established, tends to be debilitating
  - o Calcium-channel blocker, diltiazem (240 mg BID) – reportedly associated with gradual resolution in a small number
  - o Surgical removal
- **General**
  - o Physical therapy, especially in children, to prevent contractures
  - o Bed rest for those with severe muscle inflammation
  - o If dysphagia, ↑ head of bed, don't eat before bedtime, occasionally need NG tube
  - o Sun avoidance and sun protective measures
  - o Prednisone+MTX→increased risk of peptic ulcer disease; monitor this carefully and consider adding a proton-pump inhibitor

Table 64 Therapeutic ladder for dermatomyositis

Systemic Therapy
Oral prednisone: 1 mg/kg/day tapered to 50% over 6 months and to zero over 2–3 year[2]
– Option to use pulse, split dose, or alternate day[2]
Methotrexate: low-dose weekly MTX[1]
Mycophenolate mofetil[2]
Azathioprine: 2–3 mg/kg/day[1]
– Combined azathioprine and methotrexate[1]
High-dose intravenous immunoglobulin[1]
Cyclosporin A[1*]
Cyclophosphamide[3]
Chlorambucil[3]
Rituximab[3]
Tumor necrosis factor α inhibitors[2]
Tacrolimus[3]
Rapamycin[3]
Efalizumab[3]
Plasma exchange – NOT helpful[1]
Cutaneous Lesions
Sunscreens – high SPF and UVA protection[3]
Topical corticosteroids[2]
Hydroxychloroquine[2]
Hydroxychloroquine+Quinacrine[3]
Low-dose weekly MTX[2]
Mycophenolate mofetil[2]
Topical tacrolimus[2]
Retinoids[3]
Rituximab[3]

(continued)

Table 64 (continued)

Cutaneous Lesions
Dapsone[3]
Thalidomide[3]
Pulsed dye therapy[3]

1 = randomized, double-blinded studies (good)
2 = clinical series (medium)
3 = anecdotal evidence (weak)
* = randomized, but not double-blinded
Reference: Used with permission from Elsevier. Jorizzo JL. Dermatomyositis. In: Bolognia JL, Jorizzo JL, Rapini RP, eds. Dermatology. New York: Mosby; 2003; p.582

Pearls and Pitfalls

- Evaluate for at least 3 years following diagnosis
- **Genitourinary malignancies, especially ovarian cancer, and colon cancer may be overrepresented** in patients with dermatomyositis
- Major causes of death are cancer, ischemic heart disease, and lung disease
- Consider the diagnosis of early dermatomyositis in patients with a very itchy scalp with some erythema
- Emphasize sun protection, particularly against UVA
- Dermatomyositis in children
  - Usually not associated with malignancy and is more often associated with calcinosis
  - Chondrodermatitis nodularis helicis in children is rarely associated with dermatomyositis and should be screened for

Discoid Lupus Erythematosus (DLE)

Etiology and Pathogenesis

- AKA – chronic cutaneous lupus erythematosus
- Autoimmune condition. Genetic factors also play a role.

Clinical Presentation

- Chronic, scarring, atrophy producing, photosensitive dermatosis
  - Lesions most common on the face, scalp, ears, but may be present anywhere
  - Unusual for lesions to present below the neck unless there are also lesions above the neck
  - Rarely – discoid lupus may occur on mucosal surfaces including the lips, nasal mucosa, conjunctivae, and genital mucosa.
  - Disfiguring scarring and dyspigmentation is often present
  - Scarring alopecia common
- < 5% progress to SLE
- Most common type of cutaneous lupus
- Rarely, squamous cell carcinoma can develop within long-standing lesions
- Unusual variant of DLE is hypertrophic DLE, characterized by thick scaling overlying the discoid lesion or occurring at the periphery of a discoid lesion. May mimic an SCC clinically.

Labs

- Some patients with DLE (approximately 20%) manifest a positive antinuclear antibody (ANA)
- Anti-Ro (SS-A) autoantibodies are present in approximately 1–3% of patients
- Antinative DNA (double-stranded or nDNA) or anti-Sm antibodies usually reflect SLE, and they may occur in some patients (<5%)
- Cytopenia or leukopenia may be present
- RF may be positive
- ↑ ESR may be present
- Complement levels may be depressed
- Urinalysis may reflect the presence of renal involvement with proteinuria

DDx – vitiligo, SCC, actinic keratosis, hypertrophic lichen planus, psoriasis, PMLE

Histology

- Epidermal atrophy or hyperplasia with vacuolar interface changes. There is a superficial and deep perivascular and periadnexal inflammatory infiltrate consisting primarily of lymphoctyes and histiocytes. Follicular plugging often present. Increase in dermal mucin.

Treatment

- Sun-protective measures, including sunscreens, protective clothing
- Cosmetic measures, such as makeup or wigs, may be suggested for appropriately selected patients. Makeup used for camouflage includes Covermark and Dermablend.
- Topical corticosteroids
- IL corticosteroids – if a patient is given 10 mL of triamcinolone 3 mg/mL, this means that the patient has received a total of 30 mg, and toxicity is the same as if it had been delivered orally or by intramuscular injection
- Antimalarials – smoking decreases the efficacy
  - Hydroxychloroquine 200–400 mg/day PO; not to exceed 6.5 mg/kg/day; 310 mg PO qd or bid for several week depending on response; 155–310 mg/day for prolonged maintenance therapy
  - Chloroquine 250–500 mg PO qd (more ocular toxicity)
- Topical calcineurin inhibitors
- Topical retinoids reported helpful
- Topical imiquimod – helpful in some cases
- Dapsone 100–200 mg PO qd; check G6PD prior
- Methotrexate (MTX) may be considered. In Dr. Callen's experience, azathioprine and, recently, mycophenolate mofetil, have been more successful than MTX, while systemic corticosteroids are rarely effective
  - Azathioprine 1 mg/kg/day PO for 6–8 week; increase by 0.5 mg/kg q 4 week until response is seen or dose reaches 2.5 mg/kg/day
  - Mycophenolate mofetil 1 g PO bid
- Efalizumab (Raptiva) has been demonstrated in an open-label study to be effective in patients with chronic CLE and SCLE (off the market in the US)
- Auranofin (Ridaura) – gold → 6 mg/day PO qd or divided bid; after 3 months, may increase to 9 mg/day divided tid; then, if no response, discontinue drug
- Thalidomide 100–300 mg PO hs aq, and >1 h pc
- Oral retinoids
  - Acitretin (Soriatane) → Initial dose: 25 or 50 mg/day PO single dose w/ main meal Maintenance dose: 25–50 mg/day PO after initial response; terminate therapy when lesions have resolved sufficiently
  - Isotretinoin → 40–60 mg/day PO for 4 months
- Interferon alfa-2a and alfa-2b – 2 million U/m^2 SC 3 times/week for 30 days

Pearls and Pitfalls

- Several cutaneous diseases have been reported, perhaps in greater frequency, in patients with DLE
  - Malignant degeneration of chronic lesions of lupus erythematosus (LE) is possible, although rare, leading to NMSC. Dark-skinned individuals may be more prone to skin cancer because of the lack of pigmentation within the chronic lesion, combined with chronic inflammation and continued sun damage.
  - Porphyria cutanea tarda appears to be overrepresented in LE patients. Often, the porphyria is discovered when antimalarials first are administered.
  - Lichen planus-like lesions may be part of an overlap between LE and lichen planus or may occur as a result of antimalarial therapy

Drug Hypersensitivity Syndrome (DRESS)

Etiology and Pathogenesis

- DRESS stands for "drug reaction with eosinophilia and systemic symptoms" but also called "drug hypersensitivity syndrome"
  - Common medications
  - Anticonvulsants → phenytoin, carbamezapine, phenobarbital, lamotrigine (especially when co-administered with valproate)
  - Sulfonamides
  - Minocycline
  - Allopurinol → especially in the setting of renal dysfunction
  - Dapsone
  - Gold salts
  - Abacavir
- Pathogenesis of disease probably involves alteration in the metabolism of specific drugs, such as a defect in the detoxification process
- Possible role of HHV-6 and HHV-7 has been proposed
- Genetic predisposition – HLA-B*5701 predisposes to drug hypersensitivity to abacavir and should not be used in these individuals. Testing is done prior to starting this HIV medication.
- Incidence may be higher in African-Americans and patients from the Caribbean basin

Clinical Presentation

- Develops 2–6 weeks after the precipitating drug is started, which is later than other immunologically mediated skin reactions
- Fever and cutaneous eruption
  - Morbilliform eruption which tends to become more accentuated around follicles
  - Facial edema – hallmark of the condition
  - May develop vesicles, tense bullae – induced by the edema
  - Patients may become erythrodermic
  - Lymphadenopathy
- Systemic involvement
  - Liver is most common organ involved – responsible for the majority of deaths
  - Cardiac – myocarditis, pericarditis, acute necrotizing eosinophilic myocarditis
  - Thyroid
  - Brain
  - Kidneys – interstitial nephritis

- **Bocquet's Criteria** (1996). Some have proposed adding HHV-6 positivity to the criteria
  - ○ Cutaneous drug eruption
  - ○ Hematologic abnormalities
    - ▪ Eosinophilia ≥ 1.5 × 10⁹/L or
    - ▪ Presence of atypical lymphocytes
  - ○ Systemic involvement
    - ▪ Lymphadenopathy ≥ 2 cm in diameter
    - ▪ or hepatitis (liver transaminases values ≥ 2x Upper limit normal)
    - ▪ or interstitial nephritis
    - ▪ or interstitial pneumonitis
    - ▪ or myocarditis

Labs

- CBC + diff → eosinophilia may not be present until later. May see lymphopenia or lymphocytosis
- LFTs → may not be elevated until later
- Thyroid function tests – usually normal until 2–3 months after eruption
- HHV-6 serologies (at time of presentation and later)
- EKG, echo – may be abnormal early or late. Get baseline EKG.

DDx – other types of drug eruptions, viral infections, idiopathic hypereosinophilic syndrome, lymphoma, pseudolymphoma, serum sickness-like reactions

Histology – dense lymphocytic infiltrate in the superficial dermis associated with eosinophils and dermal edema.

Treatment

- High-dose systemic corticosteroids are first-line
- Topical corticosteroids
- Other treatments – IVIG, mycophenolate mofetil, azathioprine, muromonab-CD3, plasmapheresis, rituximab
- If cardiac involvement – start standard therapies for heart failure (cardiology)

Pearls and Pitfalls

- The cardiac involvement is an increasingly recognized entity that is often missed. Get a baseline EKG and counsel patient to go to ER immediately if any chest pain or SOB. Get cardiology involved early if any symptoms.
  - Ventricular assist devices can be helpful and life-saving in severe cardiac involvement (early consultation with cardiothoracic surgery)
  - Even with myocardial biopsy, there are sampling errors due to the patchy nature of the inflammation and necrosis; can thus get a negative result
- Check thyroid studies 2–3 months after eruption
- This can be a very difficult to control disease, and relapses are common. Often need patients on immunosuppressive therapy for months.
- The mortality is high if cardiac or liver involvement; otherwise it is around 10%

References:

Bourgeois GP, Cafardi JA, Groysman V, Hughey LC. A review of DRESS-associated myocarditis. J Am Acad Dermatol. 2011 Jun 7. [Epub ahead of print].
Fulminant myocarditis as a late sequela of DRESS: two cases.
Bourgeois GP, Cafardi JA, Groysman V, Pamboukian SV, Kirklin JK, Andea AA, Hughey LC. J Am Acad Dermatol. 2011; 65(4): 889–90.

Dyshidrotic Eczema

Etiology and Pathogenesis

- AKA – "Pompholyx" which derives from *cheiropompholyx*, which means "hand and bubble" in Greek
- Etiology unclear but appears to be multifactorial from combination of exogenous and endogenous factors ….
  - Genetic – some familial forms
  - Atopy – As many as 50% of patients with dyshidrotic eczema have reportedly had personal or familial atopic diathesis
  - Nickel sensitivity – both topical and ingested
    - Low-nickel diets reportedly decrease frequency and severity of flares in some
  - Id reaction – to chemicals, metals, or to a distant dermatophyte infection
  - Fungal infection – such as tinea pedis
- Emotional stress

Clinical Presentation

- Recurrent or chronic relapsing form of vesicular palmoplantar dermatitis of unknown etiology
- Typically affects the fingers, palms, and soles and is characterized by a sudden onset of deep-seated pruritic, clear "tapioca-like" vesicles. Large bullous and pustular lesions may be present.
- Later – see scaling fissures and lichenification
- Spontaneous remission may occur in 2–3 weeks
- Tend to have recurrent episodes

Labs – rule out tinea (KOH), rule out scabies (scabies prep), bacterial cultures and sensitivities

DDx – scabies, inflammatory tinea pedis or tinea manus, palmopustular psoriasis, langerhans cell histiocytosis (in babies), acropustulosis of infancy (in babies), herpes simplex, impetigo, allergic contact dermatitis, bullous erythema multiforme, dyshidrosiform pemphigoid

Histology – spongiosis and intraepidermal edema with intraepidermal vesicles

Treatment

- For "weeping" lesions …
  - Domeboro's soak – put packet in basin of lukewarm water. Put gauze in water and then on bullae. Leave on for 20–30 min. Repeat BID-TID.
- Topical corticosteroids are mainstay of treatment – class I initially
  - Ointments penetrate skin better than creams
- Consider prednisone taper if very severe presentation
- Topical calcineurin inhibitors – such as tacrolimus or pimecrolimus
- Hand/foot UVA therapy 3x/week
- Severe, refractory dyshidrosis – azathioprine, methotrexate mycophenolate mofetil, cyclosporine, or etanercept may be helpful
- Tap water iontophoresis with pulsed direct may be helpful as adjuvant treatment
- Botulinum toxin A injections may be helpful in some patients
- For nickel-sensitive patients, consider a nickel-free diet for 3–4 weeks
  - Foods rich in nickel: canned foods, foods cooked in nickel-plated utensils, herring, oysters, asparagus, beans, mushrooms, onions, corn, spinach, tomatoes, peas, whole grain flour, pears, rhubarb, tea, cocoa, chocolate, and baking powder
- For cobalt-sensitive patients, consider a cobalt-free diet
  - Avoid: apricots, beans, beer, beets, cabbage, cloves, cocoa, chocolate, coffee, liver, nuts, scallops, tea, and whole grain flour
- PO antihistamines

Pearls and Pitfalls

- The nickel-free and cobalt-free diets are difficult to follow, and are not typically recommended first-line. It may be a consideration in difficult cases where other treatments have been exhausted, where there is any suggestion of a diet-triggered eruption or if the patient is motivated to try one of these diets.

Epidermolysis Bullosa Acquisita (EBA)

Etiology and Pathogenesis

- Immune-mediated disease where IgG autoantibodies target the basement membrane of stratified squamous and other complex epithelia
  - React with Type VII collagen, the major component of anchoring fibrils in the lamina densa and sublamina densa region. Autoantibodies commonly target the NC1 domain of the protein, but reactivity with the central collagenous domain or the NC2 domain have been rarely observed.
- Genetic susceptibility → DRB1*1501 and DR5 and DRB1*13

Clinical Presentation and Types

- Usually seen in adults, although children can develop EBA
- Cutaneous
  - Non-inflammatory bullous disease which favors the acral surfaces. Lesions heal with atrophic scarring, milia, and hyper- or hypopigmentation
  - Bullae may be serous or hemorrhagic
  - Acral involvement may be mutilating – "mitten deformity of the digits", syndactyly, nail dystrophy, and complete nail loss.
  - Scalp involvement occurs in up to 20% and may lead to a scarring alopecia
  - Mucous membrane involvement is variable. Erosions and vesicles may be seen in mouth, larynx, and esophagus.
  - Ocular involvement reported and may lead to blindness
- Clinical Variants
  - **Mechanobullous form** → see above
  - **Bullous pemphigoid-like** → widespread vesicles and bullae involving intertriginous areas that heal without milia or scars.
  - **Cicatricial pemphigoid-like** → may develop a Brunsting–Perry pemphigoid phenotype with scarring alopecia
- Diseases associated → inflammatory bowel disease (especially Crohn's), myeloma, SLE, rheumatoid arthritis, thyroiditis, diabetes

Labs – Consider CBC+diff, complete metabolic profile, thyroid studies, fasting glucose, ANA, RF, porphyrin studies. Screen for tuberculosis prior to starting immunosuppressives.

DDx – bullous pemphigoid, cicatricial pemphigoid (including the Brunsting–Perry type), epidermolysis bullosa (inherited forms), linear IgA bullous dermatosis, porphyria cutanea tarda, pseudoporphyria, bullous SLE

Histology

- Subepidermal bulla without acantholysis. There is a variable inflammatory infiltrate composed of neutrophils, eosinophils, or lymphocytes in the BP-like and CP-like forms. Little to no infiltrate in the mechanobullous form.
- DIF (perilesional) → continuous, rather broad, linear pattern along the epidermal BMZ. Less commonly see linear deposits of C3, IgA, or IgM
- IIF → circulating anti-BMZ antibodies detected in about 50% of patients, primarily of IgG class but IgA also reported.
- Indirect IF on salt-split skin → circulating antibodies bind to the dermal side of the blister

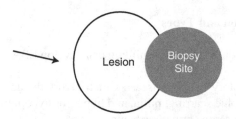

Fig. 11 Where to biopsy SKIN lesions of epidermolysis bullosa acquisita for DIF

Treatment

- Treatment is difficult and unsatisfactory
- Systemic corticosteroids
- Colchicine often used first
- Other – azathioprine, mycophenolate mofetil, methotrexate, cyclophosphamide for the BP-like presentations
- Dapsone, IVIG, cyclosporine, gold, extracorporeal photochemotherapy – may be helpful

Pearls and Pitfalls

- Prognosis is variable, but usually not life-threatening
- **EBA in children** → treatment often is a combination of dapsone and prednisolone

Erythema Annulare Centrifugum (EAC)

Etiology and Pathogenesis

- Pathogenesis of EAC unknown, but probably due to a hypersensitivity reaction; Some cases associated with:
  - **Underlying systemic disease** (e.g., liver disease, Sjögren syndrome, systemic lupus erythematosus, Graves disease, hypereosinophilic syndrome, appendicitis, sarcoid)
  - **Drug** – reports of medication-associated EAC exist (most commonly antimalarials, cimetidine, spironolactone, gold, salicylates, piroxicam, penicillin, and amitriptyline)
  - **Arthropod bites**
  - **Infections**
    - Bacterial – *E. coli*, Strept
    - Mycobacterial – tuberculosis
    - Viral – EBV
    - Fungal – Dermatophyte, *Malassezia,* Candida
    - Parasites – *Ascaris lumbricoides, Phthirus pubis*
    - Filarial
  - **Ingestion** (blue cheese *Penicillium*)
  - **Malignancy** (anecdotal associations) – SCC, nasopharyngeal CA, AML, myeloma, Hodgkin, prostate CA, ovarian CA, malignant histiocytosis, peritoneal carcinomatosis
- The disappearance of EAC after interferon suggests that TNF-α and IL-2 may play a role in its pathogenesis

Clinical Presentation

- Classified as one of the figurate or gyrate erythemas
- Lesions begin as firm pink papules that expand centrifugally and subsequently develop central clearing. There is typically desquamation at the inner margins ("trailing scale")
  - Plaques may appear as incomplete arcs or polycyclic bands
  - Vesicles occasionally develop at the peripheral margin
- Mean duration of EAC is 11 months

Labs and Imaging to consider

- KOH – to rule out tinea, candida
- Lyme antibody titer if appropriate history of travel to endemic area
- ANA, pregnancy test

- PPD to rule out tuberculosis
- CBC+diff – to rule out eosinophilia with parasite, leukocytosis with bacterial infection
- Stool exam for ova and parasites
- CXR – tuberculosis, sarcoid, malignancy, lymphoma

DDx – CTCL, erythema gyratum repens, granuloma faciale, SCLE, annular urticaria, erythema migrans, erythema marginatum rheumaticum, tinea corporis, linear IgA bullous dermatosis (if vesicles/bullae are present at peripheral margin)

Histology – occasional focal spongiosis or parakeratosis. Sharply demarcated "coat-sleeve" lymphocytes densely arranged around dilated superficial and deep blood vessels.

Treatment

- Topical steroids
- Systemic or injection steroid therapy is effective, but the eruption returns once these drugs are withdrawn
- EAC associated with hypereosinophilic syndrome – reports of the eruption resolving after treatment with ketoconazole, dapsone, and trimethoprim–sulfamethoxazole
- Interferon alpha therapy – reports of success
- Reports of response to hyaluronic acid, metronidazole, and calcipotriol
- Case reports of TNF-alpha inhibitors have been tried for prolonged, chronic cases (etanercept)

Pearls and Pitfalls

- Always look at their feet. Tinea pedis is a very common association/cause of EAC.
- Always review the medication list
- Malignancies are only anecdotally associated, but should be a consideration in recalcitrant cases or if other symptoms (unexplained weight loss, generalized pruritus, constitutional symptoms)

Erythema Dyschromicum Perstans (EDP)

Etiology and Pathogenesis

- AKA – Ashy dermatosis
- Etiology unclear but majority of patients are from Latin America
- Postulated to be a cell-mediated immune reaction to an ingestant or a contactant that leads to localized areas of pigment incontinence. In most patients, a trigger is never found.
- HLA-DR4 allele may be risk factor for EDP in Mexican patients
- Has been occasionally associated with:
  - Ingestion of ammonium nitrate, oral x-ray contrast media
  - Medications (benzodiazepines, penicillin)
  - Exposure to pesticides and fungicides
  - Endocrinopathies such as thyroid disease
  - Whipworm
  - HIV infections

Clinical Presentation

- Usually presents in second to third decade, but may present in children or in elderly
- Asymptomatic
- Oval or circular, irregularly shaped macules and patches that are slate-gray to blue-brown in color
- Symmetrical
- Distribution – initially on trunk with subsequent spread to neck, upper extremities, and occasionally the face. Includes sun-protected areas.
- Active lesions may have a thin, raised border which tends to resolve over a few months
- Peripheral hypopigmentation may be seen in older lesions

DDx – lichenoid drug eruption, minocycline-induced pigmentation (or other medication), lichen planus pigmentosa, generalized fixed drug eruption, macular urticarial pigmentosa, post-inflammatory hyperpigmentation, and less likely, leprosy or pinta.

Histology

- Active lesions → vacuolar degeneration of basal cell layer, perivascular mononuclear cell infiltrate in upper dermis and increased epidermal melanin and dermal melanophages. Colloid bodies and dermal hemosiderin may be present.

- Inactive lesions→ minimal mononuclear cell infiltrate, increased number of dermal melanophages

Treatment

- No consistently effective treatment. Anecdotal reports of treatment success with:
  - Oral corticosteroids, antibiotics, antimalarials, isoniazid, griseofulvin, UV light, laser therapy
  - Small series → dapsone and clofazamine successful
- Topical corticosteroids and hydroquinone not effective
- High rate of spontaneous remission in children (2/3 of cases)
- Tends to progress in adults

Erythema Elevatum Diutinum (EED)

Etiology and Pathogenesis

- Etiology *(Not fully established)*, but thought to be due to immune complex deposition
  - Bacterial – Strept
  - Viral – Hep B, HIV
  - Autoimmune conditions – such as lupus, Wegener's, inflammatory bowel dz, relapsing polychondritis, rheumatoid arthritis
  - B-cell Lymphoma
  - Hematologic disease – (most common factor associated) – myelodysplasia, myeloproliferative dz, hair cell leukemia, polycythemia vera
  - Plasma cell dyscrasias – IgA gammopathy (common), multiple myeloma
  - Drugs – erythropoietin

Clinical Presentation

- Rare type of LCV characterized by symmetric red-violaceous, brown, or yellow papules, plaques, or nodules
  - Distributed on extensor surfaces – especially over joints
  - Lesions can be completely asymptomatic, painful, or cause a sensation of burning or itching. Symptoms can be exacerbated by cold. Arthralgias may be present.
  - Some may note that lesions enlarge during the day and return to previous size overnight
- Several studies have shown an association of EED with ocular abnormalities – including nodular scleritis, panuveitis, autoimmune keratolysis, and peripheral keratitis.

Labs and Imaging

- Immunoelectrophoresis (IEP) can be used to identify possible gammopathies
- Antineutrophil cytoplasmic antibodies of IgA class may become a helpful para-clinical marker of disease
- Elevated ESR

DDx – acute febrile neutrophilic dermatosis, erythema induratum, EM, granuloma faciale, granuloma annulare, multicentric reticulohistiocytosis, pyoderma gangrenosum, xanthomas

Histology

- Biopsy consistent with leukocytoclastic vasculitis with a neutrophilic infiltrate in the upper and mid dermis (some eosinophils) in early lesions, which is followed by fibrotic replacement of the dermis in older lesions. Extracellular cholesterol deposits are classic in late-stage lesions.
- DIF – complement as well IgG, IgM, IgA, and fibrin around the damaged vessels

Treatment

- Dapsone 50–300 mg QD; check G6PD prior
- Other therapies–Sulfapyridine, NSAIDs, colchicine, niacinamide 100 mg PO tid, tetracyclines, chloroquine, IL steroids
- Intermittent plasma exchange (PLEX) was shown to control IgA paraproteinemia associated with EED. The IgA levels responded to PLEX treatment, followed by consolidative doses of cyclophosphamide. This treatment might be promising for the control of severe EED that is not controlled by dapsone.

Pearls and Pitfalls

- Always check for monoclonal gammopathy or hematologic abnormality

Table 65 Diseases associated with monoclonal gammopathies

Type	Disease
IgA	EED, pyoderma gangrenosum, subcorneal pustular dermatosis, IgA pemphigus, POEMS, Sweet's syndrome
IgM	Schnitzler syndrome, Waldenstrom macroglobulinemia
IgG	NXG (IgG κ), scleredema (IgG $\kappa > \lambda$), scleromyxedema (IgG $\lambda > \kappa$)

Erythema Multiforme (EM)

Etiology and Pathogenesis

- Considered a manifestation of a distinct skin-directed immune reaction that occurs in the setting of infection or predisposed individuals.
- HLA associations – HLA-DQw3 (specifically DQB1*301 split), DRw53, and Aw33

Table 66 Causes of erythema multiforme

Infectious	Viral – HSV (2/3 of cases due to HSV), adenovirus, cat-scratch, coxsackie, echovirus, hepatitis, EBV, CMV, parvovirus, influenza A, paravaccinia, parapoxvirus (orf), polio, vaccinia (smallpox vaccine), varicella zoster, variola, HIV Bacterial – *Mycoplasma pneumoniae*, *chlamydophilia*, *salmonella*, *Mycobacterium tuberculosis*, BCG vaccine, diphtheria, gonorrhea, *Streptococcus hemolyticus*, leprosy, pseudomonas, staphylococcus, syphilis, tularemia, *Vibrio parahemolyticus*, yersinia Fungal – *Histoplasma capsulatum*, dermatophytes
Physical	Cold, x-ray, trauma, UV irradiation, poison ivy
Endocrine	Menses, pregnancy
Drugs	Allopurinol, antibiotics (especially penicillin and sulfa), anticonvulsants (especially phenytoin), antipyretics, analgesics, aspirin, corticosteroids, gold, hydralazine, mercury, nickel, NSAIDs, phenolphthalein, phenylbuta-zone, sulfonamides, sulfonylureas, tetracycline
Neoplasia	Internal malignancy, leukemia, lymphoma, multiple myeloma, myeloid metaplasia, polycythemia
Rheumatologic	Dermatomyositis, SLE (Rowell's syndrome), polyarteritis nodosa, rheumatoid arthritis, Wegener's granulomatosis , inflammatory bowel disease, Behçet's
Contact	Fine sponge, poison ivy and oak, primula allergens
Miscellaneous	Beer drinkers, tooth extraction, food (margarine emulsifiers), Reiter's syndrome

Clinical Presentation and Types

- Acute, self-limited skin disease characterized by abrupt onset of symmetrical fixed red papules which evolve into target lesions. Two types of target lesions (favor acral sites):
  - Typical, with at least three different zones
  - Atypical papular with only two different zones and/or poorly defined border
- Lesions may be bullous
- The two spectra are now divided into (1) EM consisting of erythema minor and major (EMM) and (2) SJS/TEN. The clinical descriptions are as follows:
  - **EM minor** – Typical targets or raised, edematous papules distributed acrally
  - **EM major** – Typical targets or raised, edematous papules distributed acrally with involvement of one or more mucous membranes; epidermal detachment involves less than 10% of total body surface area (TBSA)

○ **SJS/TEN** – Widespread blisters predominant on the trunk and face, presenting with erythematous or pruritic macules and one or more mucous membrane erosions; epidermal detachment is less than 10% TBSA for SJS and 30% or more for TEN

Labs

- CBC – ↑ WBC with atypical lymphocytes (if ↑↑, consider infection). Eosinophil may be ↑. Mild ↓ in Hgb/Hct may be present.
- Electrolytes values may be abnormal with severe skin and mucous membrane involvement due to fluid losses. These values are useful to guide volume and electrolyte replacement therapy.
- BUN and creatinine tests are indicated to screen for renal involvement and dehydration in severe cases requiring hospitalization
- LFTs may be abnormal with hepatic involvement
- ESR may be ↑ but is nonspecific
- Cultures are indicated in severe cases and should be obtained from blood, sputum, and mucosal lesions
- CXR if pulmonary symptoms

DDx – SJS/TEN, fixed drug eruption (in some cases), allergic contact dermatitis, bullous pemphigoid, paraneoplastic pemphigus, drug eruption, urticarial vasculitis, lupus

Histology – findings are not specific but are useful for ruling out other conditions

- Necrotic keratinocytes with basal layer liquefaction (sometimes subepidermal blister)
- Edema in papillary dermis with perivascular or interface lymphocytes (rarely eosinophils)
- Sometimes see spongiosis with intraepidermal vesicles

Treatment

- Prophylaxis for recurrence of herpetic-associated EM should be considered in patients with more than five attacks per year
  ○ Low-dose acyclovir (200 mg qd to 400 mg bid) can be effective for recurrence of HAEM, even in subclinical HSV infection. In children, the dosage of 10 mg/kg/day may be considered.
  ○ Prophylaxis may be required for 6–12 months or longer
  ○ If unresponsive, continuous therapy of valacyclovir (500 mg bid) has been reported to be effective

- Alternative treatments include dapsone, antimalarials, azathioprine, cimetidine, thalidomide
- For all forms of EM: symptomatic treatment, including oral antihistamines, analgesics, local skin care, and soothing mouthwashes, is of great importance. Topical steroids may be considered.
  - Oral involvement – triamcinolone dental paste may be helpful
- Systemic corticosteroids given in severe cases

Pearls and Pitfalls

- Stevens–Johnson syndrome (SJS) was considered an extreme variant of EM for many years, while toxic epidermal necrolysis (TEN) was considered a different entity
  - However, in 1993, a group of medical experts proposed a consensus definition and classification of EM, SJS, and TEN based on a photographic atlas and extent of body surface area involvement. According to the consensus definition, SJS was separated from the EM spectrum and added to TEN. Essentially, SJS and TEN are considered severity variants of a single entity

Erythema Nodosum (EN)

Etiology and Pathogenesis

- Currently, the most common cause of EN is streptococcal infection in children and streptococcal infection and sarcoidosis in adults
- **Bacterial infections** – streptococcal, tuberculosis, *Yersinia, Mycoplasma pneumoniae*, lymphogranuloma venereum, *salmonella, campylobacter*, brucellosis, *E. coli, chlamydia pneumonia* or *trachomatis*
- **Mycobacterial infections** – tuberculosis, EN leprosum (is a LCV)
- **Fungal infections** – coccidioidomycosis (good prognosis), histoplasmosis, blastomycosis
- **Viral** – upper respiratory infection, hepatitis B, HIV
- **Drugs** – oral contraceptives, sulfonamides, gold, sulfonylureas, penicillin, bromides, iodides
- **GI** – Crohn's disease > ulcerative colitis, giardiasis
- **Heme/onc** – Hodgkin disease and lymphoma; reports of EN preceding the onset of acute **myelogenous** leukemia have been published
- **Sarcoid** – most common cutaneous presentation is EN
  - Lofgren syndrome – characteristic form of acute sarcoidosis involves the association of EN, hilar lymphadenopathy, fever, arthritis, and uveitis. Good prognosis with complete resolution within several months in most patients.
- **Pregnancy** – especially in second trimester
- **Other** – syphilis, idiopathic, neutrophilic dermatoses (Sweet's syndrome, Behçet's)

Clinical Presentation

- Symmetric, acute, nodular, erythematous eruption that usually is limited to the extensor aspects
  - Usually occur on legs > thighs or forearms > trunk, neck, and face
  - Unlike other forms of panniculitides, ulceration is not a feature
  - Can get systemic symptoms, particularly with the eruptive phase – arthralgias (or may precede eruption), fever, malaise (not necessarily related to a systemic disease)
- Findings suggestive of a systemic cause for erythema nodosum
  - Synovitis
  - Diarrhea
  - Abnormal CXR
  - Preceding upper respiratory infection
  - Positive PPD
  - ↑ antistreptolysin O and/or anti-DNase B titers

Labs – ESR (often high), antistreptolysin titer (ASO), throat culture to exclude group A beta-hemolytic strept, stool exam if GI complaints, CXR (sarcoid, TB eval), PPD

DDx – cellulitis, erythema induratum (nodular vasculitis), insect bites, pseudolymphoma, urticaria, thrombophlebitis, other panniculitides

Histology

- Septal panniculitis of lymphocytes, histiocytes, neutrophils, and/or eosinophils. Multinucleated giant cells in older lesions, without caseation.
- Miescher's microgranulomas is seen in early lesions → characteristic if not pathognomonic
- Septal fibrosis in older lesions.
- Occasionally see mild fat necrosis with foamy histiocytes

Treatment

- Treat underlying cause; d/c causative medications.
- Symptomatic relief – **NSAIDs**, cool wet compresses, elevation, bed rest
  ○ Naproxen 275 mg PO q 6–8 h
- **Corticosteroids** are effective but seldom necessary in self-limited disease
- Saturated solution of potassium iodide (**SSKI**) may relieve lesional tenderness, arthralgia, and fever
  ○ 150–300 mg PO TID for 3–4 week. Mask with juice (bitter aftertaste).
  ○ Do not to exceed 15 gtt TID
  ○ Do not use during pregnancy. Caution in thyroid disease.
  ○ Acute SE – nausea, excessive salivation, urticarial, angioedema, vasculitis
  ○ Chronic SE – enlargement of salivary and lacrimal glands, acneiform eruption, iododerma, hypothyroidism, ↑ potassium, occasionally hyperthyroidism
- **Colchicine** has been used in a few refractory cases with good results
  ○ 0.5–1.2 mg PO initially, followed by 0.5–0.6 q 1–2 h or 1–1.2 mg q 2 h until response is satisfactory; not to exceed 4 mg/day
- Dapsone
- Hydroxychloroquine
- Mycophenolate
- Other – infliximab (if inflammatory bowel disease), cyclosporine (especially in setting of Behçet's)

Pearls and Pitfalls

- Discard SSKI if solution turns yellow-brown. Crystallization may occur with cold temperatures, but rewarming and shaking dissolves these crystals.
- There are reports of SSKI triggering erythema nodosum

Erythrasma

Etiology and Pathogenesis

- Chronic superficial infection of the intertriginous areas of skin – *Corynebacterium minutissimum*
- Coral red fluorescence of scales seen under Wood light is secondary to the production of porphyrin by these diphtheroids

Clinical Presentation

- Pink-red, well-defined patches that are covered with fine scaling and wrinkles. Color fades to brown with time. Most are asymptomatic but mild pruritus may be seen.
- **Distribution** – common on inner thighs, crural region, scrotum, and toe webs. Less common –axillae, submammary area, periumbilical region, and intergluteal fold. Toe web lesions appear as maceration.
- **Risk factors**
  - Heat, occlusion, humidity, hyperhidrosis, warm climate, advanced age, poor hygiene, obesity, diabetes (especially if recurrent erythrasma), immunocompromised state
- **Variant** – a generalized "discform" variant may occur outside the typical intertriginous areas. This form can be the presenting manifestation of type-2 diabetes mellitus

Labs – Wood's light examination reveals **coral-red fluorescence** of lesions; Gram staining reveals gram-positive filamentous rods

DDx – acanthosis nigricans, cutaneous candidiasis, allergic contact dermatitis, irritant contact dermatitis, intertrigo, psoriasis, seb derm, tinea corporis, tinea cruris, tinea pedis, tinea versicolor, pruritus ani

Histology – Filamentous bacteria seen in stratum corneum with Giemsa stain

Treatment

- Erythromycin EES (drug of choice)
  - 250 mg PO qid or 500 mg PO BID for 7–10 days
  - 2–4% solution: Apply to affected area BID for 4–6 week

- Clarithromycin (Biaxin)
  - 1 g PO once
  - Peds: 15 mg/kg PO once
- Miconazole cream 2% – apply BID for 2 weeks (Lotrimin)
- Benzoic acid 6%, salicylic acid 3% (Whitfield's ointment) – apply BID for 4 weeks
- Clindamycin 2% soln – TID × 1 week
- *C. minutissimum* is generally susceptible to penicillins, first-generation cephalosporins, erythromycin, clindamycin, ciprofloxacin, tetracycline (250 mg QID for 14 days), and vancomycin. However, multiresistant strains have been isolated.

Pearls and Pitfalls

- Results of Wood's light examination may be negative if the patient bathed prior to presentation
- Antibacterial soaps may be used initially and prophylactically once infection has cleared

Erythroderma

Etiology and Pathogenesis

- May be the end result of any number of dermatoses
- SCALP DIG: Seb derm, scabies, CTCL, contact dermatitis, atopic dermatitis, lymphoma/leukemia, psoriasis, PRP, drug reaction, idiopathic, GVHD
  - Also – ichthyoses, pemphigoid, pemphigus, dermatophytosis, lichen planus, Leiner disease, sarcoid, connective tissue disease such as dermatomyositis
- **Neonates and infants** – ichthyoses, immunodeficiencies, psoriasis, staphylococcal scalded skin syndrome, drug induced
- **Common drugs** – allopurinol, beta-lactam antibiotics, antiepileptic meds, gold, phenobarbital, sulfasalazine, sulfonamides, zalcitabine

Clinical Presentation

- Scaling erythematous dermatitis involving 90% or more of the cutaneous surface
- Erythema often begins on the trunk and expands within a few days to weeks. Erythema is followed by scaling.
- Pruritus is most common complaint and varies with cause (severe in atopic dermatitis and Sézary syndrome)
- Lymphadenopathy common
- Hepatomegaly in 20% of patients
- Complications of erythroderma
  - Temperature dysregulation (resulting in heat loss and hypothermia) and possible high-output cardiac failure (especially in the elderly)
  - Fluid loss by transpiration is increased in proportion to the basal metabolic rate
  - Marked loss of exfoliated scales occurs that may reach 20–30 g/day. This contributes to the hypoalbuminemia commonly observed in ED. Hypoalbuminemia results, in part, from decreased synthesis or increased metabolism of albumin.
  - Edema and alopecia
  - Immune responses may be altered – ↓ CD4, ↑ IgE
  - Secondary *Staphylococcus aureus* infection

Labs

- Frequent – ↑ ESR, anemia, hypoalbuminemia, hyperglobulinemia
- ↑ IgE may be seen in ED when caused by atopic dermatitis
- Peripheral blood smears and bone marrow exam may be useful in leukemia workup

- Immunophenotyping, flow cytometry, and particularly, B- and T-cell gene rearrangement analysis may be helpful in confirming Dx if lymphoma strongly suspected
- Skin scrapings may reveal hyphae or scabies mites
- Cultures may show bacterial overgrowth or the herpes simplex virus
- Consider HIV testing (PCR instead of ELISA – detect seroconversion)
- Decreased CD4$^+$ T-cell count was observed in patients without HIV disease

Histology – Histopathologic features of the underlying disease are seen in 2/3 of patients, but may be subtle

Treatment

- Discontinue unnecessary meds
- Carefully monitor and control fluid intake
  - Patients can dehydrate or go into cardiac failure
  - Risk of hypernatremic dehyrdation
- Monitor body temp – risk of hypothermia
- Monitor nutrition – consider nutrition consult or eval
- Wet wraps; change q 2–3 h. Apply intermediate-strength topical steroids (triamcinolone cream 0.1%) beneath wet dressings.
- Dry skin care
- Initiate systemic antibiotics if signs of secondary infection are observed
- Control pruritus – antihistamines, emollients, etc.
- Systemic steroids (prednisone 1–2 mg/kg) may be helpful – avoid in suspected cases of psoriasis, SSSS
- Further treatment based on likely underlying cause of erythroderma (Ex: PRP → Soriatane; Psoriasis → cyclosporine, etc.)
- Consider IVIG in severe cases

Pearls and Pitfalls

- When to hospitalize:
  - Consider in the elderly – higher risk of high-output cardiac failure
  - Neonates
  - Severe thermoregulatory dysfunction
  - Any patient showing signs of malnutrition, severe electrolyte imbalances
  - If secondary infection
- If splenomegaly is seen on exam, consider possibility of lymphoma
- Due to increased transcutaneous absorption (not to mention irritation), avoid topical salicylic acid and topical lactic acid

Folliculitis

- **Infectious folliculitis**
  - Multiple small papules and pustules on an erythematous base that are pierced by a central hair, although the hair may not always be visualized. Deeper lesions manifest as erythematous, often fluctuant, nodules.
  - Sometimes, a patterned folliculitis occurs in areas that were shaved or occluded. Any hair-bearing site can be affected, but the sites most often involved are the face, scalp, thighs, axilla, and inguinal area.
  - Superficial
    - Impetigo of Bockhart → staph
    - Sty → occurs on eyelid; staph
  - Deep
    - Folliculocentric dermal abscess
      - When the condition occurs on the face, it is referred to as sycosis barbae (vulgaris)
      - If it occurs elsewhere, it is referred to as a furuncle (or boil). A confluence of several furuncles results in a carbuncle
- **Herpetic folliculitis**
  - Infection by herpes simplex viruses 1 and 2 and is found in areas adjacent to a primary cold sore. It is spread by shaving.
  - These lesions appear as grouped or scattered vesicles
  - Treatment – responds to valacyclovir, famciclovir, or acyclovir
- **Demodex folliculitis**
  - Occurs as a result of either overgrowth of *Demodex folliculorum* mites or an acquired hypersensitivity to the mite
  - Clinical – perifollicular scaling or rosacea-like erythematous follicular papules and pustules with a background of erythema on the face
  - Treatment – permethrin cream, ivermectin
- **Pityrosporum folliculitis**
  - Young adults, with a slight female predominance
  - Intensively pruritic small uniform papules and pustules on the back, chest, shoulders
  - It occurs more often in warm, humid climates and may be more frequent in immunocompromised patients or in patients on long-term antibiotics
  - This eruption is due to follicular infection by *Malassezia furfur,* which is a lipophilic yeast
  - Treatment
    - Initially responds to topical antifungals – ketoconazole cream or shampoo but often associated with relapses
    - For relapses, systemic antifungals should be tried

- **Gram-negative folliculitis**
  - Primarily occurs in patients on long-term antibiotic therapy, often antibiotics given for the treatment of acne
  - This type of folliculitis arises from disequilibrium of the normal skin bacteria in favor of gram-negative organisms such as *Enterobacter, Klebsiella, Escherichia, Serratia,* and *Proteus* species
  - These lesions manifest as multiple small pustules that are most pronounced in the perinasal region and can spread to the chin and cheeks
  - Treatment – isotretinoin
- **Actinic folliculitis** – sun-induced, rare
- **Eosinophilic folliculitis– Three Types**
  - **Ofuji disease**
    - Arises in Japanese males at an average age of 30 years
    - Lesions begin as discrete papules and pustules that eventually coalesce to form circinate plaques composed of a peripheral rim of pustules with central clearing
    - These lesions appear cyclically on the face, back, and extensor surfaces of the arms and spontaneously resolve in 7–10 days. Often, peripheral eosinophilia is present
  - **HIV-AIDS related**
    - Seen most often in adult males with a CD4$^+$ count of less than 250–300 cells/µL
    - Persistent and does not form an annular pattern
    - Lesions tend to favor the face, scalp, and upper trunk
  - **Infantile form**
    - Usually within the first 24 h to first few weeks of life
    - More common in male infants and usually is self-limited; however, as in Ofuji disease, it may follow a cyclic course lasting months to years
    - Lesions primarily affect the scalp and eyebrows
    - This form may also be associated with peripheral eosinophilia
  - Treatment (in no particular order)
    - Topical corticosteroids – useful for initial tx
    - Tacrolimus – also useful for initial tx
    - Pimecrolimus
    - Indomethacin – 50–75 mg/day; use short term (< 1 week) – can cause peptic ulcers
    - Metronidazole – 250 mg TID
    - Pruritus → Cetirizine – 20–40 mg/day, cyproheptadine 2–4 mg/day
    - PUVA or UVB phototherapy → phototherapy tends to help only while on tx; disease flares when tx stopped
    - Itraconazole – start at 200 mg/day and increasing to 300–400 mg/day
    - Isotretinoin – 1 mg/kg/day
    - Acitretin – 0.5 mg/kg/day
    - Cephalexin
    - Doxycycline or Minocycline – 100 mg PO BID

- Dapsone – 50–100 mg BID
- Cyclosporine 5 mg/kg/day
- Topical 5% permethrin
- Interferon (IFN)-alpha-2b
- IFN-gamma
- Transdermal nicotine patches also reported to help eosinophilic folliculitis
  o Notes on Treatment (HIV-associated eosinophilic folliculitis)
- Clinicians should be aware that EF may develop within 3–6 months of initiation antiretroviral therapy
- Paradoxically, although EF may develop with initiation of HAART, it also responds well to HAART – tends to dissipate once CD4 gets above 250–300
- EF does not respond well to tx unless immune system is being restored

References:

(1) Ellis E and Scheinfeld N. Eosinophilic pustular folliculitis: a comprehensive review of treatment options. Am J Clin Dermatol. 2004; 5(3): 189–97.
(2) Nervi SJ, Schwartz RA and Dmochowski M. Eosinophilic pustular folliculitis: A 40 year retrospect. JAAD 206; 55(2): 285–9.

Flushing

Etiology and Pathogenesis

- Increase in cutaneous blood flow occurs with relaxation of vascular smooth muscle and may be triggered by the autonomic nervous system, endogenous vasoactive agents (such as histamine, serotonin) or exogenous agents
- Can be episodic or constant. Episodic attacks are generally mediated by release of endogenous vasoactive mediators or by drugs. Repetitive flushing over long periods (persistent flushing) may produce fixed facial erythema with telangiectasias and a cyanotic tinge.
  - Dry Flushing → usually results from agents that act directly on vascular smooth muscle
  - Wet Flushing – associated with sweating → indicates autonomic hyperactivation
- Causes
  - **Physiologic**
  - **Exogenous agents**
    - **Medications** → ACE-inhibitors, calcium-channel blockers, calcitonin, chlorpropamide, cholinergic agents such as pilocarpine, cyclosporine, disulfiram, flutamide, fumaric acid esters, gold, hydralazine, IV contrast dye, leuprolide, methylprednisolone, metoclopramide, nicotine, nicotinic acid, nitrates, opiates, prostaglandins, sildenafil, tadalafil, vancomycin, vardenafil, tamoxifen
      - □ **Chemotherapy** → doxorubicin, mithramycin, dacarbazine, cisplatin, interferon-alpha 2
    - **Food** → MSG, sodium nitrite, sulfites, spoiled scomboid fish
    - **Alcohol** → may result from both direct effects and from cutaneous vasodilation from elevated blood levels of acetaldehyde (seen in alcohol dehydrogenase deficiency and common in Asians). Tyramine may also lead to flushing and is in some fermented alcoholic drinks
  - **Menopause**
  - **Neurologic disorders** → anxiety, autonomic dysfunction, tumors, migraine, Frey syndrome, multiple sclerosis, Parkinson's disease, trigeminal nerve damage, Horner syndrome
  - **Systemic diseases** → Carcinoid syndrome (flushing, bronchospasm, diarrhea, right-sided cardiac dysfunction, hypotension, peptic ulcers), mastocytosis, pheochromocytoma, medullary thyroid carcinoma, thyrotoxicosis, POEMS syndrome, pancreatic cell tumor (VIP tumor), prostaglandin-secreting renal cell carcinoma

Clinical Presentation

- Sensation of warmth accompanied by visible reddening of the skin
- "Classic carcinoid flush" – seen in 10% of midgut tumors (small intestine, appendix, proximal colon), lasts minutes, and consists of erythema and pallor as well as a cyanotic hue. Liver metastases are required.
  - Type III gastric carcinoid tumors – associated with a pruritic patchy bright red flush admixed with white patches, which is probably mediated by histamine
  - Hindgut tumors (distal colon, rectum) are rarely, if ever, associated with carcinoid syndrome and flushing, even with liver metastases
- Bronchial tumors are associated with a prolonged (hours to days) intensely red to purple flush

Labs and Imaging to Consider

- CBC + diff and thyroid function tests
- Serum tryptase, histamine → **Mastocytosis**
- Chromogranin A levels → elevated in **neuroendocrine tumors, pheochromocytoma, pancreas and prostate CA, carcinoid syndrome, diabetes,** plasma free metanephrines
- UPEP/SPEP and/or urine/serum IFE
- Urinalysis → hematuria may be present with **renal cell carcinoma**
- Elevated vasoactive intestinal peptide (VIP) → elevated with **pancreatic cell carcinoma**
- Elevated calcitonin (+ thyroid nodule) → **medullary thyroid carcinoma**
- 24 h urine collection for:
  - Serotonin metabolites such as 5-hydroxyindole acetic acid (5-HIAA) → **Carcinoid**
  - Fractionated metanephrines (metanephrine, normetanephrine, total metanephrine), norepinephrine, VMA, catecholamines → **pheochromocytoma**
  - PDG2 metabolites, histamine metabolites such as methylimidazole acetic acid (MIAA) → **Mastocytosis**
- CT/MRI scans; somatostatin receptor scintigraphy (using radiolabeled analogue of somatostatin)

DDx – rosacea, photodamage, photosensitive disorder, autoimmune connective tissue disease

Treatment and Management

- History, physical exam
  - Ask patient to keep a diary for 2 weeks. Document the timeline of . . .
    - Flushing reactions, their qualitative aspects, associations (dyspnea, bronchospasm, lightheadedness, hypoglycemia, tachycardia, abdominal cramps, diarrhea, HA, urticaria, pruritus) and all exogenous agents (food, drugs, physical exertion, alcohol, emotion, stress, occupational exposures)
  - Exclude suspected drugs and food additives if triggers
- If associated urticaria and pruritus, consider a histamine-mediated reactions (such as mastocytosis, vancomycin, and other mast cell-degranulation agents)
- Medical management
  - Non-selective beta-blockers – propranolol, nadolol
  - Clonidine
  - Menopausal flushing → clonidine or SSRIs

Pearls and Pitfalls

- Check for associated symptoms – sweating, urticarial, diarrhea, bronchospasm
- Consider referral to endocrine (if endocrine abnormalities) or allergy (if anaphylaxis may be present)
- Potential mast cell degranulators
  - Meds – aspirin, opiates, dextromethorphan, NSAIDs, amphotericin B, thiamine, polymyxin B, tetracaine, procaine, iodine-containing contrast media, D-tubocurarine, scopolamine, gallamine, pancuronium, decamethonium
  - Venoms – bee stings, jellyfish, snakebites
  - Foods – egg whites, crayfish, lobster, chocolate, strawberries, tomatoes, citrus, alcohol
  - Physical – exercise, heat, hot baths, hot beverages, cold exposure, sunlight, stress

Genital Ulcers – Infectious Etiologies

Table 67 Genital ulcer diseases – infectious causes (Excluding herpes simplex – see "herpes" section)

	Primary syphilis	Chancroid	Granuloma inguinale	Lymphogranuloma venereum
Causative organism	*T. pallidum*	*H. ducreyi*	*Klebsiella granulomatosis (formerly Calymmatobacterium granulomatosis)*	*Chlamydia trachomatis L1, L2, L3*
Characteristic clinical features	**Painless** chancre with "ham-colored" base and sharply defined, indurated border Chancre has cartilage-like consistency and exudes clear fluid Bilateral	Soft, **painful** chancre with ragged edges "School of fish" on Gram or Giemsa stain Plate quickly b/c organism only survives 24 h on swab Culture can be difficult – use two different media	Primary lesion: papule, subcutaneous nodule (pseudobubo), or ulcer Four clinical forms: ulcerovegetative (most common – especially in genital area), nodular, hypertrophic, and cicatricial **Donovan bodies ("safety pin"** shaped intracytoplasmic inclusions in macrophages) seen on microscopy	**Painless,** soft erosion that heals spontaneously Secondary inguinal adenopathy with fluctuant, tender nodes above and below Poupart's ligament – "Groove sign" (can be bilateral) Serologic diagnosis by complement fixation test
Treatment	Penicillin	Azithromycin Ceftriaxone Ciprofloxacin Erythromycin	TMP-SMX Doxycycline Erythromycin Ciprofloxacin	Doxycycline

Pearls and Pitfalls

- In the HIV population (particularly in MSM), consider
  - Consider penile amebiasis on your differential of penile ulcerations
  - HIV as an etiology
  - Herpes simplex (resistance to acyclovir becoming more common)
  - CMV (in the anal area)
- Knife-cut fissures in the groin/genital area are classic for cutaneous Crohn's disease. GI involvement may or may not be present with cutaneous Crohn's (i.e., the absence of GI involvement does NOT rule out cutaneous Crohn's)
- Scrotal, penile, or labia edema – consider Crohn's, sarcoid, or even hidradenitis (if a lot of drainage)

Granuloma Annulare (GA)

Etiology and Pathogenesis

- Etiology unknown, but reported inciting factors have included: insect bites, trauma, tuberculin skin testing, sun exposure, PUVA therapy, viral infections
- May be a delayed hypersensitivity reaction to an unknown antigen

Clinical Presentation and Types

- Very common in children
- Benign, usually self-limited skin disease that presents as arcuate to annular plaques
  ○ Plaques may be pink-violaceous in color and are often made up of small papules
- Distribution – often on the extremities (hands/arms > legs and feet > both upper and lower extremities > trunk. Facial lesions are rare.
- **Variants**
  ○ **Localized GA (most common)**
  ○ **Subcutaneous/deep GA** – large, painless, skin-colored nodules. Typically on palms, hands, anterior tibial surfaces, and feet and buttocks. Rarely see scalp and eyelid involvement. 50% also have classic GA lesions.
  ○ **Perforating GA** – small papules with central umbilications, crusts, or focal ulcerations
  ○ **Generalized GA** – pink to violaceous papules coalescing into larger plaques and covering a large body surface area
  ○ **Patch GA** – patches of erythema on extremities and trunk. Symmetrical lesions on the dorsum of the feet usually present as "patch GA".
  ○ Some consider **actinic granuloma** (annular elastolytic giant cell granuloma) to be a subset of GA.

Labs – Consider lipid prolife and fasting glucose in generalized GA.

DDx

- **DDx Localized GA** → annular lichen planus, erythema annulare centrifugum, erythema elevatum diutinum, erythema migrans of Lyme disease, Hansen's disease, necrobiosis lipoidica diabeticorum
- **DDx Generalized GA** → cutaneous mets, cutaneous paraneoplastic syndrome, lichen myxedematous, lichen planus, sarcoidosis

- **DDx Subcutaneous/Deep GA** → epithelioid sarcoma, rheumatoid nodule
- **DDx Perforating GA** →elastosis perforans serpiginosa, molloscum contagiosum, perforating collagenosis
- **DDx Actinic granuloma** → erythema annulare centrifugum, necrobiosis lipoidica diabeticorum, sarcoidosis

Histology

- Normal epidermis
- In the dermis, see palisading granulomas around small foci of mild connective tissue degeneration (necrobiosis) and mucin accumulation
- Often see single-filing or subtle interstitial pattern of histiocytes or giant cells between collagen bundles
- Perivascular lymphocytes and eosinophils sometimes
- Perforating GA → Exhibits transepidermal elimination of degenerating collagen

Treatment

- **Localized GA**
  - Not often symptomatic and tends to resolve → reassurance
  - Spontaneous resolution within 20 years in 50% of cases. Recurrence in 40%.
  - Potent topical steroids +/− occlusion for 4–6 weeks
  - IL steroids
  - Cryotherapy (but can get secondary dyschromia) – not helpful for deep GA
  - Tacrolimus/pimecrolimus
  - Imiquimod cream
- **Generalized GA**
  - Rare spontaneous resolution, poor response to treatment and frequent relapses
  - Isotretinoin – this and light tx tend to be first-line treatment
  - Phototherapy → PUVA
  - Dapsone
  - Systemic corticosteroids
  - Pentoxifylline
  - Hydroxychloroquine
  - Cyclosporine
  - Potassium iodide
  - Nicotinamide

Pearls and Pitfalls

- Generalized GA → may be associated with lipid abnormalities, diabetes
- Classic GA and perforating GA – may occur in herpes zoster scars
- Atypical variants have been associated with HIV infection
- GA has been described as a paraneoplastic phenomenon – solid organ tumors, Hodgkin disease, non-Hodgkin lymphoma, and granulomatous mycosis fungoides. Clinical pattern is usually atypical, lesions are painful and in unusual locations (including the palms and soles).

Granuloma Faciale

Etiology and Pathogenesis

- Immunofluorescence microscopy has demonstrated IgG, IgA, IgM, and C3 within blood vessels, which supports a role for immune complexes. Exact pathogenesis unknown.

Clinical Presentation

- Solitary or, more commonly, multiple, soft, elevated, well-circumscribed papules or plaques
- Color varies from shades of dull red to brown, blue-violaceous
- Lesions have a smooth surface with peau d'orange appearance; may see telangiectasias
- Lesions vary in size from a few millimeters to several centimeters in diameter
- Distribution – Most common on face. Extrafacial lesions typically on – scalp, the trunk, and the upper and lower extremities. Common for the extrafacial lesions to involve sun-exposed areas.
- Usually asymptomatic, but may be tender, pruritic, or have a stinging sensation

DDx – fixed drug eruption, acute febrile neutrophilic dermatosis, alopecia mucinosa, amyloidosis (nodular, localized cutaneous), angiolymphoid hyperplasia with eosinophilia, CTCL, pseudolymphoma, Jessner's, DLE, lymphocytoma cutis, sarcoid, foreign body granuloma, leprosy

Histology

- Below the grenz zone ("border") is a dense, polymorphous inflammatory infiltrate (neutrophils, lymphocytes, eosinophils, monocytes, and, occasionally, mast cells) in the papillary, mid dermis.
- Vasculitic changes, including perivascular inflammation with nuclear dust and vessel wall damage, are often observed.
- Extravasated RBCs, hemosiderin deposition (may contribute to the color of the lesions).
- Later, lesions may show considerable fibrosis around venules.
- **DIF** – IgG, fibrin, and occasionally IgM, at basement membrane zone and around vessels.

Treatment

- *Notoriously difficult to treat*
- Pulsed Dye Laser (585 nm) – some recommend trying this first because if they respond (and many do), then the patient is not committed to indefinite systemic treatment
- Topical corticosteroids and/or intralesional steroids
- Anecdotal reports of success with – antimalarials, PUVA, tacrolimus ointment 0.1% BID, dapsone 25–200 mg/day (check G6PD prior), clofazamine (lamprene) 50–300 mg/day, oral bismuth

Pearls and Pitfalls

- Extrafacial granuloma faciale can be difficult to distinguish from erythema elevatinum diutinum (EED), both clinically and histologically
  - ○ Clinically – EED usually presents on the extensor extremities and typically affects the skin overlying joints
  - ○ Histologically – EED typically lacks a grenz zone. The vasculitis is usually more pronounced and neutrophils predominate over eosinophils in EED. Prominent lipid-laden macrophages may be seen in EED, but not in granuloma faciale

Hand Dermatitis

- Patterns of hand dermatitis
  - *Hyperkeratotic* – "Tylotic Eczema" (2%)
    - Painful fissures
    - 40–60 year olds
  - *Atopic* (22%)
    - Volar wrist
    - Dorsal hand
  - *Nummular Eczema*
    - Asymmetric
    - Distal fingers, dorsal hands
    - Can be associated with positive patch test
  - *Dyshidrotic Eczema* (Pompholyx)
    - Marked outbreaks and healing
    - Risks: Tinea pedis, AD, ACD to nickel/cobalt, stress
  - *Chronic Vesicular*
    - Unknown etiology
    - Debilitating
    - Radiation tx may be effective
    - Huge negative effect on quality of life
  - *Frictional Hand Eczema* – "Pressure Dermatitis"
    - Absence of vesicles and pruritus
    - Protected areas spared
    - Common risks – handling small metal objects, paper, cardboard, driving
      - Paper handlers – see on first three fingers
  - *Irritant Contact Dermatitis* (30%)
    - Can precede ACD
    - Quickly occurs with reexposure
    - Combination risks: irritation, friction, high/low humidity
  - *Allergic Contact Dermatitis*
    - Involvement of dorsal hand > than in ICD > AD
    - Dorsal fingers > ICD > AD
    - Type IV hypersensitivty
    - Symptoms worsen 8–96 h post challenge
    - ACD more common in patients who already have an irritant dermatitis (can start as one and morph into another)
  - *Psoriasis*
    - Assess for skin, nail changes
    - Some forms pustular
- **Reasons to patch test**
  - Worsening endogenous dermatitis (atopy, psoriasis)
  - Changing pattern of dermatitis
  - High index of suspicion

- o If **no** itching, consider *not* patch testing
  - ■ Itching → ACD
  - ■ Burning → irritant dermatitis
- **Clues to Occupational or Avocational ACD**
  - o One hand worse than another
  - o Determine dominant handedness
- Know what gloves protect against what chemicals
  - o www.contactderm.org → shows you what gloves protect against what chemicals and what gloves contain
    - ■ Need to be a member
- Allergens missed by TRUE test (not a complete list)
  - o Occupational chemicals
  - o Corticosteroids (A, B)
  - o Dyes
  - o Preservatives
  - o Detergents
  - o Balsam of Peru
  - o Bacitracin
  - o Acrylates used in dentistry, artificial nails, and printing
  - o Pesticides
  - o Plastics, glues, rubbers
  - o UV protectants
- Treatment
  - o Detailed history – occupational, cosmetics, hobbies
  - o Consider patch testing
  - o Topical corticosteroids
  - o Dry skin care
  - o Emollients – Vaseline, CeraVe, Cetaphil
  - o Antihistamines
  - o Protopic, Elidel
  - o Tar-containing products – Balnetar soaks, etc.
  - o Light therapy
    - ■ UVA – hand/foot box – 3x/week
    - ■ Topical PUVA 3x/week
    - ■ NBUVB
  - o Methotrexate
  - o Steroid-sparing immunosuppressants (rarely use)
  - o Disulfiram: Occasionally, an individual who is highly allergic to nickel with severe vesicular hand dermatitis benefits from treatment with disulfiram (Antabuse). The chelating effect of disulfiram is helpful in reducing the body's nickel burden. Alcohol ingestion may produce severe adverse reactions in patients taking disulfiram.

Herpes Simplex

Etiology and Pathogenesis

- Two types exist: type 1 (HSV-1) and type 2 (HSV-2)
  - HSV belongs to the family Herpesviridae and to the subfamily Alphaherpesvirinae, and is a double-stranded DNA virus
- The reactivation and replication of latent HSV can be induced by a variety of stimuli (e.g., fever, trauma, emotional stress, sunlight, menstruation), resulting in overt or covert recurrent infection and peripheral shedding of HSV
- HSV-1 and 2 can both be present in either oral or genital locations; HSV-1 more likely to reactivate in oral region and HSV-2 more likely to reactivate in genital location

Clinical Presentation

- Herpes simplex infections are asymptomatic in as many as 80% of patients
- **Acute herpetic gingivostomatitis** – manifestation of primary HSV-1
  - Children ages 6 months to 5 years, from saliva of adult or another child
  - Adults can develop this – less severe, presents as pharyngitis
  - Incubation of 3–6 days; abrupt onset of fever (102–104), anorexia, striking gingivitis, vesicular lesions in mouth, tender lymphadenopathy
  - Acute sx resolve in 5–7 days; course usually completed in 2 weeks
- **Acute herpetic pharyngotonsillitis**
  - In adults, oropharyngeal HSV-1 causes pharyngitis and tonsillitis more often than gingivostomatitis
  - Vesicles rupture to form ulcerative lesions with grayish exudates on the tonsils and the posterior pharynx
  - Fever, malaise, headache, sore throat
- **Herpes labialis**
  - Most common manifestation of recurrent HSV-1
  - Prodrome of pain, burning, and tingling often occur at the site, followed by the development of erythematous papules that rapidly develop into tiny, thin-walled, intraepidermal vesicles that become pustular and ulcerate
  - In most patients, fewer than two recurrences manifest each year, but some individuals have monthly recurrences
  - Maximum viral shedding is in first 24 h of the acute illness but may last five days
- **Primary genital herpes**
  - Can be caused by both HSV-1 and HSV-2; More recurrences with HSV-2
  - The incubation period is 3–7 days (range = 1 day to 3 week)
  - Painful genital ulcers

- o Can be associated with constitutional symptoms include fever, headache, malaise, and myalgia (prominent in the first 3–4 days); local symptoms include pain, itching, dysuria, vaginal and urethral discharge, and tender lymphadenopathy
- o Women tend to have more severe symptoms and more complications; shed virus for mean of 12 days
- **Recurrent genital herpes**
  - o In one study, 90% of patients reactivated within the first 12 months
  - o For HSV-2 infection, 38% had six recurrences in 1 year, and 20% had more than ten recurrences in the first year
  - o Lesions are often very painful. Fever and constitutional symptoms are uncommon. Lesions heal in 8–10 days and viral shedding lasts an average 5 days
- **Subclinical genital herpes**
  - o The majority of primary genital HSV infections are asymptomatic, and 70–80% of seropositive individuals have no history of symptomatic genital herpes. Nevertheless, they experience periodic subclinical reactivation with virus shedding, thus making them a source of infection.
  - o This is important in neonatal herpes because most mothers have no signs and symptoms of genital herpes during pregnancy

Labs

- Viral culture is gold standard, but a lot of false negatives → best to aspirate fluid from intact vesicle
- Tzanck smear – does not differentiate between VZV and HSV
  - o Positive result is the finding of multinucleate giant cells
  - o *See section on Tzanck Smear for instructions on how to perform*

DDx – candidiasis, chancroid, syphilis, hand-foot-mouth disease, apthous ulcers, erosive lichen planus, Behçet's

Treatment – *See Herpes Zoster section*

Pearls and Pitfalls

- Virus readily inactivated at room temp and by drying; hence, aerosol and fomitic spread rare
- Can cause increased morbidity and mortality in immunocompromised patients
- Herpes vegetans – verrucous plaques that often signify acyclovir resistance. Seen in immunocompromised patients, especially in HIV.
- Herpes labialis may precipitate a herpes folliculitis on the face in immunocompromised patients on chemotherapy, etc.

Herpes Zoster (HZ)

Etiology and Pathogenesis

- Airborne droplets are usual route of primary varicella (chickenpox), although contact with HZ vesicles is another mode of transmission. During primary varicella infection, viremia follows an initial 2–4 days of replication within regional lymph nodes. A secondary viremia occurs after a second cycle of replication in the liver, spleen, and other organs and seeds the entire body. Skin lesions occur after the virus travels to capillary endothelial cells approximately 14–16 days post exposure. VZV subsequently travels from cutaneous and mucosal lesions to invade the dorsal root ganglion, where it remains until reactivation at a later date.
  - Reactivation may occur spontaneosly or be associated with stress, fever, radiation therapy, tissue damage, or immunosuppression.
  - During herpes zoster outbreak, the virus continues to replicate in the affected dorsal root ganglion and produces severe pain.

Clinical Presentation

- Erythematous papules and plaques develop in a linear, dermatomal distribution. These lesions subsequently progress to grouped vesicles on erythematous bases which later become erosions. Severe pain often *precedes* the skin lesions and is a helpful clue to the diagnosis.
- Rarely crosses the midline (exceptions can occur in HIV patients and the immunocompromised)
- **Complications**
  - **Post-herpetic neuralgia** → more common after age 50
  - Secondary bacterial infection
  - Scarring and depigmentation of hair (in affected area)
  - **Ramsay–Hunt** → due to reactivation of VZV infection of the geniculate ganglion, and in addn to vesicles of the ear canal, tongue and/or hard palate, patients may have acute facial nerve paralysis, pain in the ear, taste loss of the anterior 2/3 of the tongue, and a dry mouth and eyes.
    - If vestibulocochlear nerve also affected → tinnitus, hearing loss, and/or vertigo
  - Meningoencephalitis secondary to herpes zoster is more likely to be seen in immunocompromised patients
  - Disseminated zoster may be seen in immunocompromised patients – hematogenous spread may result in the involvement of multiple dermatomes and organs

- **Variations/other findings**:
  - ○ **Zoster sine herpete** – pain and paresthesias along the dermatome without the development of visible cutaneous involvement
  - ○ **Hutchinson's sign** – Lesions on the tip of the nose signify involvement of the nasociliary nerve; this finding mandates slit-lamp examination with fluorescein stain to look for the dendritic corneal lesions of herpetic keratitis

Labs

- Tzanck smear – does not differentiate between HSV and VZV
- Diagnosis can be confirmed by sending swabs to the laboratory (false negatives); don't delay treatment waiting for culture
  - ○ Lift the top of the lesion and swab the exposed base. The swab should then be rolled across a sterile glass side, which is air dried and sent to the laboratory for staining with immunofluorescent antibodies.
  - ○ The swab can also be placed in viral transport medium for detection of viral DNA by polymerase chain reaction

DDx – allergic contact dermatitis, photoallergic eruption, bullous impetigo, erysipelas, necrotizing fasciitis

Histology – Identical to HSV on routine H&E.

- Intraepidermal vesicle or ulceration
- Epidermal necrosis and ballooning degeneration: Enlarged and pale keratinocytes with steel-gray nuclei, marginization of chromatin at the edge of the nucleus, sometimes with pink intranuclear inclusions surrounded by artifactual cleft (Cowdry type A inclusions, Lipschutz bodies), acantholysis, and multinucleated giant cells

Treatment

- **Topical Medications**
  - ○ **Aluminum Acetate** (Burows' solution, Domeboro powder) – Functions as an astringent (contraction of tissue, decrease of secretions)
    - ▪ Rx: Dissolve one packet of powder or tablet in a pint of water (1:40 solution). Moisten gauze with this solution and apply to affected area. Leave on for 15–20 min, then remove and pat dry.
    - ▪ Avoid topical antivirals – don't work well and may cause irritation

- **Oral Medications (Immunocompetent Host)**
  - Refer to: Dworkin RH, Johnson RW, Breuer J, et al. Management of Herpes Zoster. CID 2007: 44 (Supplement 1).
  - GOALS
    - Decrease viral replication (and subsequent nerve damage) and reduce pain
    - Ideal to give antivirals within 72 h of rash; however, there may still be benefit in giving the med after 72 h to decrease risk of PHN. Give if patient continues to develop new vesicles.
  - **Analgesics**
    - **Gabapentin (Neurontin)** – 300 mg QHS or 100–300 mg TID. Increase by 100–300 mg TID every two days as tolerated. Max dose is 3,600 mg (1,200 mg TID). Reduce if renal impairment. May help decrease PHN.
    - **Pregabalin (Lyrica)** – 75 mg QHS or 75 mg BID. Increase by 75 mg BID every 3 days as tolerated. Max 600 mg QD (300 mg BID). Reduce if renal impairment. May help decrease PHN.
    - NSAIDs, acetaminophen, opioid analgesics (give round the clock, not prn; give preemptive stool softener)
    - TCAs – **Amitriptyline** or **Nortriptyline** (latter preferred) 25 mg PO QHS (can increase by 25 mg QD every 2–3 days as tolerated for max of 150 mg QD.) Baseline EKG for patients > 40. Start 10 mg in elderly.
    - Lidocaine 5% patch – don't give in acute vesicular phase. Useful only for PHN
  - **Antivirals**
    - Acyclovir (may be less effective and not recommended if the other meds are an option), valcyclovir, famciclovir

Table 68 Treatment of herpes infection

	Famciclovir (Famvir)	Valcyclovir (Valtrex)	Acyclovir (Zovirax)
GH – initial episode	Not indicated	1 gm BID – 10 days	200 mg 5x per day – 10 days
Recurrent GH – Episodic	125 mg BID – 5 days (1,000 mg BID for 1 day) HIV patients – 500 mg BID for 7 days	500 mg BID – 3–5 days	200 mg 5x per day – 5 days
Recurrent GH – Suppression	250 mg–500 mg BID	500 mg QD (≤ nine outbreaks per year), 1 gm QD (> none outbreaks per year)	400 mg BID (up to 1 year)
GH – Reduction of Transmission	Not indicated	500 mg QD	Not indicated
GH – for HIV-infected patients	Recurrent 500 mg BID – 7 days	Suppression 500 mg BID	Not indicated

Table 68   (continued)

	Famciclovir (Famvir)	Valcyclovir (Valtrex)	Acyclovir (Zovirax)
Cold sores – for immunocompetent patients	1,500 mg QD or 750 mg BID for 1 day	2 gm BID – 1 day	Not indicated in oral formulation
Herpes Zoster	500 mg TID – 7 days	1 gm TID – 7 days	800 mg 5x QD for 7–10 days

GH = genital herpes

- **Prednisone** – controversial
  - May help by decreasing incidence of post-herpetic neuralgia
  - Dose: 60 mg daily × 7 days, decrease to 30 mg QD × 7 days, then decrease to 15 mg QD × 7 days, and then discontinue
  - Does not contribute to reducing prolonged pain, but may have beneficial effects on acute pain and some cutaneous end points
- **Oral Medications (Immunocompromised Host)**
  - Setting of malignancy or organ transplantation
    - R/o systemic disease – look for fever, etc.
    - PO Valcyclovir, Famciclovir, or Acyclovir – coupled with close clinical observation, is reasonable
  - HIV patients
    - PO Famciclovir or Acyclovir. Valcyclovir not studied
    - Can develop chronic VZV encephalitis, rapidly progressive herpetic retinal necrosis (RPHRN), post-HZ myelitis
- **Complicated Presentations of Herpes Zoster**
  - HZ ophthalmicus and VZV retinitis
    - Famciclovir or Valacyclovir for 7–10 days (especially within 72 h) – to resolve acute dz and inhibit late inflammatory recurrences
    - Pain meds and cool to tepid wet compresses
    - Antibiotic ophthalmic ointment and lubricating artificial tears
    - Urgent ophthalmology consult – will likely give topical steroids, etc.
    - PO Steroids – in event of moderate-to-severe pain or rash, if significant edema. May need IV ABX if retinitis – defer to ophthalmology.
  - Frail elderly
    - Pain – makes patient vulnerable to inactivity, poor PO intake
    - Start at lower doses of meds, adjust for decreased renal clearance, warn about sedation
  - Pregnancy
    - Safety of antivirals in pregnancy not firmly established
    - Tx in cases in which benefits outweigh potential risk to fetus

Pearls and Pitfalls

- Recent studies suggest that patients with recent herpes zoster or herpes zoster ophthalmicus may be at risk for stroke. Antivirals do not seem to have an effect.
  - *Neurology 2010 Mar 9; 74(10)* and *Stroke 2009 Nov; 40(11)*
- **Herpes Zoster Vaccination (Zostavax)** – *per Dr. John Gnann (UAB), 2008 AAD Lecture*
  - Vaccine ↓ incidence of HZ by 51%, ↓PHN in 66.5% overall (Oxman et al. NEJM 2005)
  - Indicated for prevention of HZ in individuals 60 years and above
  - Protects for at least 5 years.
  - No contraindication to giving it to age<60, but insurance probably won't cover it. Also, will likely need a booster vaccination at some point (unclear when).
  - Is vaccine indicated if patient previously had HZ?
    - Risk of second case of HZ is small (an episode of HZ boosts one's immunity)
    - ACP recommends vaccination whether or not patient reports prior episode of HZ
    - If HZ in the past year or two, they probably won't benefit, but unclear when immunity would wane
  - Can give this in conjunction with other vaccinations
  - Contains replicating VZV → **contraindicated in immunocompromised** per pkg insert
    - If on prednisone 20 mg QD>2 weeks → safety concern with live viruses. Wait 1 months after stopping prednisone before vaccination.
    - Gray areas – those on low-dose MTX, those on TNF-α inhibitors, and other immunomodulators
  - Immunization before immunosuppression – 4 weeks is fine, 2 weeks before *may* be ok

Hidradenitis Suppurativa (HS)

Etiology and Pathogenesis

- Thought to represent an inflammatory disorder originating from the hair follicle. Rupture of the follicle allows introduction of its content (keratin, bacteria) into the surrounding dermis → vigorous chemotactic response and abscess formation. Epithelial strands are generated (possibly from the ruptured follicles) and form sinus tracts.
- Those of African descent seem to have higher incidence than those of European descent
- Women > Men (3:1)

Clinical Presentation

- Inflammatory nodules and sterile abscesses which tend to develop in the axillae, groin, perianal, and/or inframammary areas. Lesions become very painful and drain purulent material. Over time, sinus tracts form and hypertrophic scars develop.
- HS is considered a component of the follicular occlusion tetrad (also includes acne conglobata, dissecting cellulitis of the scalp, pilonidal sinus)
- Three key elements required to diagnose: **typical lesions**, **characteristic distribution**, and **recurrence**
- Complications of HS
  - Anemia, secondary infection, lymphedema, fistulae formation (to urethra, bladder, peritoneum, rectum), hypoproteinemia, nephrotic syndrome, arthropathy, SCC
- Associated with Other Disorders
  - Fox–Fordyce disease, acanthosis nigricans, pityriasis rubra pilaris (PRP), steatocystoma multiplex, Dowling–Degos disease, SAPHO, Crohn's
  - HIV-associated PRP is characterized by the cutaneous lesions of PRP and a variable association with the lesions of acne conglobata, HS, and lichen spinulosus. This disease can be designated by the wider term *HIV-associated follicular syndrome.*

Labs

- Culture purulent drainage
- Consider tissue culture if concern for deep fungal infection or mycobacterial infection
- Most patients have normal androgen levels

DDx – Cutaneous Crohn's, ulcerative colitis, granuloma inguinale, lymphogranuloma venereum, infected cyst, abscesses, cutaneous TB, lymphadenitis, cat-scratch disease, actinomycosis

Histology – Frequently see ruptured pilosebaceous unit with perifollicular infiltrate of neutrophils, lymphocytes, plasma cells, histiocytes, and/or multinucleated giant cells. Can see follicular plugging, sinus tracts, fibrosis.

Treatment

- Difficult and frustrating condition to treat. Often associated with depression in affected patients.
- Local – Hygiene and care, loose-fitting clothing, antiperspirants/deodorants, drysol
- Wide **surgical excision** with margins beyond the active borders – often need flaps, grafts
- Anti-inflammatory antibiotics – tetracycline, doxycycline, minocycline
- **Clindamycin + Rifampin**
  - ○ Clindamycin 150 mg TID-QID (or can do 300 mg PO BID)
  - ○ Rifampin 300 mg PO BID
- Isotretinoin – 1 mg/kg PO qd or divided bid (Preg Category X) – disease recurs when stopped
- Dapsone 100 mg PO QD; check G6PD prior
- IL corticosteroids
- Hormonal – Preg Category X
  - ○ Cyproterone acetate (Androcur) 50 mg PO bid on days 5–14 of menstrual cycle
    - ■ +30 μg/day estrogen ethinyl estradiol – administer with cyproterone acetate
  - ○ Finasteride (5 mg/day for 3 months), inhibitor of 5-alpha reductase type II isoenzyme, may be beneficial
- Immunosuppressants (TNF-α inhibitors): Infliximab >>adalimumab or etanercept
  - ○ **Infliximab** 3–5 mg/kg per infusion q 6–8 week; start with induction at week 0, 2, 4, 6, then q 8 weeks
- Nd:Yag Hair Laser (JAAD 2010)
- CO_2 Laser
- Botox may be useful in hyperhidrosis is a large aggravating factor

Pearls and Pitfalls

- Of the TNF-α inhibitors, infliximab seems to work the best (perhaps because it is weight-based)
- Encourage weight loss
- Encourage smoking cessation
- Rifampin has a lot of drug interactions – be sure to check
- Lithium has been reported to aggravate HS
- Consider referral to psychiatry if depression is a major issue as a result of this chronic skin condition

Histochemical Staining

Table 69 Histochemical staining

Stain	Purpose
Hematoxylin-Eosin	Routine
Masson trichome	Collagen
Verhoeff–von Gieson	Elastic fibers
Pinkus acid orcein	Elastic fibers
Silver nitrate	Melanin, reticulin fibers
Fontana–Masson	Melanin
Methenamine silver	Fungi, Donovan bodies, Frisch bacilli, basement membrane
Grocott	Fungi
Periodic acid-Schiff (PAS)	Glycogen, neutral MPS, fungi
Alcian blue, pH 2.5	Acid MPS
Alcian blue, pH 0.5	Sulfated MPS
Toluidine blue	Acid MPS
Colloidal iron	Acid MPS
Hyaluronidase	Hyaluronic acid
Mucicarmine	"Epithelial" mucin
Giemsa	Mast cell granules, acid MPS, myeloid granules, *Leishmania*
Fite	Acid-fast bacilli
Perls potassium ferrocyanide	Hemosiderin
Alkaline Congo Red	Amyloid
Von Kossa	Calcium
Scarlet red	Lipids
Oil red O	Lipids
Dopa (unfixed tissue)	Tyrosinase
Warthin–Starry	Spirochetes
Dieterle and Steiner	Spirochetes, bacillary angiomatosis

Table 70 Histochemical staining – Immuno

Epidermal	
Cytokeratin 20	Merkel cell carcinoma
Cytokeratin 7	Paget's disease
EMA	Eccrine, apocrine, sebaceous glands
CEA	Metastatic adenocarcinoma, extramammary Paget's, eccrine/apocrine gland
Mesenchymal	
Desmin	Muscle (all 3 types)
Vimentin	Cells of mesenchymal origin
Actin	Muscle
CD31	Endothelial tumors: angiosarcoma
CD34	DFSP: CD34+, XIIIa– (DF: CD34–, XIIIa+, ST3+)
Neuroectodermal	
S100	Melanocytes, nerve, Langerhans, eccrine, apocrine, chondrocytes (desmoplastic melanoma S100–)
HMB-45	Premelanosome vesicles, melanocytic nevi and MM (desmoplastic melanoma HMB-45-)
MART-1	Melanocytic nevi and malignant melanoma
Hematopoietic	
CD45 (LAC)	CD45RO: memory T-cell; CD45RA: B cells, naïve T-cell
CD20	Pan B-cell marker
CD43 (Leu-22)	Pan T-cell marker
K and λ	Mature B cells and plasma cells
CD30 (Ki-1)	Stains activated T and B cells, Reed–Sternberg cells, large cell, anaplastic CTCL, Lymphomatoid papulosis type A
CD68 (Kp-1)	Marker for histiocytes
Factor XIIIa	Platelets, macrophages, megakaryocytes, dendrites
Miscellaneous	
BCL2	Follicular center lymphoma (B origin), BCC (bcl2+)
CD1A (Leu-6)	Langerhans cells
CD3	Pan T-cell marker
CD4	T helper cell
CD8	T cytotoxic suppressor cells
CD20	Pan B-cell marker
CD31	Endothelial cell marker
CD34	Endothelial cells, dermal spindle cells
CD56	NK cells and angiocentric T-cell lymphoma
CD68	Histiocytes

Hyperhidrosis

Etiology and Pathogenesis

- **Primary** – focal, visible excessive sweating present for 6 months or more without a secondary cause. Have at least two of the following: bilateral and symmetric, impairs activities of daily life, at least one episode per week, age of onset <25 years, positive family history, stops during sleep.
- **Secondary** – sweating that is caused by or associated with another systemic disorder. May be localized or generalized. Many causes and categorized by cause – cortical, hypothalamus, medullary, spinal, or localized.
  - **Cortical** – isolated sweating of palms/soles. Due to cortical excitation by emotional or sensory stimuli. Associated with hereditary palmoplantar keratodermas in some cases and other genodermatoses.
  - **Hypothalamic** – hypothalamus responsible for thermoregulation

Table 71   Causes of hypothalamic hyperhidrosis

Drugs/Toxins	Alcohol
	Arsenic toxicity
	Mercury toxicity (acrodynia)
	Opioid withdrawal
Infection	Acute febrile illnesses
	Brucellosis
	Malaria
	Subacute bacterial endocarditis
	Tuberculosis
Metabolic	Acromegaly
	Gout
	Hyperthyroidism
	Hypoglycemia
	Menopause
	Obesity
	Phenylketonuria
	Porphyria (acute intermittent)
	Pregnancy
Neurologic	Cerebrovascular accidents
	Cold-induced sweating syndrome
	Episodic spontaneous hypothermia with hyperhidrosis
	Familial dysautonomia
	Parkinson's disease
	Postencephalitic
	Tumors
Tumors	Lymphoma
	Pheochromocytoma
	Carcinoid

Table 71 (continued)

Vasomotor	Acrocyanosis
	Autoimmune connective tissue disease
	Cold injury
	Congestive heart failure
	Myocardial ischemia
	Raynaud's phenomenon
	Reflex sympathetic dystrophy
	Symmetrical lividity of palms and soles
Other	Coffee/Tea
	Compensatory hyperhidrosis in association with miliaria, diabetes
	POEMS syndrome
	Speckled lentiginous nevus syndrome
	Mitochondrial disorders
	Pressure and postural hyperhidrosis

- ○ **Medullary (gustatory)** – any food or drink that stimulates the taste buds may induce sweating in normal individuals, especially on certain parts of the face
  - ■ Spicy foods, citrus fruits, alcohol, condiments
  - ■ **Frey's syndrome** – typically occurs after injury to parotid gland (usually from surgery, usually in adults). Salivary stimulation elicits localized sweating in the parotid area. Can rarely be seen in children and can be mistaken for food allergy.
- ○ **Spinal** – spinal disorders may result in lack of thermal sweating below the injury as well as unusual forms of hyperhidrosis. Mass reflex sweating may occur around the injury area.

Labs and Workup

- Patients who do not fit the classic pattern of primary hyperhidrosis should undergo further workup
- Starch-Iodine test
  - ○ Iodine solution is applied to clean, shaved skin and allowed to dry, then starch powder (e.g., cornstarch) is brushed onto the area. Mixture turns blue-black in sites with sweating.
- Labs to consider as history and exam directs – complete metabolic profile, TSH, free T4, PPD screening for tuberculosis, chest x-ray, complete blood count, sedimentation rate, antinuclear antibodies, urinary catecholamines

Treatment

- Topical 20% aluminum chloride (Drysol) QHS
- 6.25% aluminum tetrachloride
- Zirconium salts
- Iontophoresis

- Anticholinergics (may cause dry mouth, urinary retention. Rarely – confusion)
  - Oxybutynin 1.25–5 mg BID
  - Glycopyrrolate 1–2 mg BID
- α_2-adrenergic agonist
  - Clonidine 0.1–0.3 mg BID → can cause hypotension, rebound hypertension, headache
- Botulinum toxin A every 4–6 months
- Sympathectomy – last resort. May get compensatory hyperhidrosis.

Pearls and Pitfalls

- Drysol can be irritating. May start by using this every other night.

Intertrigo

Etiology and Pathogenesis

- Inflammatory condition of skin folds induced or aggravated by heat, moisture, maceration, friction, and lack of air circulation. With ↑moisture, the stratum corneum becomes eroded.
- Condition frequently is worsened or colonized by infection, which most commonly is candidal but also may be bacterial, fungal, or viral

Clinical Presentation

- Macerated, erythematous patches commonly distributed in the inframammary region, axillae, groin, or under a pannus/abdominal folds

Labs – KOH, Wood's light, bacterial culture, consider biopsy if poor response to treatment

DDx – inverse psoriasis, erythrasma, candida, cellulitis, contact dermatitis (allergic or irritant), Hailey–Hailey disease, acanthosis nigricans, acrodermatitis enteropathica, granuloma inguinale, impetigo, lymphogranuloma venereum, Paget's disease, seborrheic dermatitis, group A streptococcus

Treatment

- Eliminate friction, heat, and maceration by keeping folds cool and dry
  - ○ Air conditioning, absorbent powders and by exposing skin folds to the air
  - ○ Skin surfaces in deep folds can be kept separated with cotton or linen cloth; however, be sure to avoid tight, occlusive, or chafing clothing or dressings
  - ○ Emphasize weight loss, diabetes control
  - ○ **Castellani paint** (carbol-fuchsin paint) also can be helpful
  - ○ Patagonia boxers
  - ○ **Zeasorb powder or drying gel**
- Anti-mycotic agent → **econazole, clotrimazole cream**
- Anti-inflammatory → **Hydrocortisone, Vytone** (hydrocortisone-iodoquinol); iodoquinol has both antifungal and antibacterial properties
- Formulations combining protective agents, antimicrobials, and topical steroids may be helpful, including the following
  - ○ Triple Paste comprises petrolatum, zinc oxide paste, and aluminum acetate (Burow) solution applied qs ad (in a sufficient quantity)

- ○ Greer Goo is composed of nystatin (Mycostatin) pwdr 4 mU, hydrocortisone pwdr 1.2 g, and zinc oxide paste 4 oz applied qs ad (in a sufficient quantity)
  ○ Barrier pastes (Desitin, ProShield Plus)
- Protopic ointment 0.1% BID
- Elidel cream

Pearls and Pitfalls

- Use caution with topical steroids in these naturally occluded areas. Use low-potency topical steroids only. Patients tend to overuse and cause striae, atophy, etc.

Kaposi's Sarcoma (KS)

Etiology and Pathogenesis

- Human herpesvirus type 8 (HHV-8) – not clear how this results in the development of KS
- Receptive anal intercourse appears to be a primary factor for transmission in MSM
- Mother-to-child transmission occurs in 1/3 of HHV-8 infected mothers in African countries
- Transmission by blood transfusion is possible
- Immunosuppression may play a role – KS common in HIV-infected patients and in some transplant patients

Clinical Presentation and Types

- Four types of KS – classic, HIV/AIDS-related, immunosuppression-associated, and African endemic
- All types typically evolve through stages as red, brown or violaceous patches, papules, plaques and nodules. Edema is often present in all types
- **Classic KS**
  - Spongy feel during early stage and become more firm with time. Typically seen on the lower legs of elderly men of Mediterranean descent
  - Lesions can later become brown, hyperkeratotic, and/or eczematous
  - Oral mucosa and gastrointestinal tract are rarely involved
  - Slow progression of disease
- **HIV/AIDS-related KS**
  - Often seen in HIV patients with low CD4 counts, can be seen with immune reconstitution (IRIS). Recent reports of well-controlled HIV patients (viral load undetectable, high CD4 counts) now developing KS.
  - More widely distributed macules, patches or plaques, which can occasionally become ulcerated
  - Oral involvement and facial lesions seen more often than in classic KS and may be one of the first indications of HIV
  - Commonly involves genitals, lungs (persistent cough, bronchospasm, dyspnea), GI tract (stomach and duodenum). 80% of AIDS patients with KS will develop GI involvement – nausea, vomiting, bleeding, perforation, and/or ileus
- **Immunosuppression-associated KS**
  - Rapid progression and dissemination unless the immunosuppressive agents are discontinued or markedly reduced
  - *Sirolimus* (rapamycin) is administered for immunosuppression in place of calcineurin inhibitors
  - Similar clinical presentation to AIDS-related KS

- **African endemic KS – Four subtypes**
  - **Nodular** – small number of well-circumscribed nodules. Usually a benign course lasting 5–8 years.
  - **Lymphadenopathic** – typically affects lymph nodes rather than skin. More common in children and young adults.
  - **Florid and Infiltrative** – large number of skin lesions. Very aggressive and may involve subcutaneous tissue, muscle, and bone.

DDx – angiosarcoma, acroangiodermatitis (pseudo-KS), bacillary angiomatosis, ecchymosis, hemangioma, pyogenic granuloma, pseudolymphoma, lymphoma, vasculitis.

Histology

- Vascular channels lined by atypical endothelial cells and surrounded by a proliferation of spindle-shaped cells
- **Patch stage** – proliferation of small, jagged, endothelial-lined spaces in the superficial dermis. These vessels may separate collagen bundles. Perivascular lymphocytic infiltrate may be seen (+/– plasma cells).
- **Plaque stage** – spindle cells infiltrate dermal collagen bundles of deeper dermis. Irregular, cleft-like vascular channels seen along with hyaline globules and hemosiderin. Perivascular lymphocytic infiltrate.
- **Nodular stage** – Well-circumscribed sheets and fascicles of spindle cells within network of slit-like vascular spaces infiltrating dermis and subcutaneous tissue. See cytologic atypia, mitoses.
- HHV-8 stain +

Treatment

Table 72 AIDS clinical trials group staging classification for Kaposi's sarcoma

	Good Risk (*all* of the following)	Poor Risk (*any* of the following)
Tumor (T)	Confined to skin, nodes, or few oral lesions	Tumor associated with edema/ulcer
Immune system (I)	CD4 count ≥ 200	CD4 cell count ≤ 200
Systemic illness (S)	No opportunistic infection/candida No B symptoms (fever, weight loss, diarrhea) Not confined to bed > 70% of time	Opportunistic infections/candida B symptoms present Confined to bed > 70% of time Other HIV-related illness

- Start HAART therapy in HIV patients – takes 9–18 months for lesions to resolve
- Localized treatment
  - Cryotherapy – for small lesions
  - Radiation – particularly useful for feet, genitals, or locally disfiguring disease
  - Topical alitretinoin
  - Intralesional interferon-α
  - Intralesional vinblastine – painful
- Systemic chemotherapy – should be considered urgent if pulmonary or rapidly progressive KS or KS with marked systemic features.
  - Vinblastine, doxorubicin, daunorubicin have traditionally been used for extensive classic and endemic KS
  - Liposomal-encapsulated anthracyclines and paclitaxel have now become first-line when systemic involvement present

Pearls and Pitfalls

- Castleman's disease and primary effusion lymphoma also associated with HHV-8
- Bacillary angiomatosis and KS can exist in the same HIV patient. Consider biopsying more than one lesion if some have different morphologies. Bacillary angiomatosis often has a collarette of scale around the base.
- Transplant patients – change regimen to include Sirolimus

References:

(1) Jessop S. HIV-Associated Kaposi's sarcoma. Dermatol Clin. 2006; 24: 509–20.
(2) Krown SE, et al. AIDS-related Kaposi's sarcoma: prospective validation of the AIDS Clinical Trials Group Staging classification. AIDS Clinical Trials Group Oncology Committee. J Clin Oncol. 1997; 15(9): 3085–92.

Keloids

Etiology and Pathogenesis

- Injury → hemostasis → inflammation → excessive synthesis of collagen by fibroblasts → keloid
- Transforming growth factor-β (TGF-β) is highly expressed in keloidal tissue
- Seen primarily in the black population

Clinical Presentation

- Raised, pink-to-purple papules that are often painful, pruritic, or both. The overlying epidermis is typically smooth.
- May be disfiguring as it grows beyond the initial tissue injury into adjacent tissues
- Recurrence after surgical removal is common and may be larger, more extensive when it recurs

DDx – hypertrophic scar (keloid extends into adjacent tissue whereas hypertrophic scar remains within the confines of the original injury), sclerotic form of xanthoma disseminatum, lobomycosis, dermatofibroma, DFSP, acne keloidalis nuchae, keloidal forms of scleroderma and morphea, keloidal plaques on lower extremities of patients with type IV Ehlers–Danlos

Histology

- Large, thick collagen fibers that are composed of multiple, closely packed fibrils. Subepidermal appendages are absent, as in all types of scars. Amorphous extracellular material surrounds the fibroblastic cells within keloids.
- Both hypertrophic scars and keloids have increased cellularity, vascularity, and connective tissue compared to normal skin.

Treatment and Management

- Prevention is key! Close surgical wounds with minimal tension. Surgical scars should not cross joints. Avoid midchest incisions. Try to follow skin lines with surgery.
- Occlusive dressings – silicone gel sheets and dressings, nonsilicone occlusive sheets
- Compression therapy

- IL corticosteroid injections – Kenalog 10–40 mg/mL administered intralesion-ally with a 25- to 27-gauge needle at 4- to 6-week intervals
- Topical corticosteroids – Cordran tape, steroid ointments
- Cryosurgery
- Excision – follow with IL corticosteroids and pressure (such as earrings); choose patients who will follow-up appropriately
- Other options – Radiation therapy (safety has been questioned), laser therapy (CO_2, argon, PDL, Nd:YAG), interferon therapy, doxorubicin, bleomycin (concentration of 1.5 IU/mL, given via multiple punctures), verapamil (study with patients treated with surgical excision and 5 tx of verapamil at 2.5 mg/mL over 2 month period. Doses varied from 0.5 to 5 mL, depending on keloid size), tacrolimus, retinoic acid, imiquimod 5% cream, tamoxifen
- 5-FU intralesional injections for keloids and hypertrophic scars – *courtesy of Dr. Alexander Zhang*
  1. Add 0.1 mL of 10 mg/mL triamcinolone acetonide to 0.9 mL of 50 mg/mL 5-FU
  2. Once-weekly intralesional injections for the average patients. For the scars that are more inflamed or more indurated can be injected up to three times per week.
  3. Injection frequency – individualize according to patient response

Pearls and Pitfalls

- I have not found imiquimod to be very helpful
- Excision more helpful on the ear, but patients must follow-up regularly

Leishmaniasis

Etiology and Pathogenesis

- Infection caused by various species of *Leishmania* protozoa, which are transmitted by bite of sandflies (vector). Sandflies are approximately half the size of mosquitoes and do not "buzz".
- *Leishmania* life cycle begins when parasites in the promastigote form are inoculated by a sandfly bite into the skin of a mammalian host. Human neutrophils first ingest the organisms → burst out → ingested by macrophages but cannot be killed.
- 90% of cutaneous leishmaniasis cases are contracted in Afghanistan, Pakistan, Syria, Saudi Arabia, Algeria, Iran, Brazil, and Peru.

Table 73 Types of leishmaniasis and associated species

Syndrome	Location	Species
Cutaneous leishmaniasis	Old World	L. major
		L. tropica
		L. aethiopica
	New World	L. Mexicana
		L. amazonensis
		L. venezuelensis
Cutaneous leishmaniasis/ mucocutaneous leishmaniasis	New World	L. braziliensis
		L. colombiensis
		L. guyanensis
		L. peruviana
Visceral leishmaniasis	Old World	L. donovani
		L. infantum
	New World	L. chagasi

Clinical Presentation and Types

- **Cutaneous leishmaniasis (CL)** – infection limited to the skin and lymphatic system, but it may affect deeper tissues in diffuse CL or recur in the mucous membranes of the mouth, nose, or pharynx in MCL.
  - Not life-threatening
  - Red papule (usually painless) → ulcerates. Typically has slightly elevated border. Can stay like this for 3–4 months and then spontaneously clears→ Scar.
  - Sporotrichoid lymphatic spread possible.
- **Mucocutaneous leishmaniasis (MCL)** – affects mucous membranes of the mouth, nose, pharynx. Typical species are *L. braziliensis, L. colombiensis, L. guyanensis, L. peruviana.*
  - 80–90% of CL resolve without sequelae, but a small percentage of leishmaniasis cases are caused by species that lead to mucocutaneous involvement

- **Visceral leishmaniasis (aka kala-azar)**

  - Typically caused by *L. donovani*. Incubation period of 1–36 months.
  - Fever, wasting, cough, lymphadenopathy, hepatosplenomegaly, nephropathy, enteritis, pneumonia. Skin findings may include papules, nodules, ulcers or purpura, hyperpigmentation, xerosis, hair discoloration.

- **Post-kala-azar dermal leishmaniasis (PKDL)** is a dermal sequela of visceral leishmaniasis (VL), reported mainly from two regions – Sudan in eastern Africa and the Indian subcontinent
  - ○ May arise several years after successful treatment of visceral leishmaniasis
  - ○ Skin lesions vary – hypopigmented macules, skin-colored nodules, malar erythema, verrucous papules
  - ○ Etiopathogenesis of PKDL is presumably due to an immunological assault on latent dermal parasites
- **Leishmaniasis recidivans** – characterized by recurrence at site of an original ulcer, usually within 2 years and often at the edge of a scar

Labs

- CDC can do PCR on formalin-fixed tissue in order to speciate
- Skin slits smear – Take a scalpel blade and split lesion from center to border. Smear on a slide and stain with Giemsa. Can see organisms in macrophages.
- Biopsy
- Culture difficult but can be done→ will change from amastigotes (without flagellate) to flagellated form. Novy–MacNeal–Nicolle medium required.
- Serologic tests are not sensitive for the diagnosis of CL.

DDx – Methicillin-resistant *Staphylococcus aureus* infection, furuncle, paracoccidioidomycosis, histoplasmosis, mycobacterial infections (*Mycobacterium marinum*, cutaneous tuberculosis, and other atypical mycobacteria), syphilis, tertiary yaws, leprosy, sarcoidosis, cutaneous neoplasms, angiocentric NK/T-cell lymphoma, Wegener's granulomatosis.

Histology

- Epidermis may be normal, atrophic, hyperplastic, or ulcerated
- Diffuse mixed granulomatous dermal infiltrate of lymphocytes, histiocytes, plasma cells, neutrophils, multinucleated giant cells; occasional caseation necrosis
- Fibrosis in older lesions
- *Amastigote organisms* usually seen in histiocytes and can be seen on H&E stains, but best with Giemsa stains. Organisms measure 2–3 microns, with a 1-micron round nucleus and a smaller rod-shaped paranucleus (*kinetoplast*)

Treatment

- **It is important to determine species, as the species leading to mucocutaneous leishmaniasis need more aggressive treatment to prevent sequelae. PCR is method of choice.**
  - CDC can speciate from formalin-fixed tissue (404-639-3670)
- Aim of treatment is: (1) prevent mucosal invasion (2) accelerate healing, and (3) prevent disfiguring scars
- Cutaneous Leishmaniasis
  - Depending on the species, anatomic location, some may opt not to treat
  - Treatment encouraged for multiple lesions or large (> 4–5 cm), if present for > 6 months or if lesions in a cosmetically sensitive area or over a joint
- Mucocutaneous Leishmaniasis – Needs to be treated

Table 74 Treatment options for leishmaniasis

Disease type	Medication	Dosing	Adverse effects and comments
Cutaneous	Sodium stibogluconate (pentavalent antimony)	20 mg antimony (Sb)/kg/day IV × 20 days	• LFTs, amylase, lipase in > 50% myalgias, arthralgias, abdominal pain, nausea, ↓ platelets
	Meglumine antimoniate (pentavalent antimony)	20 mg Sb/kg/day IV or IM × 20 days	• EKG changes and cardiac toxicity (< 25%). Avoid in patients with cardiac problems, prolonged QT. Dilute in 120 mL of 5% dextrose and infuse over 2 h. Patients with cardiac dz and hypokalemia at risk. Hospitalization during tx justified as cardiac monitoring recommended during infusion. • Baseline – CMP, CBC, amylase, EKG • Note that pentavalent antimony comes in two forms: sodium stibogluconate and meglumine antimoniate
	Intralesional antimony	50 mg/0.5 mL q 2–3 weeks × 12 weeks	• Injection painful • Used in Non-American CL only • Consider in patients where parenteral tx contraindicated
	Miltefosine	2.5 mg/kg/day PO × 28 days (max 150 mg/day)	• Nausea, vomiting, diarrhea, ↑ Creatinine ↑ LFTs (<25%) • Teratogenic in animals • Consider in cases resistant to pentavalent antimony
	Pentamidine	2–3 mg/kg/day IV or IM QD or QOD × 4–7 doses	• Nausea and vomiting in > 50% • Consider in cases where pentavalent antimony contraindicated. Few side effects.
Other options for CL – cryotherapy, imiquimod, photodynamic therapy, allopurinol, azoles (ketoconazole, itraconazole) have been evaluated both alone and in combination with pentavalent antimony (sodium stibogluconate and meglumine antimoniate). Ointment containing 15% paromomycin and 12% methylbenzethonium chloride can be compounded – BID × 20 days. Do not recommend these alternatives for spp., which may lead to mucosal involvement.			

Table 74 (continued)

Disease type	Medication	Dosing	Adverse effects and comments
Mucosal	Meglumine antimoniate	20 mg/kg/day IV or IM × 28 days	See above
	Amphotericin B	2–3 mg/kg/day IV QD or QOD until lesion healing	• Infusion-related reactions in > 50% • Azotemia • Anemia, hypokalemia in < 25% • Liposomal formulation should be used – less renal toxicity compared with deoxycholate
	Pentamidine	2–4 mg/kg/day QD until lesion healing	See above

Pearls and Pitfalls

- The sandfly's biting apparatus cannot penetrate clothing and thus clothing can be protective
- Sandflies can penetrate mosquito netting; however, one can spray the netting with permethrin spray (available at sporting goods stores) and this will last through a few washes and can be effective
- Insect repellant helpful in prevention – recommend long-lasting repellant such as Ultrathon (contains DEET)
- May see in returning military personnel and in returning travelers
- Not really contagious to others, although one could purposely take tissue and inoculate another individual and give them a lesion. Mothers in the third World will do this on their children's buttocks to prevent scarring of the face.
- Montenegro or leishmanin skin test utilized in endemic countries – diameter > 5 mm in 48–72 h considered positive. Not available in US.
- Surgery can reactivate dormant parasites after area has been treated so plastic surgery is discouraged.

References:

(1) David CV and Craft N. Cutaneous and mucocutaneous leishmaniasis. Dermatol Ther 2009; 22: 491–502.
(2) Schwartz E, et al. New world cutaneous leishmaniasis in travellers. Lancet Infect Dis 2006; 6: 342–49.

Lichen Planus (LP)

Etiology and Pathogenesis

- May be a T-cell-mediated autoimmune disease that targets basal keratinocytes expressing altered self-antigens on their surface
- Associations with hepatitis C, HHV-6 and -7, HSV, VZV, vaccines, bacteria (*Helicobacter pylori*), contact allergens, drugs
  - Drugs commonly implicated → captopril, enalapril, labetalol, methyldopa, propranolol, chloroquine, hydroxychloroquine, quinacrine, hydrochlorathiazide, gold salts, penicillamine, quinidine
- LP may arise in patients with other immunologically mediated disorders, including alopecia areata, dermatomyositis, LsA, morphea, myasthenia gravis, primary biliary cirrhosis, ulcerative colitis, and vitiligo

Clinical Presentation

- Flat-topped violaceous papules and plaques that favor the wrists, forearms, genitalia, distal lower extremities, and presacral areas.
  - Lesions prone to friction (such as the genital area) may become eroded
- Buccal mucosa may have a network of fine white lines called "Wickham's striae". May also see small gray-white puncta. Oral lesions seen in over 50% of patients and may be the only site of involvement.
- Koebner phenomenon commonly seen
- **Variants**
  - **Actinic LP** – red-brown plaques with annular configuration, but melasma-like hyperpigmented patches have been observed. Onset is in spring or summer on sun-exposed areas.
  - **Acute LP (or eruptive)** – widely distributed lesions that disseminate rapidly. May be the result of a drug.
  - **Annular LP** – papules spread peripherally and the central area resolves. Annular edge is slightly raised and typically purple to white in color, while central portion is hyperpigmented or skin-colored. May resemble granuloma annulare.
  - **Atrophic LP** – May be a resolving form of LP. See thinning of the epidermis that mimics lichen sclerosus or morphea.
  - **Bullous LP and LP pemphigoides** – Bullae may form within preexisting LP lesions or more randomly, including on previously uninvolved skin
  - **Hypertrophic LP** – pruritic, thick hyperkeratotic plaques seen primarily on the shins or dorsal feet and may be covered by a fine adherent scale. SCC has been reported to arise within these lesions.
  - **Inverse LP** – lesions appear in intertriginous areas (axillae>inguinal and inframammary folds). Lesions may be violaceous or hyperpigmented.

o **LP Pigmentosus** – presents in skin types III and IV as brown to gray-brown macules in sun-exposed areas of face and neck, often with no preceding erythema. Evolves into diffuse or reticulated pigmentation. Involvement of intertriginous sites is occasionally seen.
o **Lichen planopilaris** – *see hair section*
o **Linear LP** – lesions appear within lines of Blaschko. May be intermediate form between LP and lichen striatus. Usually seen in patients in their late 20s and 30s.
o **LP-lupus overlap** – Clinical and histological findings (including DIF) show features of both LP and lupus
o **Nail LP** – seen in approximately 10% of LP patients. Nail abnormalities include lateral thinning, longitudinal ridging, and fissuring, which can lead to scarring and dorsal pterygium. Considered a nail emergency.
o **Oral LP** – can appear in at least seven forms, which occur separately or simultaneously → atrophic, bullous, erosive, papular, pigmented, plaque-like, and reticular. Gingival involvement common. Erosive LP more commonly associated with Hepatitis C.
o **Ulcerative LP** – can occur within preexisting LP lesions, especially on the soles. Intensely painful and often recalcitrant to typical therapies. Risk of SCC.
o **Drug-induced LP** – see list above
o **Vulvovaginal LP** – erosive disease is most common and can lead to scarring. Follow closely as risk of malignancy within scars.

Labs to consider – Hepatitis C Ab, HIV-1 and -2

DDx – GVHD, lichen nitidus, lichen simplex chronicus, pityriasis rosea, guttate psoriasis, plaque psoriasis, tinea corporis, syphilis

Histology

- **H&E** – wedge-shaped hypergranulosis, irregular acanthosis with "saw-toothed" rete ridges. Colloid bodies often seen. Liquefaction degeneration of the basal layer and lichenoid infiltrate of lymphocytes in the papillary dermis. Melanin incontinence common.
- **DIF** (not necessary to perform) – Direct immunofluorescence study reveals globular deposits of immunoglobulin M (IgM) and complement mixed with apoptotic keratinocytes

Treatment

- Localized Involvement
  - Class I or II topical steroids
  - IM triamcinolone 40–80 mg q 6–8 weeks
  - Oral acitretin has been effective – published studies
- Widespread Involvement – NbUVB, PUVA
- Oral Involvement
  - Triamcinolone acetonide 0.1% in 1% carboxy cellulose for dental paste QID (stays on well)
  - Betamethasone 0.5 mg tab – Dissolve in 10–15 mL of water; Use as a mouth rinse for 1 min, TID-QID, until erythema or erosions resolve
  - Ointments work best in mouth – can be combined with Orabase. For example, 15 g of clobetasol ointment with 15 g of Orabase; this mixture should be indicated on the prescription
  - Corticosteroid inhalant typically used to treat asthma (Beclovent, Vanceril): Use MDI with 50 mcg per puff. Direct inhaler to sites of greatest erythema or erosion.
  - Protopic or Elidel
  - Topical cyclosporine – may be less effective, more expensive than clobetasol
  - Topical retinoids
  - PO retinoids
  - Biopsy persistent oral ulcerations – malignant degeneration can occur
  - Consider antifungals if concomitant candida
  - Topical anesthetic – Orabase-B (OTC) contains 20% benzocaine
  - Adjustments in food/hygiene
    - Eliminate foods that can easily traumatize (hard breads, tough steaks); acidic foods may also aggravate
    - Consider ruling out allergy to metals (such as certain tooth fillings) if only one localized area
    - Eliminate tobacco, alcohol (both can aggravate)
    - Patients should see dentist regularly to ensure they are achieving proper dental hygiene (can be difficult with sores in the mouth)
    - Some dermatologists recommend Ultreo toothbrush → gentle microbubble toothbrush
- **Recalcitrant disease**
  - Hydroxychloroquine
  - Azathioprine – 1 mg/kg/day PO for 6–8 week; increase by 0.5 mg/kg q 4 week until response or dose reaches 2.5 mg/kg
  - Mycophenolate mofetil, dapsone, systemic corticosteroids
  - Alternative therapies – itraconazole, griseofulvin
- **Hypertrophic LP** – oral retinoids often required

Pearls and Pitfalls

- TNF-α inhibitors have been known to cause lichen planus and lichen planus-like drug eruptions (JAAD 2009)

Lichen Planus – Mouthwashes

Table 75 **Mouthwashes commonly used to treat and alleviate oral lesions in a variety of conditions**

Mouthwash	Ingredients
Benacort-Tetrastat	Nystatin suspension, 60 ml + Diphenhydradmine cough syrup, 180 ml + Tetracycline powder, 60 mg *Disp:* 240 ml *Sig:* Swish 5–10 ml up to QID. Expires in 6 months
Xyloxylin *Sugar-free mix*	Diphenhydramine HCl, USP 0.14 g + Lidocaine 1% injectable, 10 ml + Spearmint water, 60 ml + Maalox Plus suspension QS, 240 ml *Disp:* 240 ml *Sig:* Shake well. Swish 5–10 ml QID. Expires in 1 year. *Note* – Each 15 ml containes diphenhydramine 8.5 mg, lidocaine 5.25 mg, Maalox plus suspension 10 ml
Xyloxadryl	Lidocaine viscous 2%, 100 ml + Diphenhydramine syrup, 100 ml + Maalox plus suspension, 100 ml *Disp:* 300 ml *Sig:* Shake well then swish 5–10 ml QID. Expires in 6 months. *Note* – Each 15 ml contains viscous lidocaine 2% 5 ml, diphenhydramine syrup 5 ml, and Maalox 5 ml
Stomafate suspension	Sucralfate powder, 24 g + Distilled water, 80 ml + Diphenhydramine syrup, 60 ml + Maalox plus suspension QS, 180 ml *Disp:* 180 ml *Sig:* Shake well, BID to QID. Refrigerate. Expires in 2 months *Note* – Each 15 ml contains sucralfate 2 g, diphenhydramine 12.5 mg, and Maalox 2.5 ml
Dr. Weisman's Philadelphia mouthwash	Maalox Plus suspension, 90 ml + Lidocaine viscous 2%, 90 ml + Diphenhydramine cough syrup, 90 ml + Distilled water, 180 ml *Disp:* 960 ml *Sig:* Shake well, BID to QID. Refrigerate. *Note* – Each 5 ml contains lidocaine 16.5 mg, diphenhydramine 1.2 mg, maalox plus suspension 3.7 ml
Radiotherapy Mixture	Maalox Plus suspension, 700 ml + Lidocaine viscous 2%, 160 ml + Diphenhydramine cough syrup, 100 ml *Disp:* 960 ml *Sig:* Shake well, BID to QID. Refrigerate. *Note* – Each 5 ml contains lidocaine 16.5 mg, diphenhydramine 1.2 mg, maalox 3. 7 ml
Mouthwash Version #1	Maalox susp, 80 ml + Lidocaine viscous 2%, 80 ml + Diphenhydramine elixir, 80 ml *Disp:* 240 ml *Sig:* Take 1 tsp TID. Refrigerate.
Mouthwash Version #2	Tetracycline 1. 5 g + Nystatin 3 million units + Hydrocortisone powder, 60 mg + Water + flavor in 8 oz *Disp:* 8 oz *Sig:* 1 Tbsp QID. Refrigerate.
Viscous Lidocaine (Swish and Spit)	Viscous lidocaine 2% *Sig:* 5 ml (1 tsp) q 6 h as needed *Disp:* 30 day supply

(1) Note: there are many versions of "magic mouthwash" out there – you need to specify to the pharmacist what you want. Typically, they have a 1:1:1 ratio of ingredients. Common ingredients include lidocaine, diphenhydramine, nystatin, maalox, tetracycline, corticosteroids.

(2) Note: With certain patients, you could give them a Rx for the ingredients (such as nystatin or viscous lidocaine) and they could add this to maalox and diphenhydramine themselves – this would eliminate the compounding fee

Lichen Sclerosus et Atrophicus (LsA)

Etiology and Pathogenesis

- AKA – Balanitis xerotica obliterans (glans penis presentation), and kraurosis vulvae (older description of vulvar presentation)
- Exact etiology unknown but genetic factors contribute. MHC class II antigen HLA-DQ7 seen in many patients.
- IgG autoantibodies against extracellular matrix protein 1 (ECM-1) seen in 80%
- Oxidative stress may play a role in the pathogenesis of LsA

Clinical Presentation

- Sclerotic, white scar-like lesions that are guttate, aggregated or coalescent into a shiny, ivory, relatively soft scar with a wrinkled surface. Lesions may have a bluish tinge. Erosions may develop, particularly in the genital area. Atrophy is common.
- May begin as papules which coalesce into patches or plaques
- Extragenital involvement
  - ○ Oral cavity (rare) on buccal mucosa or tongue
  - ○ Neck, shoulders, flexoral wrists, sites of physical trauma or continuous pressure (e.g., shoulder or hip)
  - ○ Periorbital area and scalp – rare
- **Complications:**
  - ○ Male genital
    - ■ Painful erections, urinary obstruction, an inability to retract the foreskin, and squamous cell carcinoma (rare)
  - ○ Female genital
    - ■ Dyspareunia, urinary obstruction, secondary infection from chronic ulceration, secondary infection related to steroid use, and squamous cell carcinoma (rare, but more common than in males). Some estimates are as high as 5% for the lifetime risk of vulvar squamous cell carcinoma in patients with LsA
      - □ Risks of SCC = older age, longer duration of disease, evidence of hyperplastic/early vulvar carcinoma in situ changes
  - ○ Extragenital: cosmetic concerns

Labs – Consider checking for hepatitis C if erosive lichen planus is on the differential

DDx – scleroderma, morphea, genital LsA may mimic erosive lichen planus, GVHD, anetoderma, atrophoderma of Pasini and Pierini, inverse psoriasis in some cases.

Histology

- Hyperkeratosis often, but usually with atrophy of the spinous layer of the epidermis
- Follicular plugging and flattened dermal–epidermal junction (advanced stage)
- Liquefaction degeneration of the basal layer and rarely can see subepidermal blister
- Edematous homogenized superficial dermis with vascular dilation
- Lichenoid lymphocytes seen in early lesions near the basal layer and later in the mid dermis (beneath the homogenized layer)

Treatment

- Local treatment
  - **Potent topical steroids**
  - Tacrolimus or Pimecrolimus have been helpful in some cases of genital LsA – tend to work slower
  - Cryotherapy has been helpful for some cases
  - Circumcision in males may help resolve LsA
- Systemic treatment
  - Phototherapy – UVA1, PUVA
  - PO Retinoids (Soriatane, Accutane) – May downregulate fibroblast activity
  - PO Antipruritics prn
- Lasers have been helpful in some cases – pulsed dye and Er:YAG lasers (non-ablative) and even CO2 laser (ablative)
- Not recommended = surgery

Pearls and Pitfalls

- Biopsy suspicious changes or ulcerations to rule out malignancy
- No evidence that topical hormonal therapies (such as estrogen) play any role in treatment and can be associated with virilization. Many doctors will still prescribe this.
- Always evaluate the genital area, even in extragenital involvement (even if the patient denies involvement of the genital area)
- If a patient is seen for another issue and they mention they have LsA, it is reasonable to examine the area to: (1) confirm the diagnosis, and (2) make sure that proper treatment is being administered such there is a high risk of scarring.
- Male genital LSA is seen almost exclusively in uncircumcised men and boys
- Genital involvement in young girls may be misdiagnosed as child abuse

Linear IgA Bullous Dermatosis (LABD)

Etiology and Pathogenesis

- An immune-mediated subepidermal vesiculobullous eruption that occurs in both adults and children. At least two distinct subtypes:
  - **Lamina lucida type (majority)** – IgA antibodies directed toward carboxy terminus of BPAG2 (in contrast to BP where IgG binds in NC16 region of BPAG2)
  - **Sublamina densa type** – target unclear but some have reported IgA antibodies binding to type VII collagen in anchoring fibrils
- **In adults, the condition is frequently medication-related**
  - Meds that can cause LABD → **vancomycin,** penicillins, cephalosporins, captopril (more than other ACE inhibitors), NSAIDs
    - Uncommon – phenytoin, sulfonamide antibiotics
    - Rare – amiodarone, ARBs, atorvastatin, carbamazepine, cyclosporine, furosemide, gemcitabine, glyburide, G-CSF stimulator, IFN, IL-2, lithium, PUVA, rifampin, somatostatin
- Some reports of association with:
  - Gastrointestinal disease – inflammatory bowel disease
  - Autoimmune diseases –SLE, dermatomyositis
  - Malignancies – B-cell lymphoma, CLL, carcinoma of the bladder, thyroid, and esophagus
  - Infections – varicella, herpes zoster, antibiotic-treated tetanus, upper respiratory infections

Clinical Presentation

- Presentation may vary:
  - Subepidermal tense bullae which may mimic bullous pemphigoid
  - Lesion often appear in a herpetiform arrangement ("string of pearls") on erythematous or normal-appearing skin
  - Some present with annular expanding plaques
  - May present with oral, ocular, nasal, pharyngeal and esophageal lesions which may mimic cicatricial pemphigoid
  - **Lamina lucida type of LABD** – no mucosal lesions, no scarring
  - **Sublamina densa type of LABD** – mucosal involvement + scarring

Labs – G6PD, CBC + diff, CMP. Consider other labs based on history and physical.

DDx – bullous pemphigoid, cicatricial pemphigoid, dermatitis herpetiformis

Histology

- Subepidermal vesicular dermatosis with neutrophils aligned along the BMZ, accompanied by vacuolar change and sometimes neutrophilic microabscesses in dermal papillae (mimicking DH).
- Eosinophils become more numerous with time
- DIF
  - LABD – lamina lucida type → Linear IgA BMZ , Wavy fibrillar
  - LABD – sublamina densa type → Linear IgA BMZ, thick
- IIF
  - LABD – lamina lucida type → IgA – epidermal side
  - LABD – sublamina densa type → IgA – dermal side

Treatment

- Majority will respond to either **dapsone** or **sulfapyridine** therapy (within 48–72 h)
  - Average dose of dapsone is 100 mg, but may need more than that
- May be necessary to add oral prednisone for some
- Antibiotics have been successful in both adults and children for some
  - Tetracycline (for those over age 8–9)
  - Erythromycin
  - Dicloxacillin
- Other therapies – IVIG, mycophenolate mofetil, azathioprine, cyclosporine

Pearls and Pitfalls

- Patients with both IgG and IgA deposits in the BMZ may be more difficult to treat
- The childhood form typically remits in 2–4 years
- There should be repeated attempts to taper medications, as the disease can spontaneously remit
- Always rule out drug-induced LABD. Vancomycin is, by far, the most common cause

Liquid Nitrogen Treatment Care

Your skin has been treated with liquid nitrogen. This produces a localized severe freezing of the skin lesion and a small area of surrounding skin. Although the freezing itself wore off within minutes, the effects which the freezing produced will not be fully seen for 24–72 h.

The stinging and burning sensation which follows the actual freezing usually last only 20–30 min and will be accompanied by redness of the area. Once this burning has stopped, you should have no further pain. The area may be tender for several days, but acetaminophen (Tylenol) will generally control any persistent pain.

Within 24 h after treatment, a blister may form in the treated area. This will probably be a deep blister with a thick cover and may not resemble the type of blister you are accustomed to seeing, such as from a burn. The blister may be bloody (red to purple in color). You should not be concerned about this. You should leave the blister alone unless it is large and in the way, and then it may be punctured with a clean needle (use alcohol) to relieve the pressure.

As long as the blister is intact, healing will occur rapidly without special attention. However, if the top of the blister is removed for any reason, you should cover the area with Polysporin ointment, which you can get without a prescription, and a bandaid for 3–4 days.

Livedo Reticularis (LR)

- Relatively common physical finding consisting of macular, violaceous, connecting rings that form a netlike pattern
- **LR Without Systemic Associations**
  - Physiologic LR/cutis marmorata
    - Appears in response to cold exposure and resolves with complete warming of affected limb. Most common in neonates (especially preterm infants) and fair-skinned females. Usually on lower extremities. Usually resolves spontaneously
    - Cutis marmorata = most common cause of LR in infants and children
  - Primary LR
    - Diagnosis of exclusion. Defined by the appearance and resolution of LR independent of ambient temp and in the absence of underlying disease. Likely from spontaneous arteriolar vasospasm.
  - Idiopathic LR
    - Persistent LR without underlying cause. Diagnosis of exclusion. Shares many features as primary LR, but differs by the persistence of the livedo pattern. Does not resolve with warming, although it may become less prominent with warming. Most typically seen in females ages 20–60. Usually asymptomatic. Tx – avoid cold.
- **LR with Systemic Associations**
  - Congenital – Cutis marmorata telangiectatica congentia (CMTC)
    - Presents at birth and localized to lower extremities. Occasionally, it is more generalized. High % have assoc anomalies – most are minor, but some major.
    - Associated anomalies
      - *Craniofacial and cutaneous* – cleft palate, micrognathia, dystrophic teeth, glaucoma, optic nerve atrophy, facial asymmetry, frontal bossing, macrocephaly, high arched palate, hyperplastic skin, aplasia cutis
      - *Neurologic and skeletal* – MR, delayed motor development, seizure, hypotonia, skeletal, syndactyly
      - *Hypertrophy of affected limb*
      - *Vascular* – local varicosities, hemangiomatous malformations, cerebrovascular malformations, Sturge–Weber, patent ductus arteriosus, atrial septal defect, double aortic arch

Table 76   Conditions associated with livedo reticularis

LR without systemic associations	Physiologic LR (cutis marmorata), primary LR, idiopathic LR
LR with systemic associations	
Congenital	Cutis marmorata telangiectatica congenita (CMTC), transplacental transient vasculitis
Hematologic, Hypercoagulable	Antiphospholipid syndrome, Sneddon's syndrome, cryoglobulinemia, Cryofibrinogenemia, multiple myeloma, cold agglutinins, polycythemia vera, essential thrombocythemia, Protein S and C deficiency, antithrombin III deficiency, DVT, disseminated intravascular coagulation, thrombocytopathy, thrombotic thrombocytopenic purpura, hemolytic uremic syndrome, small vessel vasculitis
Medium vessel vasculitis	Polyarteritis nodosa, rheumatoid vasculitis, Wegener's granulomatosis, microscopic polyangitis, nodular vasculitis, thromboangiitis obliterans
Large vessel vasculitis	Takayasu's arteritis, temporal arteritis
Connective tissue disease	Dermatomyositis, SLE, systemic sclerosis, Still's disease, Sjögren's syndrome, Sharp's syndrome
Emboli/Vessel wall deposition	Cholesterol embolization syndrome, septic embolization, carbon dioxide arteriography, calciphylaxis, hyperoxaluria, atrial myxoma, primary amyloidosis, ventilator gas embolism, fat emboli, nitrogen (decompression sickness)
Medications	Amantadine, minocycline, gemcitabine, heparin, thrombolytics, interferon-β, erythromycin/lovastatin interactin, catecholamines, bismuth, quinidine
Infectious disease	Hepatitis C, mycoplasma pneumonia, brucella, coxiella burnetti, parvovirus B19, tuberculosis, meningococcemia, streptococcemia, rickettsial, rheumatic fever, typhus fever, "viral infections", syphilis, endocarditis
Neoplasia	Renal cell carcinoma, inflammatory breast cancer, lymphomas (MF, angiotrophic), acute lymphocytic leukemia
Neurologic	Reflex sympathetic dystrophy, midline catheter insertion, diabetes mellitus, pernicious anemia, multiple sclerosis, encephalitis, poliomyelitis, Parkinson's disease, brain injury
Endocrine/Nutritional	Hypercalcemia, hypothyroidism, pheochromocytoma, carcinoid, Cushing's disease, Pellagra
Miscellaneous	Chronic pancreatitis, primary fibromyalgia, congenital hypogammaglobulinemia, cardiac failure, neurofibromatosis

- Workup of Livedo Reticularis
  - Evaluate every patient carefully – comprehensive history and physical
    - Location of LR, exacerbating and alleviating factors (e.g., ambient temperatures), duration of attacks and cutaneous symptoms
    - Questions regarding symptoms of autoimmune CT disease
    - Personal or family hx of thrombosis or hypercoagulability
    - New neurologic symptoms and general review of systems
    - Recent vascular procedures
    - Medical history – Renal failure? Medications? Risk factors for hepatitis C?
  - Physical Exam
    - Ulcerations or nodules present? (can suggest a vasculitis)

- ○ Labs – should be directed by history and physical exam; with few exceptions, extensive screening panels are unlikely to be useful
  - **Lupus anticoagulant panel** – reasonable to consider in all patients with LR that is not clearly and exclusively related to cold exposure
    - □ Note – risk of thrombosis in patients with aPLs who don't have recurrent thrombosis but do have LR is unknown → benefit of tx with anticoagulant is uncertain
  - Skin biopsy may be useful. The proper area to biopsy → may be either the bluish areas forming the outer portion of the circle or the blanched area in the center of the circle. May be best to obtain two biopsies – one from each area.
    - □ If nodules or fixed purpuric areas are present, these should be biopsied.

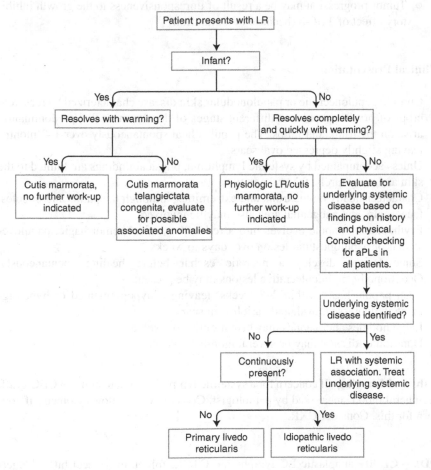

Fig. 12 Algorithm for evaluation of patient presenting with livedo reticularis (LR). *aPLs,* Antiphospholipid antibodies; *N,* no; *Y,* yes
Reference: Used with permission from Elsevier. Gibbs MB, English JC III, and Zirwas MJ. Livedo Reticularis: An update. J Amer Acad Dermatol 2005; 52(6): 1009–19

Lymphomatoid Papulosis (LyP)

Etiology and Pathogenesis

- LyP is part of a spectrum of CD30 (Ki-1)–positive cutaneous lymphoprolifera-
  tive diseases (CD30$^+$ LPDs), including LyP, primary cutaneous anaplastic large
  cell lymphoma (pcALCL), and borderline CD30$^+$ lesions
- Initiating event is unknown, but possibly viral
- Exact pathogenesis unknown but it has been suggested:
  - That interactions between CD30 and its ligand (CD30L) may contribute to
    apoptosis of the neoplastic T cells and the subsequent regression of the skin
    lesions, but the exact mechanism is yet unknown
  - Tumor progression may be a result of unresponsiveness to the growth inhibi-
    tory effect of TGF-β (because of a mutation)

Clinical Presentation

- Chronic papulonecrotic or papulonodular skin disease characterized by recurrent
  crops of pruritic papules at different stages of development that predominantly
  arise on the trunk and limbs. The papules heal spontaneously over 1–2 months
  leaving slightly depressed oval scars.
- Unless accompanied by systemic lymphoma, physical findings are limited to the
  skin and, very rarely, the oral cavity
- Characteristically on the trunk and extremities, although the palms and/or soles,
  face, scalp, and anogenital area also may be involved
- Erythematous papule evolves into a red-brown, often hemorrhagic, papulove-
  sicular or papulopustular lesion over days to weeks
- Some lesions develop a necrotic eschar before healing spontaneously.
  Occasionally, noduloulcerative lesions may be present
- Each papule heals within 2–8 weeks, leaving a hypopigmented or hyperpig-
  mented, depressed, oval, and varioliform scar
- Large nodules and plaques may take months to resolve
- Duration of disease may be several months to years

Labs and Imaging– If concern for a systemic lymphoma or leukemia → CBC + diff,
peripheral blood smear read by pathologist. Consider CTCL flow cytometry if concern for this. Consider CXR.

DDx – CD30+ anaplastic LC lymphoma, CTCL, folliculitis, insect bites, langerhans cell histiocytosis, leukemia cutis, lymphocytoma cutis, papular drug eruption,
papular MF, PLEVA, 1° or 2° cutaneous B-cell lymphoma, primary or secondary
cutaneous Hodgkin's disease

Histology – extremely variable

- Low-power →wedge-shaped dense dermal infiltrate of lymphoid cells with numerous eosinophils, neutrophils, and atypical lymphocytes. As much as 50% of the infiltrate shows the atypical lymphocytes. Epidermotropism of lymphoid cells may occur. Dermal vessels may show endothelial swelling, fibrin deposition, and RBC extravasation.
- Histologically, LyP is divided into the following three subtypes:
  - **Type A** – characterized by large (25–40 μm) CD30⁺ atypical cells intermingled with a prominent inflammatory infiltrate. Large tumor cells have polymorphic convoluted nuclei with a minimum of one prominent nucleolus and resemble Reed–Sternberg cells when binucleate, as is seen in HD. Type A is the most common histologic variant and accounts for 75% of all LyP specimens.
  - **Type B** – characterized by smaller (8–15 μm) atypical cells with hyperchromatic cerebriform nuclei resembling the atypical lymphocytes in MF. CD30⁺ large cells are rare, but epidermotropism is more common in this variant. There is some concern that Type B LyP may be better classified as a papular variant of MF.
  - **Type C** – characterized by sheets of CD30⁺ anaplastic large cells indistinguishable from ALCL, with the exception of the minimal subcutaneous invasion. Lesions resolve spontaneously and are therefore classified as LyP; however, some authorities view this histologic variant as borderline ALCL.

Treatment

- Some authorities currently are more inclined to treat lesions with systemic or more aggressive topical therapies, including phototherapy, to suppress the disease and the possibility of progression to MF, ALCL, or HD
- Low-dose weekly methotrexate (MTX) – 5 mg PO q week; may require up to 25 mg/week
  - Safe and effective treatment for suppressing LyP; however, the disease recurs within 1–2 weeks after discontinuing the medication
- PUVA
- Topical carmustine
- Topical nitrogen mustard
- Imiquimod cream
- Intralesional interferon
- Low-dose cyclophosphamide
- Chlorambucil
- UVA-1 therapy
- Excimer laser therapy
- Dapsone

Pearls and Pitfalls

- Most patients have a chronic, indolent course
- Overall survival rate was 92% at 5 and 10 years
- Long-term follow-up recommended in all patients as there is a potential risk for systemic lymphoma

Mastocytosis

Etiology and Pathogenesis

- Alterations in KIT structure and activity are central to the pathogenesis of some forms of mastocytosis. Point mutations in *c-kit* proto-oncogene cause constitutive activation of KIT, leading to continued mast cell development.
- Stem cell factor (SCF), which is the ligand for KIT, may also play a role in the pathogenesis.

Clinical Presentation and Types

- **Childhood mastocytosis** (75% of all cases appear in childhood)
  - All three of the childhood forms may display vesicular or bullous variants, which is related to histamine release.
  - **Darier's sign** – hallmark of the disorder and seen in 90%. Rubbing the lesion leads to erythema, edema, and urticarial wheals. Develops within a few minutes of the stimulus and may persist for 30 min. May be negative in patients with entirely flat lesions.
  - **Solitary mastocytoma** – solitary tan or red-brown or yellow-tan nodule or plaque. May present at birth or arise in infancy. Represent 15–20% of all childhood mastocytosis. Location often on distal extremities and often spares the central face, scalp, palms, and soles.
  - **Urticaria pigmentosa** – most common presentation. See numerous tan or red-brown papules and nodules distributed over body. Most cases of UP in children resolve spontaneously by ages 3–5, although acute extensive degranulation rarely can cause life-threatening episodes of shock.
  - **Diffuse cutaneous mastocytosis** – rare in children. Characterized by diffuse infiltration of the skin by mast cells, leading to skin that may appear grossly normal, thickened, doughy, and reddish-brown (or peau d'orange texture). Present with extensive bullous eruptions. This form has the highest frequency of systemic disease. May also develop pruritus, flushing, temp elevation, vomiting, diarrhea, abdominal pain, GI ulceration, or respiratory distress and shock.
  - **Telangiectasia macularis eruptiva perstans (TMEP)** – rare in children; usually seen in adults. Have an eruption of small, red-brown, telangiectatic macules on the trunk and extremities. Little or no tendency toward urtication.
  - **Systemic mastocytosis** – markedly more common in adults than in children. Can develop symptoms involving GI (abdominal pain, diarrhea, nausea, vomiting, hemorrhage), pulmonary (bronchospasm and respiratory distress), kidneys, lymph nodes, cardiac liver, spleen, bone marrow, and skeletal (radio-opacities, radiolucencies).
  - Risk of hematologic malignancy is a major concern for adults with mastocytosis but the risk in childhood is extremely low.

- **Adult mastocytosis** (peak ages 30–49)
  - ○ **Telangiectasia macularis eruptiva perstans (TMEP)** – Have an eruption of small, red-brown, telangiectatic macules on the trunk and extremities. Little or no tendency toward urtication.
  - ○ **Diffuse cutaneous mastocytosis** – Characterized by diffuse infiltration of the skin by mast cells, leading to skin that may appear grossly normal, thickened, doughy, and reddish-brown (or peau d'orange texture).
  - ○ **Numerous mastocytomas** – most common and appear as red-brown macules or papules. Usually located on the trunk and proximal extremities. May resolve spontaneously and reappear.
  - ○ Adult-onset systemic mastocytosis has a malignant transformation rate as high as 30%
    - ▪ Mast cell leukemia or hematologic malignancy
- WHO criteria for diagnosis of systemic mast cell disease
  - ○ Need 1 major + 1 minor OR 3 minor
  - ○ **Major** – Multifocal dense infiltrates of mast cells in bone marrow or other extracutaneous organs (>15 mast cells aggregating)
  - ○ **Minor**
    - ▪ Mast cells in bone marrow, or other extracutaneous organs show abnormal (spindling) morphology (>25%)
    - ▪ Codon 816 *c-kit* mutation D816V in extracutaneous organs
    - ▪ Mast cells in bone marrow express CD2, CD25, or both
    - ▪ Serum tryptase values greater than 20 ng/mL

Labs and Imaging to Consider

- CBC – may reveal anemia, ↓ plts, ↑plts, ↑ WBC, and ↑ Eos in systemic mastocytosis
- Plasma or urinary histamine level: Patients with extensive cutaneous lesions may have 24-h urine histamine excretion at 2–3 times the normal level
- Urinary *N*-methylhistamine (NMH) and *N*-methylimidazoleacetic acid levels – may be more sensitive and specific than urinary histamine levels
  - ○ NMH levels decrease with age; therefore, consider the patient's age when interpreting results
- Total tryptase level (marker of mast cell degranulation released in parallel w/ histamine)
  - ○ Total tryptase levels in plasma correlate with the density of mast cells in UP lesions in adults with systemic mastocytosis
  - ○ Patients with only CM typically have normal levels of total tryptase
  - ○ Seems to be a more discriminating biomarker than urinary methylhistamine for the diagnosis of systemic mastocytosis
  - ○ May be more useful than histamine levels, because histamine can be elevated in hypereosinophilic states

- Urinary prostaglandin D$_2$ metabolite level (not widely available)
  - May range from 1.5 to 150 times higher than normal levels even during asymptomatic periods
- Bone marrow biopsy and aspirate: Consider in patients with UP if peripheral blood test abnormalities, hepatomegaly, splenomegaly, or lymphadenopathy to determine if they have an associated hematologic disorder
- Bone scan and radiologic survey
  - Obtain a bone scan and radiologic survey in nonpediatric patients or if the CBC count is abnormal in a young child. If a patient has skeletal system symptoms, perform a bone scan and radiologic survey to identify lytic bone lesions, osteoporosis, or osteosclerosis.
- GI workup (upper GI series, small bowel radiography, CT scanning, endoscopy)
  - If patient has GI symptoms, order workup to ID peptic ulcers, abnormal mucosal patterns, or motility disturbances

DDx – bullous disorders may be considered, urticaria, arthropod bites, herpes simplex, bullous impetigo, nodular scabies, Spitz nevi, pseudolymphomas, and juvenile xanthogranulomas.

Histology

- NOTE on **Biopsy**: Inject an anesthetic agent **without** epinephrine adjacent to, not directly into, the lesion chosen as the biopsy specimen to avoid mast cell degranulation, which makes histologic examination difficult.
- Perivascular or diffuse dermal mast cells, often with a few eosinophils. See dermal edema or subepidermal bullous formation (occasionally). Mast cells can be recognized on H&E stain, but are better demonstrated with Giemsa, Leder, toluidine blue, or tryptase stains. Mast cells can have a "fried egg" appearance with granules in the cytoplasm.
- Immunohistochemical staining available → CD117 (KIT)

Treatment

- Advise patients to avoid agents that precipitate mediator release, such as aspirin, NSAIDs, codeine, morphine, alcohol, thiamine, quinine, opiates, gallamine, decamethonium, procaine, radiographic dyes, dextran, polymyxin B, scopolamine
- H1 and H2 antihistamines decrease pruritus, flushing, and GI symptoms
  - **Hydroxyzine** 25–100 mg PO hs or divided QID
    - Peds → <6 years: 0.7 mg/kg/dose PO tid, >6 years: 50–100 mg/day PO in divided doses
  - **Cimetidine** (Tagamet) 300 mg PO QID with meals and hs
    - Peds → 20–40 mg/kg/day PO in divided doses

- PO disodium cromoglycate may ameliorate cutaneous symptoms, such as pruritus, whealing, and flushing, as well as systemic symptoms, such as diarrhea, abdominal pain, bone pain, and disorders of cognitive function
  - **Gastrocom** 200 mg PO qid 0.5 h ac and hs
    - Peds → <2 years: 20 mg/kg/day PO divided qid (attempt only in severe dz), 2–12 years: 100 mg PO qid 0.5 h ac and hs
- Aspirin to inhibit prostaglandin synthesis and maintain mast cell degranulation
  - May be beneficial for patients with dz resistant to H1 and H2 antagonist tx alone
  - Start with small doses, slowly titrate to reach plasma level of 20–30 mg/100 mL
  - Initiate this treatment regimen in a controlled environment, because aspirin can induce mast cell mediator release and subsequent cardiovascular collapse
- Corticosteroids may be helpful if limited area of involvement
- PUVA – may be used for TMEP; risk of skin cancer if > 200 tx
  - Reserve for severe, unresponsive cases in adults
- UVA-1 tx
- Interferon-α-2b has been used with some success in aggressive forms
- Imatinib mesylate (Gleevec®) – effective in treating other tumors with KIT mutations. Check for KIT mutation prior to using.
- Other
  - Medical alert bracelets should be made available
  - Epinephrine self-injector demonstration should be performed and self-injector prescribed for patients with systemic mastocytosis
  - General anesthesia may be problematic in patients with systemic mastocytosis, although more recent studies suggest otherwise as long as patient monitored by anesthesiologist
- Hematology Evaluation in:
  - "B findings" – Indicative of a high systemic mastocytosis burden
    - Greater than 30% bone marrow mastocytosis burden
    - Serum tryptase level greater than 200 ng/mL
  - Additional "C findings" diagnostic for the presence of aggressive disease
    - Absolute neutrophil count less than 1,000/μL
    - Hemoglobin value less than 10 g/μL
    - Platelet count less than 100,000/μL
    - Hepatomegaly with ascites and impaired liver function
    - Palpable splenomegaly with hypersplenism
    - Malabsorption with hypoalbuminemia and weight loss
    - Large-sized osteolysis or severe osteoporosis causing pathologic fractures or life-threatening organopathy in other organ systems definitively caused by an infiltration of the tissue by neoplastic mast cells

Pearls and Pitfalls

– Cromolyn sodium helpful in GI symptoms are present
– Ketotifen, a mast cell stabilizer, has shown promise in alleviating symptoms
– Always give out a handout with list of things that can precipitate histamine release by mast cells and educate patient/parent about this.
– Patients should be prescribed an EpiPen or EpiPen Jr., which they should keep with them at all times for emergency use.

Melanoma

Etiology and Pathogenesis

- *NRAS* or *BRAF* mutations seen in nearly 80% of cell lines; also found in nevi
- *CDKN2A* mutations most frequent in melanoma cell lines; some families have *CDKN2A* mutations and can see familial melanoma
- Minor role for *p53* mutations in cutaneous melanoma

Clinical Presentation and Types

- Risk factors – fair skin, large numbers of common nevi, family history of melanoma (especially if *CDKN2A* mutation), history of sunburns, use of tanning, melanocortin-1 receptor (MC1-R) gene
- **Superficial Spreading Melanoma**
  - Accounts for 70% of all cutaneous melanomas. Median age is 30–50 years.
  - Location (men) – trunk; Location (women) – lower extremities
  - Asymmetric patch or plaque with variations in color and border irregularity
  - Papular or nodular component suggests deeper invasion
  - Can arise from preexisting nevi
- **Nodular Melanoma**
  - Accounts for 15% of all cutaneous melanomas. Median age is 40–50
  - Distribution similar to superficial spreading melanoma, but onset more rapid
  - Papule or nodule with colors ranging from red to blue/black. Occ ulcerated.
  - Precursor moles not usually associated
- **Acral Lentiginous Melanoma**
  - Accounts for 10% of all cutaneous melanomas. Median age is 60–65.
  - This is the predominant presentation in Asians, African-Americans
  - Etiology is not sun related – trauma?
  - Distribution is on palms/sole or nail apparatus
  - See dark brown/black macular lesion with foci of plaque or nodule formation. Can develop ulceration. Borders often very ill-defined.
- **Lentigo Maligna (premalignant lesion)**
  - Slowing growing. Not actually a melanoma. Between 5% and 30% become melanoma.
  - Usually located on head/neck
  - Macular lesion with variation in color and irregularity of border
- **Lentigo Maligna Melanoma**
  - Accounts for 5–10% of all cutaneous melanomas. Median age is 65–70.
  - Usually related to cumulative sun exposure and occurs on sun-exposed areas
  - Typically has both a macular component and a papular or nodular component

- **Amelanotic Melanoma**
  - Melanomas lacking pigment, which can be seen in any type of melanoma. May be mistaken for warts, SCC. Amelanotic melanomas do not differ from pigmented melanomas in terms of prognosis or therapy.
- **Nevoid Melanomas – Two types**
  - **Spitzoid Melanoma** – histologic features suggestive of a spitz nevus with overall symmetry and epithelioid melanocytes. Do not mature with progressively deeper extension. See mitotic figures at base. Very difficult to distinguish from a Spitz Nevus.
  - **Melanoma with small nevus-like cells (small cell melanoma)** – contains variably sized, large nests of small melanocytes with hyperchromatic nuclei and prominent nucleoli. Mitoses found throughout.
- **Malignant Blue Nevus**
  - Rare dermal tumor of melanocytes, usually located on the head or scalp and is generally > 1 cm in diameter. Appears blue-black.
  - Histologically, see elements of a blue nevus but areas of atypical spindle-shaped melanocytes, mitotic figures, necrosis, and melanophages. High rate of recurrence and metastasis.
- **Desmoplastic/Spindled/Neurotropic Melanoma**
  - Skin-colored, red or brown-black nodule or plaque, usually in sun-exposed area
  - Metastases to lymph nodes is uncommon, but tumor is highly infiltrative and locally aggressive
  - Tend to be deep at time of diagnosis and conventional T staging tends to overestimate the likelihood for metastasis
- **Clear Cell Sarcoma: Melanoma of Soft Parts**
  - Usually presents on distal extremities of adolescents and young adults
  - Arise in association with tendons, aponeuroses. Composed of oval to spindled cells with vesicular nuclei, basophilic nucleoli, and eosinophilic to clear cytoplasm.
  - Immunohistochemical studies suggest this is a melanoma, but clinical course tends to follow that of other soft tissue sarcomas → high likelihood of regional and distant metastasis
- **Animal-Type Melanoma** (so named b/c it resembles melanocytic neoplasms seen in white or gray horses)
  - Characterized by nodules and fascicles of epithelioid melanocytes with pleomorphic nuclei, striking hyperpigmentation, dendritic cells, numerous melanophages, and sometimes a lymphocytic infiltrate.
  - Metastases have been seen in some.
- **Ocular Melanoma**
  - Primary ocular melanomas are rare (5% of all melanomas) and are divided → conjunctival melanomas, uveal melanomas
  - Patients with numerous dysplastic nevi have increased number of conjunctival, uveal nevi
  - Patients with nevus of Ota may be at higher risk for uveal melanoma
  - Prognostic features and treatment differs from those of cutaneous melanoma

- **Mucosal Melanoma**
  - Account for < 4% of all melanomas. Many are amelanotic.
  - Rare lesions that occur in the mouth, nasopharynx, larynx, vagina, and anus
  - Tend to occur near the mucocutaneous junctions of squamous and columnar epithelia
  - These tumors tend to be diagnosed at an advanced stage
- **Childhood Melanoma**
  - Very rare. Approximately 2% of melanomas occur in patients < age 20 and only 0.3% in those < age 14. Risk factors are same as in adults.
  - Rare conditions such as xeroderma pigmentosa and giant congenital nevi contribute minimally to the prepubertal incidence

Labs – elevated serum lactate dehydrogenase (LDH) at the time of diagnosis portends a particularly dismal outcome. Currently, if the LDH is elevated at the time of diagnosis (regardless of site or number of metastases), it automatically places the patient into the worst prognostic category, stage M1c.

DDx – many conditions can simulate melanoma, either clinically or histologically – spitz nevi, dysplastic nevi, seborrheic keratoses, blue nevi, pyogenic granuloma, etc.

Histology – can vary somewhat depending on the type of melanoma
- Epidermis may be normal, atrophic, hyperplastic or ulceration (latter = worse prognosis)
- Poorly defined, asymmetrical proliferation of melanocytes
- Atypical melanocytes – small, spindled, or epithelioid – arise at the dermal–epidermal junction and invade the dermis. Cytologic atypia may be slight or severe.
- Poor maturation of the melanocytes (deeper cells just as large, atypical as the superficial ones)
- Pagetoid melanocytes and melanocytes above the DEJ
- Regression sometimes present – vascular fibrous tissue in papillary dermis, +/− melanophages.
- Special stains → S-100 (most sensitive, but not specific), HMB-45, and Mart-1 (more specific, less sensitive and tend to be negative in spindle cell melanoma).

Treatment

- If untreated, cancer will likely metastasize – spreads to draining lymph nodes → distant sites
- Primary melanoma
- Surgery

Table 77 Surgical treatment of primary melanoma[a]

Thickness	Excision margins (cm)	Comments
In situ	0.5	No randomized studies, lentigo maligna of the face might be treated with radiotherapy in specialized centers
≤ 1 mm	1.0	AAD task force suggests 1 cm margin for melanoma <2 mm
1–4 mm	2.0	AAD task force suggests 2 cm margin for melanoma ≥2 mm
> 4 mm	2.0–3.0	No randomized studies

[a]With new 2010 AJCC staging, it is recommended that a SLNB be performed for T1b (Breslow depth ≤ 1 mm with ulceration or mitoses ≥ $1/mm^2$), T2, T3 and T4

- Lymph Node Disease – Interferon α-2A
- Distant internal disease – nothing very effective
  - ○ Chemotherapy with **dacarbazine**
  - ○ **Ipilimumab** – Yervoy™ (Bristol–Meyers Squibb) – A fully human monoclonal antibody against cytotoxic T-Lymphocyte antigen4 (CTLA-4 antagonist). Dosed as a 3-mg/kg infusion over 90 min every 3 weeks for a total of four doses (12 weeks).
    - ■ FDA-approved labeling of ipilimumab only discusses monotherapy, although it has been studied in combination with dacarbazine, temozolomide, carboplatin, and fotemustine. The only combination therapy for which there is currently evidence of benefit is ipilimumab plus dacarbazine, which improves the overall survival, compared with either drug alone.
  - ○ Immunotherapy with interleukin-2
  - ○ Vaccine trials

Staging of Melanoma

- Stage I, II → local disease
- Stage III → regional disease
- Stage IV → distant disease
- American Joint Committee on Cancer (AJCC) revised melanoma staging criteria in 2010
  - ○ Sentinel lymph node biopsy (SLNB) is recommended for: T1b, T2, T3, and T4
  - ○ SLNB is a recommended requirement for inclusion in clinical trials
  - ○ Mitotic rate has replaced Clark level for stratification of thin melanomas
  - ○ Tumor thickness and ulceration remain significant in staging.

Table 78   2010 TNM staging system for cutaneous melanoma (AJCC)

Primary tumor (T)	
TX	Primary tumor cannot be assessed (e.g., curettage or severely regressed primary)
T0	No evidence of primary tumor
Tis	Melanoma in situ
T1	≤ 1 mm a: without ulceration and mitoses < 1/mm² **b: with ulceration or mitoses[3] 1/mm²** – *SLNB recommended at this point*
T2	1.01 – 2 mm a: without ulceration b: with ulceration
T3	2.01 – 4 mm a: without ulceration b: with ulceration
T4	> 4 mm a: without ulceration b: with ulceration
Regional lymph nodes (N)	
NX	Patients in whom the regional lymph nodes cannot be assessed (e.g., previously removed for another reason)
N0	No regional metastases detected
N1	1 lymph node a: micrometastases b: macrometastases
N2	2–3 lymph nodes a: micrometastases b: macrometastases c: in-transit met(s)/satellite(s) without metastatic lymph nodes
N3	Four or more metastatic lymph nodes, or matted lymph nodes, or in-transit met(s)/satellite(s) with metastatic lymph node(s)
Distant metastasis (M)	
M0	No detectable evidence of distant metastases
M1a	Metastases to skin, subcutaneous, or distant lymph node, normal serum LDH
M1b	Lung metastases, normal LDH
M1c	Metastasis to other visceral organs with a normal LDH, or any distant metastases and an elevated LDH
Micrometastases=diagnosed after SLN biopsy and completion lymphadenectomy (if performed)	
Macrometastases=defined as clinically detectable lymph node metastases confirmed by therapeutic lymphadenectomy or when nodal metastasis exhibits gross extracapsular extension	

2010 TNM stage groupings for cutaneous melanoma

Stage	Primary tumor (T)	Regional lymph nodes (N)	Distant metastasis (M)
Clinical staging			
Stage 0	Tis	N0	M0
Stage IA	T1a	N0	M0
Stage IB	T1b	N0	M0
	T2a		
Stage IIA	T2b	N0	M0
	T3a		
Stage IIB	T3b	N0	M0
	T4a		
Stage IIC	T4b	N0	M0
Stage III	Any T	N1, N2, or N3	M0
Stage IV	Any T	Any N	M1
Pathologic staging			
Stage 0	Tis	N0	M0
Stage IA	T1a	N0	M0
Stage IB	T1b	N0	M0
	T2a		
Stage IIA	T2b	N0	M0
	T3a		
Stage IIB	T3b	N0	M0
	T4a		
Stage IIC	T4b	N0	M0
Stage IIIA	T1-4a	N1a	M0
	T1-4a	N2a	
Stage IIIB	T1-4b	N1a	M0
	T1-4b	N2a	
	T1-4a	N1b	
	T1-4a	N2b	
	T1-4a	N2c	
Stage IIIC	T1-4b	N1b	M0
	T1-4b	N2b	
	T1-4b	N2c	
	Any T	N3	
Stage IV	Any T	Any N	Any M

Pearls and Pitfalls

- 5-year survival for patients with lymph node disease is about 30%
- 5-year survival for patients with internal organ disease is < 10%
- Discuss ABCDE's with patients → Asymmetry, border irregularity, color varie-gation, diameter > 5–6 mm, evolving
- Encourage monthly self-skin exams
- Epidemiology → in 2005, one in 34 people get invasive or in situ melanoma. Incidence of melanoma is increasing.

Melasma

Etiology and Pathogenesis

- Exact pathogenesis unknown. UV irradiation causes hyperfunctional melano-cytes to produce increases melanin compared to uninvolved skin. Genetic and ethnic factors also play a role, as does skin type and hormones (estrogen and possibly progesterone)
- Other potential aggravating factors – phenytoin-related anticonvulsants, photo-toxic drugs, autoimmune thyroid disease.

Clinical Presentation

- Presents as symmetric hyperpigmented macules, which can be confluent or punctate. The cheeks, the upper lip, the chin, and the forehead are the most common locations, but it can occasionally occur in other sun-exposed locations.
- Lesions fade during winter months
- May be more common in light brown skin types, especially Hispanics and Asians, from areas of the world with intense sun exposure
- **Distribution** – one of three patterns: centrofacial, malar, or mandibular. Rare pattern confined to forearms is seen in women receiving exogenous progesterone and in Native American Indians
- **Examination with Wood Lamp** – excess melanin can be visually localized to the epidermis or the dermis by use of a Wood lamp (wavelength, 340–400 nm).
  - Epidermal pigment is enhanced during examination with a Wood light, whereas, dermal pigment is not
  - Clinically, a large amount of dermal melanin is suspected if the hyperpigmentation is bluish black
  - In individuals with dark-brown skin, examination with a Wood light does not localize pigment, and these patients are thus classified as indeterminate

Labs – consider checking thyroid function, but usually no labs necessary

DDx– Addison disease, drug-induced photosensitivity, drug-induced hyperpigmentation, DLE, mastocytosis, poikiloderma of Civatte, actinic lichen planus, linear morphea, phytophotodermatitis, PIH, EDP, pigmented contact dermatitis, cutaneous mercury deposits, erythromelanosis follicularis faciei et colli

Histology

- Increased melanin deposition in all layers of epidermis. An increased number of melanin-containing dermal macrophages (melanophages) may also be seen. Epidermal melanocytes are normal to increased in number and are enlarged with prominent dendrites.

Treatment

- Sun-protection key in effective therapy and preventing relapses →broad-spectrum sunscreen, hats, clothing (if extra facial). Without strict adherence, any treatment regimen will fail.
- Most common regiment=**hydroquinone (2–4%)+tretinoin (0.05–0.1%)+corticosteroid (Class V–VII)**. May need 2–6 months of treatment.
- Hydroquinone-based therapy – apply BID; may cause an irritant or contact derm
  - **Claripel 4% cream** → contains HQ 4%+avobenzone sunscreen
  - **Lustra** → HQ 4%, vitamins C an E, moisturizers, glycolic acid
  - **Lustra AF** → HQ 4%, vitamins C an E, moisturizers, glycolic acid+sunscreen
  - **Lustra-Ultra** → HQ 4%, vitamins C an E, moisturizers, + Retinol 0.3%, (no glycolic acid)
  - **Tri-Luma** → fluocinolone acetonide 0.01%, HQ 4%, tretinoin 0.05%
  - **Melanex**
  - **EpiQuin Micro**→ HQ 4% and retinol 0.15%, incorporated into patented porous microspheres for delayed release – may help to minimize irritation
  - **EpiQuin Micro XD**
  - **Solaquin Forte 4% cream or gel** – apply BID
  - **Other** – Alphaquin HP, Alustra, Eldopaque, Eldopaque Forte, Eldoquin, Eldoquin Forte, Esoterica, Esoterica Sensitive Skin, Glyquin, Glyquin-XM, Melanex, Melanol, Melpaque HP, Melquin HP, Melquin-3, Nuquin HP, Viquin Forte
- Tretinoin – Slower response than with HQ (takes 6+ months) and may not work as well
- Azelaic acid – available as a 20% cream-based formulation; appears to be as effective as 4% HQ and superior to 2% HQ in the treatment of melasma
- Kojic acid
- Ascorbic acid
- Licorice extract (Glabridin)
- Salicylic acid and glycolic acid peels can be used as adjunctive therapy
- Deeper chemical peels, laser therapy, and dermabrasion have led to mixed results and are associated with side effects such as scarring and dyspigmentation
  - Lasers may include – Intense Pulse Light (IPL), Fraxel

Pearls and Pitfalls

- Hydroquinone can be very irritating and can lead to an allergic contact dermatitis or irritant contact dermatitis, which can then lead to worsening of the pigmentation (from a superimposed post-inflammatory hyperpigmentation)
- Exogenous ochronosis is rare and is usually due to prolonged use (years) of hydroquinone at a concentration > 2%. Nonetheless, always discuss this rare side effect with patients.

Merkel Cell Carcinoma (MCC)

Etiology and Pathogenesis

- Controversial whether MCC arises from the normal Merkel cell, which is a specialized mechnoreceptor in the epidermal basal cell layer or if it arises from pluripotent stem cells that later differentiate in a neuroendocrine direction.
- Merkel cell polyomavirus integrates into band 3p14 at the human protein tyrosine phosphatase, receptor type, G gene, a tumor suppressor gene.

Clinical Presentation

- Median age is 68–70 (may occur at younger age in immunosuppressed)
- Very aggressive neoplasm that usually present as a solitary, asymptomatic, firm, rapidly growing nodule found most commonly on sun-exposed areas of the head and neck
  - ○ Less commonly found on lower extremities, upper extremities, trunk, buttock, and vulva
- Most common color was reddish-pink , followed by bluish-violaceous hue and flesh-colored hue
- AEIOU – **A**symptomatic, **E**xpanding rapidly (3 months or less), **I**mmunosuppression, **O**lder than 50 years, location on **U**ltraviolet-exposed site
- Risk factors – history of PUVA, arsenic exposure, immunosuppression (chronic lymphocytic leukemia, HIV, solid organ transplant patients)

DDx – cyst, acneiform lesion, adnexal tumors, lipoma, dermatofibroma or fibroma, vascular lesion such as pyogenic granuloma, nonmelanoma skin cancer, lymphoma, leukemia cutis, metastatic carcinoma, sarcoma, carcinoid, neuroblastoma, retinoblastoma

Histology

- Ill-defined dermal mass comprised of small round blue cells with multiple mitoses, speckled dense nuclear chromatin, sparse cytoplasm, and high apoptotic index that aggressively invades the subcutaneous tissue
- Three histologic patterns (bear no impact on the prognosis): Intermediate (most common), small cell, and trabecular
- MCC can mimic metastatic neuroendocrine tumors including small cell lung carcinoma. Certain immunohistochemical stains helpful.

Table 79   Immunohistochemical stains to distinguish Merkel cell carcinoma from small cell lung carcinoma

Immunohistochemical stain	Merkel cell carcinoma	Small cell lung carcinoma
CK-20	+	+
Thyroid transcriptase factor-1 (TTF-1)	–	+
CK-7	–	+
Neuron-specific enolase (NSE)	+	–
Synaptophysin	+	–
Chromogranin A	+	–
Kit receptor tyrosine kinase (CD117)	+	–

Treatment

Table 80   AJCC staging system

T	N	M
T1: < 2 cm	N0: no regional lymph node involvement	M0: no distant metastasis
T2: > 2 cm	N1: regional lymph node involvement	M1: distant metastasis
Stage TNM		
1 T1N0M0		
2 T2N0M0		
3 Any T, N1M0		
4 Any T, Any N, M1		

- **Stage 1 and 2**
  - Surgery (Mohs or wide local excision to fascia or pericranium). Excision margins of 2–3 cm have been used historically. Guidelines now are 1 cm margin for stage 1 disease, 2 cm margins for stage 2.
  - Sentinel lymph node biopsy should ideally be performed to evaluate for lymph node involvement and to appropriately stage the disease
  - Radiation – controversial in Stage 1 but recommended in Stage 2. Also consider radiation to primary site, in-transit lymphatics, and regional lymph node basins if SLNB has not been performed.
- **Stage 3 (Tumor board recommended)**
  - SLNB + → complete lymph node dissection recommended. If CLND not possible, radiation as monotherapy may be considered.
  - Imaging recommended in patients with clinically positive nodal disease to determine extent of metastatic disease
  - Chemotherapy not recommended – morbidity associated with this and no change in survival
- **Stage 4 (Tumor board recommended)**
  - Imaging recommended for patients with metastases
  - Chemotherapy, surgery, radiation therapy, and clinical research trials may be considered; however, surgery and radiation therapy are regarded as palliative at this stage
  - Chemotherapy agents typically platinum-based such as cisplatin or carboplatin, doxorubicin, etoposide, or topotecan

Pearls and Pitfalls

- Mortality rate of 33%, which is over twice that of melanoma
- Median survival in patients with metastases is 9 months. Follow patients very closely.
- Most often mistaken for a cyst

References:

(1) Heath M, et al. Clinical characteristics of Merkel cell carcinoma at diagnosis in 195 patients: The AEIOU features. J Am Acad Dermatol 2008; 58: 375–81.
(2) Lien MH, et al. Merkel cell carcinoma: clinical characteristics, markers, staging and treatment. J Drugs Dermatol 2010; 9(7): 779–84.

Morphea

Etiology and Pathogenesis

- Etiology unknown but there is an increased prevalence of anti-single strand (ss) DNA, topoisomerase IIα, -phospholipid, -fibrillin 1, and –histone antibodies in morphea patients
  - Anti-ssDNA especially common in linear morphea
  - Remainder of antibodies common in generalized form
  - High ANA titers seen in juvenile patients with linear morphea and in generalized form
- Sclerosis of the skin thought to involve: (1) vascular damage, (2) activated T cells, and (3) altered connective tissue production by fibroblasts

Clinical Presentation and Types

- AKA – "Localized Scleroderma" – a disorder characterized by excessive collagen deposition leading to thickening of the dermis, subcutaneous tissues, or both
- Unlike systemic sclerosis, morphea lacks features such as sclerodactyly, Raynaud's phenomenon, and internal organ involvement
- Types of Morphea
  - **Plaque-type morphea** – most common and benign morphea subtype
    - Includes guttate and keloidal (nodular) variants. Atrophoderma of Pasini and Pierini is thought to be an abortive form of plaque-type morphea
    - Relatively superficial, primarily involving the dermis
  - **Generalized morphea**
  - **Linear morphea**
    - Variants – En coup de sabre and Parry-Romberg
    - Often qualifies as deep morphea (albeit in a linear pattern), involving the deep dermis, subcutaneous fat, muscle, bone, and even underlying meninges and brain
  - **Deep morphea** – aka subcutaneous morphea or morphea profunda
    - Variants – eosinophilic fasciitis (Schulman syndrome) and disabling pansclerotic morphea of children
    - Primarily involves the subcutaneous fat and underlying structures such as fascia
    - "Groove Sign" may be present in late disease
  - **Bullous morphea** – rare variant; tense subepidermal bullae develop overlying plaque-type, linear, or deep morphea lesions
    - This phenomenon may result from stasis of lymphatic fluid due to the sclerodermatous process or coexisting lichen sclerosus

Labs and Imaging to Consider

- CBC → usually normal. May see eosinophilia in early morphea or eosinophilic fasciitis. Anemia and thrombocytopenia occasionally develop in patients w/ eosinophilic fasciitis
- ESR → usually normal, but it may be elevated in patients with eosinophilic fasciitis or extensive, active morphea
- IgG and IgM → Polyclonal increases in both antibody types may occur, especially in patients with linear and deep morphea. This finding correlates with disease activity and the development of joint contractures in linear morphea
- RF is positive in 15–40% of morphea pts, most often children with linear morphea
- ANA positive in approximately 50% of morphea pts, typically with a homogeneous pattern
- Anti-ssDNA → positive in 25% of plaque-type, 75% of generalized, 50% of linear; levels correlate with extensive, active dz and joint contractures
- Antitopoisomerase 2-alpha antibodies are present in 75% of morphea patients
- MRI of the brain and skull in patients with en coup de sabre and Parry-Romberg syndrome may reveal abnormalities such as cortical atrophy, subcortical calcifications, white matter lesions, ventricular dilatation, leptomeningeal enhancement, anomalous intracranial vasculature, and skull atrophy, even in the absence of neurological symptoms
- MRI is useful in the diagnosis of eosinophilic fasciitis. Typical findings include diffuse edema of the subcutaneous tissues with thickening, increased signal intensity on T2-weighted images, and contrast enhancement of the fascial planes

DDx – amyloidosis (primary systemic), atrophoderma of Pasini and Pierini, Eosinophilia-Myalgia syndrome, eosinophilic fasciitis, GVHD, LsA, nephrogenic systemic fibrosis (NSF), scleredema, linear lupus erythematosus panniculitis, linear melorheostosis, linear atrophoderma of Moulin, lipodermatosclerosis, radiation fibrosis, scleromyxedema, Stiff skin syndrome, morpheaform DFSP, sclerodermoid conditions caused by chemical/toxin exposures (polyvinyl chloride, epoxy resins, pesticides, dry cleaning solvents, silica dust), sclerodermoid conditions caused by iatrogenic agents (bleomycin, taxanes, gemcitabine, uracil-tegafur, melphalan isolated limb perfusion, L-tryptophan, vitamin K injections, pentazocine injections, silicone or paraffin implants), interstitial mycosis fungoides

Histology – specimens must include subcutaneous fat and it is important to note whether biopsy site is inflammatory border or fibrotic center
- **Early stage** – vessel walls show endothelial swelling and edema. Capillaries and small arterioles surrounded by lymphocytic infiltrate but may contain eosinophils, plasma cells, and mast cells

- **Later stage** – minimal inflammatory infiltrate, except in some areas of the fat. Epidermis normal, but rete ridges diminished. Homogeneous collagen bundles with decreased space between the bundles replace most structures. Eccrine glands appear atrophic and are "trapped" by collagen. Biopsy looks very square – "pencil eraser sign"

Treatment

- Corticosteroids (superpotent) – topical and intralesionals
- Topical calcipotriene may also be beneficial, especially when nightly occlusion (with plastic wrap) is used to increase penetration of the medication
- Tacrolimus 0.1% ointment (with occlusion) – may decrease lesional erythema and induration
- Imiquimod – may decrease lesional erythema and induration
- Systemic corticosteroids + weekly low-dose MTX for rapidly progressive morphea
- MTX alone can also be effective
- Scattered reports have described responses of severe morphea to second-line systemic agents → cyclosporine, mycophenolate mofetil, and oral retinoids
- Little documentation of success in literature – hydroxychloroquine, azithromycin, penicillin, tetracycline
- UVA, UVA-1, PUVA – Regimens combining UV therapy with topical corticosteroids or calcipotriene may be superior to either method alone
- Photodynamic therapy using topical 5-aminolevulinic acid was also effective in a small series
- In one case report, treatment of plaque-type morphea with the 585-nm pulsed dye laser led to substantial improvement
- Other
  - Physical therapy to maintain range of motion and function – especially with linear type
  - Ophthalmology evaluation if periocular area involved
  - Neurologist if neuro symptoms

Pearls and Pitfalls

- Eosinophilic fasciitis is often a consideration if disease is extensive. Excisional biopsy (including the fascia) can help differentiate this from extensive morphea or systemic sclerosis

Mycology

Table 81 Subcutaneous mycoses

Subcutaneous mycoses	Organism	Transmission	Clinical	Histo/KOH	Treatment
Sporotrichosis	Sporothrix schenckii	Inoculation Inhalation	SubQ nodules; lymphatic spread	"cigar bodies" or round yeast	Itraconazole, potassium iodide, ampho B
Mycetoma	**Eumycotic:** Pseudo-allescheria boydii **Actino-mycotic:** Nocardia	Penetrating wound in foot (70%) > hand, thorax, scalp	Triad: tumefaction, draining sinuses, grains (aggregates of organisms)	Grains + thick hyphae (eumycotic) and thin filaments (actinomycotic)	**Eumycotic:** Excision, itraconazole **Actino:** Sulfa
Chromoblastomycosis	Fonsacaea pedrosoi (>90%)	Direct inoculation to foot/LE; farmers	Verrucous or granuloma-tous plaque or nodule with central clearing	"Copper pennies" (AKA – medlar or sclerotic bodies)	Excision, Cryotherapy Itraconazole CO_2 laser
Lobomycosis (Keloidal blastomycosis)	Lacazia loboi (formerly Loboa loboi)	Water, soil, dolphins; Brazil, Caribbean	Painless keloids, nodules, verrucous lesions on face, UE, ear	Thick-walled spherical org in "chain of coins". Cx not possible	Excision. Antifungals not effective

*See also tinea, tinea pedis, tinea capitis, onychomycosis

Subcutaneous mycoses – deeper penetration into dermis or subQ usually after trauma (inoculation) > inhalation

Table 82 Dimorphic fungi

Dimorphic fungi	Organism	Transmission	Clinical	Histo/KOH	Treatment
Histoplasmosis	H. capsulatum var capsulatum (US)	Inhalation of spores from soil >>1° inoculation	1° pulm: pneumonitis → arthritis and EN in 10%; rare skin lesions with dissemination. Eye involvement (macular) in some	Tiny yeast forms within cytoplasm of macrophages; no capsule **2–4 microns**	Itraconazole Ampho B for severe
Blastomycosis	Blastomycosis dermatitidis	Inhalation of spores from soil	Well-demarcated papules and pustules and plaques. May mimic Sweet's syndrome	Broad-based budding yeast **8–15 microns**	Itraconazole Ampho B
Paracoccidiomycosis	Paracoccidioides brasiliensis	Inhalation of spores from soil; male agriculture workers	Nasal/oral mucosal ulcers. May be verrucous. May destroy cartilage	"Mariner's wheel" or "Mickey Mouse"	Itraconazole Ketoconazole Ampho B
Coccidiomycosis	Coccidioides immitis	Inhalation of spores from soil	Facial pink papules, verrucous nodules of SQ abscesses; EN	Spherules containing endospores **10–80 microns**	Itraconazole Ampho B Fluconazole (meningitis)

Dimorphic = molds in nature, yeast in living tissue

Table 83 Opportunistic Infections

Opportunistic	Organism	Transmission	Clinical	Histo/KOH	Treatment
Cryptococcus	C. neoformans var. neoformans	Inhalation of spores or 1° cutaneous, ↑ dissem in AIDS	Ulceration, cellulitis, molloscum-like	Mucinous, encapsulated yeast	Fluconazole Ampho B + Flucytosine (HIV)
Penicilliosis	Penicillium marneffei (dimorphic)	Inhalation of spores from bamboo rats	Molloscum-like skin lesions	Oval yeast w/cross walls; parasitized macrophages	Itraconazole Ampho B Excision
Fusariosis	Fusarium sp.	**Neutropenia** Burn patients Trauma Water may be a source	Toenail paronychia common, sinus infection. ↑mortality if neutropenic	Septate hyphae 45° branching. **Cannot distinguish from aspergillus on H&E**	Ampho B+5FC Voriconazole +/− terbinafine
Aspergillosis	1°cutaneous: A. flavus Disseminated: A. fumigatus	Transplant GVHD Neutropenia Aflatoxins Burn patients	IV catheter, necrotic nodules	Septate hyphae 45° with phialides+conidia in chains. Splendore-Hoeppli. Tends to be angio-invasive. **Ident to fusarium on H&E**	Ampho B Voriconazole Itraconazole (nail dz)
Zygomycosis	• Rhizopus • Mucor • Absidia	Diabetes Burns Neutropenia Transplant Malnutrition	Ulceration, cellulitis, and necrotic abscesses; sinuses, unilat facial edema	Wide angle 45–90°. Branching non-septate broad hyphae; Rhizopus → sporangia	Excision Ampho B
Phaeohyphomycosis	• Alternaria • Exophilia • Phialophora • Curvularia • Bipolaris	Invasive dz in immunocompromised; cutaneous dz in immune-competent	SQ cysts, ulcerated plaques, hemorrhagic pustules, necrotic papules and nodules	Dematiaceous dark yeast w/ pseudohyphae-like elements; Alternaria – hand grenade; Fontana-Masson +	Excision Itraconazole
Rhinosporidiosis	Rhinosporidium seeberi (protozoa)	Direct inoculation	Wart-like lesion in nasal mucosa, eye, mouth	BIG raspberry-like spherules	Excision Dapsone
Protothecosis	Prototheca wickerhamii (algae)	Direct inoculation after trauma	Various skin **Olecranon bursitis**	Morula (sphere of endospores) like "soccer ball"	Ampho B Excision

Necrobiosis Lipoidica (NL)

Etiology and Pathogenesis

- Previously called "necrobiosis lipoidica diabeticorum" but name somewhat misleading since not all have diabetes and less than 1% of diabetic patients have this condition
- Cause unknown and no HLA linkage. Theories include: immune complex vasculitis, collagen degeneration and inflammation as a result of microangiopathic vessel changes, primary disease of collagen (inflammation is secondary)

Clinical Presentation

- Yellow-brown, atrophic, telangiectatic plaques surrounded by raised, violaceous rims, typically in the pretibial region
  - Rarely seen on upper extremities, face, scalp (may be more annular or serpiginous and less atrophic in these regions)
  - More common in females compared to males (3:1)
- Skin lesions may begin as small, firm, red-brown papules which collesce into larger plaque with central epidermal atrophy
- Usually bilateral, symmetrical
- Ulcerations may occur in about 30% and often due to trauma
- Decreased sensation to pinprick, fine touch. Also see hypohidrosis and alopecia
- **Complications** – SCCs have been reported in older lesions
- **Relationship to diabetes**
  - Can precede diabetes in some
  - Presence or progression of NL does not correlate with how well the diabetes is controlled
  - Less than 1% of diabetics have this condition

Labs – check fasting glucose level

DDx – granuloma annulare, necrobiotic xanthogranuloma, sarcoid, diabetic dermopathy, stasis dermatitis. Morphea, lichen sclerosus, sclerosing lipogranuloma, panniculitis, granulomatous infections (deep fungal infection, leprosy) may be considered

Histology – diffuse, palisaded, and interstitial granulomatous dermatitis with "layered" tiers of granulomatous inflammation aligned parallel to the epidermis. Epidermis may be normal or atrophic. See superficial and deep perivascular infiltrate that is mostly lymphocytic but also contains plasma cells and occasionally eosino-phils. Granulomatous inflammation includes multinucleated giant histiocytes but no asteroid bodies

Treatment

- No treatment has been shown effective in large, randomized controlled clinical trials
- First line → potent topical steroids for early lesions and IL steroids to active borders. Has little effect on atrophic lesions that are burnt out and may cause further atrophy
- Ulcerated NL
  ○ Tacrolimus ointment 0.1%
  ○ Topically applied bovine collagen
  ○ Cyclosporine 2.5 mg/kg/day
- Aspirin and dipyridamole have some benefit
- Increasing fibrinolysis or decreasing platelet aggregation in order to decrease microangiopathy
  ○ Pentoxifylline
  ○ Stanozolol
  ○ Inositol niacinate
  ○ Nicofuranose
  ○ Ticlopidine hydrochloride
  ○ Perilesional heparin injections
- TNF-α inhibitors (etanercept, infliximab, thalidomide) – case reports of success
- PUVA, UVA-1
- Tretinoin may help diminish the atrophy
- PDL to treat telangiectasias
- Excision and grafting but recurrence can occur

Pearls and Pitfalls

- Although not always associated with diabetes, it is important to screen patients for diabetes and to follow them as some develop diabetes (perhaps 1/3)
- Necrobiosis lipoidica may occur in children and its presence suggest a higher risk for diabetic nephropathy and retinopathy
- Encourage diabetics to control blood glucose, but no evidence that this will help with treatment of necrobiosis lipoidica (may/can prevent many other diabetic complications)
- Spontaneous remission may occur

Nephrogenic Systemic Fibrosis (NSF)

Etiology and Pathogenesis

- Previously called "nephrogenic fibrosing dermopathy" (NFD) but is now called "nephrogenic systemic fibrosis" (NSF) as this disease can involve both the skin and internal organs
- NFD/NSF occurs (with the exception of one report in two transplant patients whose organ donors' histories were not noted) in patients with renal insufficiency who have had imaging studies (e.g., MRI) with gadolinium. Gadolinium can be found in tissue samples of NFD/NSF
  - 90% of proven NSF cases are related to gadodiamide (Omniscan) and some to gadopentetate (Magnevist)
- Relationship between epoetin alfa (Epogen) and NSF controversial – epoetin upregulates bone marrow and may stimulate increased production of fibroblasts and other cells

Clinical Presentation

- Patients present with ill-defined, thick, indurated plaques that are symmetrically distributed
- Lesions are usually on extremities and trunk
- Lesions are erythematous to hyperpigmented and can have an irregular advancing edge
- **Complications**
  - Confluent involvement on extremities often results in joint contractures
  - Within weeks of disease onset, many pts become dependent on a wheelchair because of contractures
  - Ambulating difficulty may lead to falls → fractures → morbidity/mortality
  - Many pts report maddening pruritus
  - Systemic involvement (heart, lungs, skeletal muscle) may lead to death
- **Risk Factors**
  - Renal dysfunction is prerequisite
  - Exposure to gadolinium
  - Type of gadolinium (Omniscan > Magnevist)
  - Acidosis
  - Erythropoietic stimulating agents
  - Major proinflammatory events (major surgery, infection/sepsis, vascular events, or thrombosis)
  - Hypercoagulable state
  - Hyperphosphatemia
  - Concomitant immunosuppression

○ Meds that could cause transmetallation of gadolinium → iron, zinc, copper, calcium, lanthanum, sevelamer
○ Other notes: Pts with severe liver disease often have overestimated GFR; children < 1 year also at higher risk due to immature renal fxn

Labs to Consider – complete metabolic profile, phosphorus, ferritin/ESR

DDx – calciphylaxis, cellulitis, DFSP, eosinophilia-myalgia syndrome, eosinophilic fasciitis, lichen myxedematosus, morphea, systemic sclerosis, PCT, scleromyxedema, Beta-2- microglobulin amyloidosis, panniculitis, sclerodermatous chronic GVHD

Histology – Deep biopsy required
• Haphazard arrangement of thickened collagen bundles, mucin deposition, and increased dermal fibroblast-like cells that stain positive for CD34 and procollagen I. Vacular proliferation and an increased number of dendritic cells are observed, but no significant lymphoplasmacytic infiltrate
• Spectroscopy can reveal gadolinium within involved tissues

Treatment and Management – Extremely difficult to manage and no cure
• Extracorporeal photophoresis
• High-dose IVig
• Immunosuppressants (cyclosporine, MTX, mycophenolate, oral and topical steroids)
• Other – Pentoxifylline, thalidomide, PDT, PUVA, UVA-1, sodium thiosulfate, ACE-inhibitors
• Topical calcipotriene (Dovonex) under occlusion – has helped some
• Gleevac (imatinib)
  ○ Tyrosine-kinase inhibitor
  ○ Efficacy in scleroderma (NEJM 2006, Baroni et al) – pts given 100 mg BID × 12 weeks (low dose). Significant improvement in lesions, lung involvement, etc. Similar reports of efficacy in NSF
  ○ SE – GI (common), edema (common – weigh pts; periorbital edema especially common), cytopenia, CHF, hepatitic dz, muscle cramps, hypopigmentation (vitiligo-like; can be permanent), skin rashes (AGEP, Sweet's, Dress, TEN)
  ○ Dose QD unless side effects
  ○ CBC, LFTs weekly × 1 month, then bimonthly
  ○ Costs $1,600–$2,300/month → limits use
  ○ Pregnancy Category D
• Physical therapy

Pearls and Pitfalls

- 24-month mortality rates of those with cutaneous involvement is 48%
- NSF registry (Yale) → http://www.pathmax.com/dermweb/
- **Prevention is key!**
    - ○ Avoid gadolinium-based studies such as MRI in pts with renal dysfunction
    - ○ If MRI required, try to use gadolinium that is not Omniscan or Magnevist
    - ○ If MRI required, dialysis ASAP! Dr. Cowper at Yale recommends immediately after. (Prognosis is horrible, so why risk it?)
    - ○ Many hospitals have switched their gadolinium to brands that are not as likely to cause NSF

Paget's Disease

Etiology and Pathogenesis

- Has a nearly 100% association with intraductal breast cancer

Clinical Presentation

- Red, scaly plaque of nipple, breast or axilla
- Peak incidence between age 50–60

DDx – eczema, allergic contact dermatitis or Bowen's disease

Histology

- Pale staining Paget's cells (often with atypical nuclei) scattered throughout the epidermis. Groups of these cells may compress and flatten the basal cells
- Usually no dyskeratosis, unlike Bowen's disease
- Paget's cells often, but not always positive for CEA, EMA, low-molecular-weight keratin such as Cam5.2 or keratin-7, PAS with and without diastase, Alcian blue, and mucicarmine
- Underlying adenocarcinoma sometimes seen within the dermis
- Invasive cancer associated with Paget's disease was more commonly estrogen and progesterone negative, with high pathological grade
- c-erbB-2 overexpression in breast carcinoma is known to be associated with an aggressive disease potential and with worse prognosis, and this marker is common in Paget's (80–90%)

Treatment

- Biopsy important for diagnosis
- Mammogram
- Refer to surgery or surgical oncology → surgical therapy combined with breast irradiation for patients with invasive and noninvasive breast carcinoma has become the treatment of first choice. To reduce the risk of local recurrence in Paget's disease, all surgical conservative approaches should include the complete nipple–areolar complex and margins of resected specimen free of tumor
- Sentinel lymph node biopsy often performed

Pearls and Pitfalls

- Paget's is an uncommon disease, but have a low threshold to biopsy rashes on the breast. A biopsy can nail down the diagnosis and give reassurance to the worried patient

Reference:

Caliskan M, et al. Paget's disease of the breast: the experience of the European institute of oncology and review of the literature. Breast Cancer Res Treat 2008; 112: 513–21.

Paget's Disease, Extramammary

Etiology and Pathogenesis

- Thought to arise from a pluripotent stem cell within the genital skin. May be primary or secondary to underlying malignancy
  - Secondary – Associated with underlying visceral malignancy (usually colorectal or urothelial, but may arise from cervix, prostate, ovary, or endometrium) in 10–20% of patients or an underlying adnexal adenocarcinoma in<5% of patients

Clinical Presentation

- Slowly expanding erythematous plaque with sharp demarcation between normal and abnormal skin. Scattered areas of white scale and erosion can give rise to a "strawberries and cream" appearance
  - Women – usually affects vulva
  - Men – perianal area commonly affected
- There may be associated pruritus or burning or it may be asymptomatic
- Examine lymph nodes for lymphadenopathy

DDx – inverse psoriasis, lichen simplex chronicus, irritant dermatitis, allergic contact dermatitis, erosive lichen planus, candidiasis

Histology

- Vacuolated Paget cells in the epidermis are distinctive, but immunohistochemical staining is necessary to exclude pagetoid melanoma and intraepithelial neoplasia, as well as to help differentiate between primary and secondary disease

Table 84 Immunohistochemistry for extramammary pagets disease (EMPD)

Favors cutaneous origin	Favors endodermal origin
Primary EMPD (>75%) or Secondary EMPD tue to underlying adnexal adenocarcinoma (<5%)	Secondary EMPD due to visceral malignancy (10–20%)
Pankeratin +	Pankeratin +
CEA/CK7 +	CEA/CK7 +
CK20–	CK20+
GCDFP-15+ (gross cystic disease fluid protein)	GCDFP–

Treatment and Management

- A thorough search for an internal malignancy should be performed
  - All – Full cutaneous and lymph node exam, colonoscopy, cystoscopy
  - Women – Pelvic exam + pelvic imaging, breast exam + mammography
  - Men – Prostate exam + prostate specific antigen (PSA) level
- Mohs surgery or wide local excision
- Other treatment options – radiation, photodynamic therapy, CO_2 laser ablation, topical 5-FU, topical imiquimod
- Long-term follow-up recommended → Recurrences are common

Pearls and Pitfalls

- Internal malignancy is about 5x more common if these is in the perianal area (as opposed to vulvar or penoscrotal involvement)

Paraneoplastic Pemphigus (PNP)

Etiology and Pathogenesis

- Bullous disorder associated with underlying neoplasms, both malignant and benign
- Desmosomal and hemidesmosomal anti-plakin and anti-desmoglein antibodies
- Also T-cell mediated

Clinical Presentation

- Intractable stomatitis, which is usually the earliest presenting sign and is the manifestation that is most difficult to treat
  - Erosions and ulcerations that affect all surfaces of the oropharynx and characteristically extend onto the vermillion border of the lip
- Cutaneous
  - Findings are polymorphic – erythematous macules, flaccid bullae and erosions, tense bullae, erythema multiforme-like lesions on the palms and soles
- Most also have a severe pseudomembranous conjunctivitis, which may progress to scarring and obliteration of the conjunctival fornices
- Esophageal, nasopharyngeal, vaginal, labial, and penile mucosal lesions may also be seen
- Some develop **bronchiolitis obliterans**, which can be fatal
- Associated neoplasms
  - **Most common in adults** – non-Hodgkin's lymphoma (40%), chronic lymphocytic leukemia (30%), Castleman's disease (10%), malignant and benign thymomas (6%), sarcomas (6%), and Waldenstrom's macroglobulinemia (6%)
  - **Most common in children** – Castleman's disease

Labs and Imaging

- CBC+diff, peripheral blood smear, complete metabolic profile
- UPEP/SPEP and/or IFE
- Chest x-ray
- CT scan of the chest, abdomen, and pelvis
- Consider bone marrow biopsy
- Age-appropriate malignancy workup indicated, but typical neoplasms not usually seen

DDx – may depend on presentation – pemphigus vulgaris, bullous pemphigoid, IgA pemphigus, Drug-induced pemphigus, Stevens–Johnson, toxic epidermal necrolysis, erythema multiforme, drug eruption, erosive lichen planus

Histology – shows interface/lichenoid dermatitis associated with dyskeratosis throughout the epidermis +/– acantholysis.

- DIF – Deposition of complement and IgG in intracellular epidermal spaces and in the basement membrane zone in linear granular lesions
- IIF to rat bladder – shows intercellular staining
- Circulating antibodies bind to different tissue sources including urinary bladder, respiratory epithelium, and desmosomal areas of myocardium and skeletal muscle
- PNP sera react to unique complex of antigens which includes desmoplakin, bullous pemphigoid antigen 1 (BPAG1), envoplakin and periplakin, desmogleins 1 and 3. Patients have antibodies to one or all of these antigens

Fig. 13 Where to biopsy SKIN lesions of paraneoplastic pemphigus for DIF

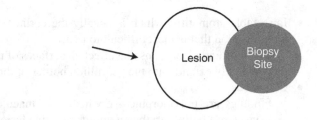

Fig. 14 Where to biopsy MOUTH lesions of paraneoplastic pemphigus for DIF

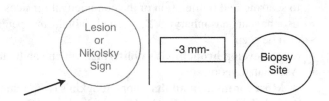

Treatment

- Treat underlying disease – may control autoantibody production and IVIG at the time of surgery may help control the disease process
- Immunosuppressive agents are required to decrease blistering, but they are often ineffective
  - High-dose corticosteroids are first-line therapy
  - Other – azathioprine, cyclosporine, and mycophenolate mofetil
- Other therapeutic options – plasmapheresis, immunophoresis, intravenous gammaglobulin, high-dose cyclophosphamide, rituximab

Pearls and Pitfalls

- High mortality
  - In general, the skin lesions of paraneoplastic pemphigus are more responsive to therapy than mucosal lesions

- CXR and/or CT scan obtained at the onset of bronchiolitis obliterans may be normal but pulmonary function tests will show small airway obstruction that does not reverse with bronchodilators
- Only pemphigus that will affect non-stratified epithelium – can get lung involvement. Nothing else can do this
- When to suspect paraneoplastic pemphigus: When it looks like …
  - Pemphigus vulgaris (PV) in extreme ages
  - PV associated with severe stomatitis: vermilion border of lip
  - PV associated with features of EM/SJS
  - PV with scarring mucositis (MMP-like)
  - PV associated with B cell lymphoproliferative neoplasm
  - Chronic progressive EM/SJS-like picture
  - Erosive lichen planus-like picture involving vermilion border of lip
  - DIF and IIF suggests pemphigus vulgaris + bullous pemphigoid
  - Histology shows Interface/lichenoid dermatitis associated with dyskeratosis throughout the epidermis +/– acantholysis
    - Lichenoid PNP – more likely to see pulmonary involvement, Castleman's disease
  - "PV refractory to therapy"

Paraneoplastic Syndromes

Table 85 Paraproteins and paraneoplastic syndromes

Clinical sign	Paraproteins
Disseminated xanthomasiderohistiocytosis	Variant of xanthoma disseminatum with keloidal-like lesions Associated with multiple myeloma
Eosinophilic fasciitis	Polyclonal hypergammaglobulinemia
Erythema elevatum diutinum (EED)	IgA monoclonal gammopathy
Necrobiotic xanthogranuloma (NXG)	IgG κ or λ
POEMS	M-protein: monoclonal gammopathy
Primary systemic amyloid	Multiple myeloma
Prominent hyperkeratosis on follicles of nose	Multiple myeloma
Pyoderma gangrenosum	IgA monoclonal gammopathy
Relapsing polychondritis	Myelodysplastic syndromes
Rosai–Dorfman	Polyclonal hypergammaglobulinemia
Schnitzler's syndromes	Monoclonal IgM κ
Scleredema	IgG multiple myeloma
Scleromyxedema (lichen myxedema)	IgG λ
Subcorneal pustular dermatosis	IgA monoclonal gammopathy
Xanthoma planum	Monoclonal gammopathy
Paraneoplastic syndromes	**Internal malignancy**
Acanthosis nigricans	Gastric adenocarcinoma
Acquired angioedema	Low C1; lymphoma

(continued)

Table 85 (continued)

Clinical sign	Paraproteins
Acquired ichthyosis	Hodgkin's lymphoma, occ–breast cancer, lung cancer, CTCL
Amyloidosis	Multiple myeloma, plasma cell dyscrasia
Anti-epiligrin cicatricial pemphigoid (laminin 5; aka laminin-332)	Any internal malignancy, non-small cell lung cancer
Carcinoid syndrome	80–85% originate in GI tract: appendix > small bowel > rectum
Cryoglobulinemia	Multiple myeloma, Waldenstroms macroglobulinemia
Cushing's syndrome	Glucocorticoid excess due to Oat Cell lung cancer
Dermatomyositis-Polymyositis	Women → ovarian and breast cancer
	Men → respiratory tract, gastric carcinoma, lymphoma
Erythema gyratum repens	Lung cancer
Erythroderma	Leukemia, lymphoma
Extramammary Paget's	In 50%, no malignancy found. Adnexal adenocarcinomas.
	GI or GU tract
Howell–Evans syndrome (AD)	Esophageal carcinoma
Hypertrichosis lanuginosa acquisita	Lung and colon cancer
Multicentric reticulohistiocytosis	30% with malignancy; no predominant type – breast, stomach, cervical
Necrolytic migratory erythema (Glucagonoma syndrome)	α-2 glucagon producing islet cell pancreatic carcinoma
Paget's disease of the breast	Always associated with intraductal breast cancer
Paraneoplastic Acrokeratosis of Bazex	Upper aerodigestive tract
	Metastatic carcinoma to lymph nodes of the neck
Paraneoplastic pemphigus	Lymphoproliferative malignancy
	Non-Hodgkin's lymphoma, CLL, thymoma, Castleman's disease (especially in kids)
Sign of Lesser-Trelat	Gastric or colon cancer
Sweet's syndrome	Hemoproliferative disorders – AML most common
	Solid: GU malignancy
Tripe palms with acanthosis nigricans	Gastric adenocarcinoma
Tripe palms without acanthosis nigricans	Lung cancer

Patch Testing

- **Before patch testing or history, perform quick exam**
  - Could the pt have contact derm or another primary dermatosis? Ask the pt to point to the area where the dermatitis first appeared
  - Pearls
    - If rash on hands, neck, face in adults → is ACD until proven otherwise
    - Don't patch test in "status eczematous"
    - Remove tape, wait 15–30 min for tape rxn to calm down
- **Dispel myths first. Educate them about …**
  - Skin allergy is a delayed-type hypersensitivity (Type IV) → doesn't cause angioedema
    - Contrast – Latex allergy is type I hypersensitivity (immediate), IgE mediated
  - Answer usage questions as "yes" even if they only use something once a month
  - Secondary allergy is common. Answer usage questions even if the medication or product was used *after* the rash started
  - Tell patients that this cannot be done with blood tests (or they may decide to go to an allergist, even though this is a different type of testing)
- **Detailed Exam**
  - Hands, face, neck
  - Fingertips, interdigital, dorsal hands
  - Photoexposed
  - Textile
  - Pantomine useful to use – ask them to show you how they do their job, apply the lotion, cut the hair, etc.
- **Stop immunosuppressives**
  - Stop topical meds to the back for 2 weeks prior to patch testing (or site of testing)
- **Decide what to test**
  - Have pts bring in their personal care products
  - Can patch test things that are meant to stay on the skin like lotion. If unclear about the product from an occupational setting, can obtain the MSD sheet. If product is NOT an irritant, is ok to patch test
- **Mark allergen sites with surgical pen and highlighter**
  - Back > anterior thigh
  - Diagram application site carefully with the patient in front of you
  - Keep back dry until the final reading
  - Keep patches in place for 48 h. Remove and note loosening of any patch. Grade the strength at 2–4 days and 5–7 days
    - Some do this differently
- **Consider photopatch testing**
- **Certain allergens peak early** (Carba, thiuram, Balsam of Peru)

- **Certain allergens peak late** (neomycin, gold, dyes, corticosteroids)
- **If patch testing negative**
  - Review for technical problems – loose patches? False negatives due to medications?
  - Reconsider irritant dermatitis, autoeczematization, drug, etc.
  - Irritant changes – appears scorched, epidermal changes, not much dermal changes
    - If any question, can have clinic volunteers wear patch as a control. If volunteers react, it is likely an irritant
  - Testing with too low of concentration?
  - Perhaps antigen is a photoallergen
  - Influence of tanning bed, immunosuppressive?
- **Patient Education**
  - Make it clear that they must avoid the allergens 100% of the time!
  - Rule of thumb – they should be 80% better in 1 month (this means they are on track)
  - Give handouts – from CARD
  - Nurse goes in after the doctor explains
    - Can ask excitedly, "What did the doctor tell you?" (can get a sense for what the pt understands). Nurse can then use this to gauze where they need to educate the pt further
- **Follow-up**
  - If no better, consider a systemic ACD – nickel, balsam of Peru, propylene glycol, copper
- Interpretation of Patch Testing

+/−	Macular erythema Red, no induration Most seem to resolve by delayed reading Difficult to assess in dark skin → equivalent to blanchable skin in dark skin
1+	Weak, vesicular Red papules May see more papules in dark skin
2+	Strong, edematous, vesicular
3+	Extreme, **spreading**, bullous, ulcerative
Irritant	Pustular, rim reaction (exception is steroid) Can have a scorched appearance, epidermal changes, but not much dermal changes Itching → favor ACD Burning → favor ICD

Delayed Read		
48 h	96 h	
+	+	allergic
−	+	allergic
+	−	irritant (although not all)
−	−	negative

Note: If positive result 2 weeks or later, we've probably sensitized the patient

Medicament Allergy

- Local anesthetics
  - ○ Benzocaine, procaine, amethocaine – often used in hemorrhoid compounds. Cross-react with sulfa, PPD
  - ○ Dibucaine – 1%
  - ○ Amide group
- Topical antibiotics
  - ○ Gentamycin cross-reacts with Neomycin
    - ▪ All aminoglycosides cross-react
    - ▪ Ear drops, eye drops, etc.
  - ○ Bacitracin (common cause, 9%) – co-reacts with neomycin
  - ○ Bag Balm (clioquinol) – can cause ACD
    - ▪ Shania Twain endorsed this product, and so people are using it more
- Corticosteroids
  - ○ If patient not getting better, suspect steroid ACD
  - ○ Type IV > type I
  - ○ A* – most allergenic (hydrocortisone) → fixocortal-21-pivalate. Usually ok with PO prednisone
  - ○ B – budesonide (everything ends in "ide") – like desonide, also triamcinolone
  - ○ C – dexamethasone – like Cloderm
  - ○ D1 – betamethasone 17-valerate – clobetasol
  - ○ D2* – hydrocortisone 17-butyrate
    - ▪ Note: A and D2 often go together
- Don't use topical antihistamines – don't work and can cause sensitization. Can result in systemic contact dermatitis
- NSAIDs
  - ○ Ketoprofen – biggest player
    - ▪ Benzophenone is the etiology – can make them sensitive to sunscreens

Table 86 Common allergic contact allergens found in rubber, shoes and tattoos

Rubber	Shoe dermatitis	Tattoos
Accelerators • Carbamates • Thiurams • Mercaptothiobenazole, mercapto mix Antioxidant • Paraphenylenediamine • Monobenzy ether of hydroquinone	Rubber • Monobenzy ether of hydroquinone • Mercaptobenzathiazole • Tetramethylthiuram • Carbamates Leather • Potassium dichromate • Formaldehyde Shoe Eyelets • Nickel Dyes • Azo dyes – may cross-react with PPD Adhesive • Paratentiary-butylphenol formaldehyde resin • Colophony (rubber adhesive	Red • Mercury sulfide (red cinnabar) • Cadmium yellow Green • Chromium Blue • Cobalt aluminate Yellow • Cadmium yellow (phototoxic rxns)

Patch Testing – Common Allergens

Table 87   Sources of common allergic contactants

Contactant	Source
2-Mercaptobenzothiazole	Adhesives, coolants, rubber
Allyl isothiocyanate	Mustard, radish
Alpha-tocopherol (vitamin E)	Topical vtiamin E, cosmetics, deodorants
Ammonium persulfate	Bleaching agent in flour, hair bleach
Antimony	Causes eczematous dermatitis. In matches, ceramics, textiles. Miners
Balsam of Peru	Fragrance, adhesives. Cross-reacts with colophony, cinnamon
Benzalkonium chloride	Baby wipes
Benzocaine	Topical anesthetics (including medications for hemorrhoids, teething, cold sores, canker sores), epilation waxes Cross-reacts with ester anesthetics, PABA, PPD, sulfonamides, procainamide
Chromate	Tanning agents for leather. Also in green tatoo, cement, matches, bleach, phosphate-containing detergents, anti-rust compounds, orange and yellow paint, glue, varnish, blueprints. "Blackjack dermatitis" – green felt on gambling tables
Cinnamic aldehyde	Perfumes, cinnamon oil and powder, cassia oil, flavoring agents, toilet soaps. May cause contact urticaria or systemic contact dermatitis. Can cross-react with Balsam of Peru
Cobalt	Often coexists with nickel in metal objects. Also in blue tattoo, glass alloy, paints, cements, pottery, ceramics. Injection of cyanocobalamine (B12) can cause flare-ups in sensitive individuals
Cocamidopropyl betaine	Amphoteric surfactant (wetting agent) frequently used in hair and bath products, shampoos, bath/shower gels
Colophony (rosin)	Adhesive tape, cosmetics, insulating tape, glossy paper, flypaper, polish, paints, inks (hand dermatitis), epilation wax, rosin bags for baseball players, varnishes, violin bows. Known as a cause of perioral dermatitis from chewing gum
Epoxy resin	Glue, adhesives, hardeners, plasticizers
Ethyl acrylate	Cross-linking agent in rubber
Ethyl cyanoacrylate	Krazy glue, super glue
Ethylene urea, melamine formaldehyde	Permanent press clothing
Ethylenediamine	Was in old Mycolog cream. Cross-reacts with aminophylline, theophylline, atarax, zinc
Formaldehyde releasers	**Quaternium-15** **Imidazolidinyl urea** Diazolidinyl urea 2-bromo-2-nitropropane-1,3-diol (Bronopol) 1,2-dibromo-2,4-dicyanobutane DMDM hydantoin
Glutaldehyde	Used for tissue fixative, antiperspirants, antiseptics, tanning agent for soft leather, embalming fluid, shampoo preservative, dentifrice, treating warts, dermatophytes, bullous diseases, hyperhidrosis, cold sterilization. Cause of ACD in x-ray techs

Table 87 (continued)

Contactant	Source
Glycerol thioglycolate	Permanent waves (perms). Common in hair dressers. Ammonium thioglycolate does NOT cross-react. Latex gloves do not protect
Hydrocortison-17-butyrate	Group B and D corticosteroids budesonide
Imidazolidinyl urea	Preservative for cosmetics, creams, lotions, hair conditioners, shampoos, and deodorants. Releases a small amt of formaldehyde
Kathon CG (methylchloroisothiazolinone)	Cosmetic preservative (formaldehyde-like). Nivea and Eucerin contain Kathon
Lanolin alcohol	Wood alcohol, wool wax, wool fat, adhesives, cosmetics, topical medications – creams, lotions, ointments, soaps. Eucerin cross-reacts. Higher incidence in venous dermatitis and ulcers
Limonene	Orange and lemon peel, tea tree oil
Methyl methacrylate	Adhesive artificial nails, dental bonding material, bone cement (used in attachment of prostheses to bone), dentures
Methylchloroisothiazolone, Methylchloroisothiazolinone	Cosmetics, skin and hair products, industrial water systems, cutting oils, jet fuel, moist paper towels
Methyldibromoglutaronitrile (20%), phenoxyethanol (80%)	Euxyl K400. Important sensitizer in facial dermatitis. Nivea, personal products
Musk	Fixative in perfume. A photosensitizing fragrance. Can cause photoallergic and non-photoallergic dermatitis
Neomycin sulfate	Topical antibiotics, first-aid creams, ear drops, nose drops. May cross-react with gentamycin and other aminoglycosides. Many also allergic to bacitracin
Nickel sulfate	Jewelry, alloys, pigments, dentures, orthopedic appliances, scissors, razors, eyeglass frames, eating utensils. Test=1% dimethylglyoxime Nickel-containing foods – beans, asparagus, pears, tomatoes, onions, carrots, nuts, whole grain flour, rye, shellfish, chocolate, beer, wine, tea
Octyl dimethyl PABA	Also called padimate O; found in sunscreens
Oxybenzone	Sunscreen (most common cause of photoallergic contact derm)
Padimate O (PABA)	Sunscreen
Paraben mix	Creams and cosmetics, industrial oils, fats and glues (common preservative). Five different parabens present – methyl, ethyl, propyl, butyl, and benzyl parahydroxybenzoates. Unna boot
Paraphenylenediamine	Hair dyes (hair dressers), inks, photodevelopers, textile dyes, temporary henna tattoos. Can cross-react with PABA, sulfonamides, benzocaine, azo dyes, HCTZ. Can cause lichenoid dermatitis on hands
Photocontact allergens	PABA Benzophenones (oxybenzone, dioxybenzone) Cinnamates (methoxycinnamate) Methoxydibenzoylmethane (Parsol 1789) Thiourea Diphenhydramine HC
Potassium dichromate	Cement, plaster, leather
Primin	Primrose

(continued)

Table 87   (continued)

Contactant	Source
Propylene glycol	5-fluorouracil, humectant, cosmetics, synalar solution, valium (contains 40%), anti-freeze, rogaine soln, EKG gel (widely used as a vehicle)
p-tert-butylphenol formaldehyde resin	Adhesive in leather/rubber products
Quaternium-15	Common preservative in cosmetics, some household cleaners and polishers
Sesquiterpene lactone mix	Oil-soluble plant oleoresin including artichoke, broomweed, chamomile, chrysanthemum, liverwort, ragweed, sagebrush. Used to detect allergy to plants of Compositae family: chrysanthemum, ragweed, artichok, chamomile, daisy, dandelion. Balsum of Peru can cross-react
Tetramethylthiuram disulfide	Rubber accelerator
Thimerisol	Piroxicam, contact soln, vaccines
Thiuram	Rubber, adhesives, certain pesticides and medications, antabuse #1 glove. Eczema flares after ingesting alcohol may be due to thiurams
Tixocortol pivalate	Group A corticosteroids
Toluenesulfonamide formaldehyde resin	Nail polish (eyelid dermatitis). Those allergic may substitute polyester resin
Triclosan	Antiseptic found in antibacterial soaps (including surgical scrub soaps), deodarants, feminine hygiene sprays, shampoos
Tuliposide A	Peruvian lily, tulip
Urushiol	Poison ivy, poison oak, poison sumac, Japanese lacquer tree, cashew nut, mango, ginkgo tree

Pemphigus Foliaceus (PF)

Etiology and Pathogenesis

- IgG (mainly IgG4 subclass) autoantibodies aginst a cell adhesion molecule, desmoglein 1 (160 kDa) which is expressed mainly in the granular layer of the epidermis
- More common in Finland, Tunisia, and Brazil

Clinical Presentation and Types

- Scaly, crusted cutaneous erosions "cornflakes", often on an erythematous base, but they do not have clinically apparent mucosal involvement even with widespread disease
- Onset of disease is subtle and initial lesions often mistaken for impetigo
- Seborrheic dermatitis distribution. Vesicles are fragile thus only the resultant crust and scale are seen
- Nikolsky sign is present
- Usually not very ill, but they do complain of burning and pain in association with the lesions
- PF has the following **six subtypes**:
  - Pemphigus erythematosus (Senear-Usher), herpetiform pemphigus, endemic PF (fogo selvagem), endemic PF with antigenic reactivity characteristic of paraneoplastic pemphigus (but with no neoplasm), immunoglobulin A (IgA) PF, and drug-induced PF
- Drug-induced PF is mostly associated with penicillamine, nifedipine, or captopril, medications with a cysteine-like chemical structure

Labs and Imaging

- Consider CXR to rule out associated thymoma
- TB skin test, CBC, blood glucose determination → prior to intiating immunosuppressives

DDx – impetigo, seborrheic dermatitis, pemphigus vulgaris, erythema multiforme, epidermolysis bullosa, allergic contact dermatitis, herpes simplex, lupus, pseudoporphyria, drug-induced bullous disorder, Hailey–Hailey, Darier's disease, Grover's disease, linear IgA bullous dermatosis, subcorneal pustular dermatosis

Histology – pemphigus foliaceos, pemphigus erythematosus, and fogo selvagem are identical histologically

- Acantholysis in the upper epidermis, within or adjacent to the granular layer. May be difficult to detect, but usually a few acantholytic keratinocytes are attached to the roof or floor of the blister
- Deeper epidermis remains intact, but secondary clefts may form
- Blister cavity sometimes contains numerous acute inflammatory cells, particularly neutrophils
- Eosinophilic spongiosis may be seen in early pemphigus foliaceous
- **DIF** → IgG in the intercellular space, mainly in the upper parts of the epidermis
- **Indirect immunofluorescence (IIF)** – monkey esophagus and guinea pig esophagus → PF stains only in upper epidermis, whereas pemphigus vulgaris stains throughout epidermis. The autoantibodies of the IgG class target desmoglein 1, its main autoantigen. IF is 90–100% sensitive. In invasive bullous or erythrodermic PF, IIF titers may be high (>1:5120)

Fig. 15 Where to biopsy SKIN lesions of pemphigus foliaceous for DIF

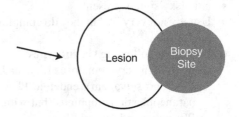

Treatment

- Therapy for PF is usually less aggressive than that of PV because of lower morbidity and mortality rates
- Topical glucocorticosteroids may be sufficient in cases of limited involvement
- Antimalarial therapy may be effective monotherapy in some patients
- In some cases, such as PE, combined therapy is beneficial with the use of corticosteroids and sulfones or antimalarial agents
  - ○ **Dapsone** 50–200 mg PO qd (check G6PD prior)
  - ○ **Plaquenil** 200 mg PO BID
- Antibiotics, such as **minocycline** 50 mg QD, may be effective
- **Nicotinamide** 1.5 g/day and **TCN** 2 g/day have also been reported to be beneficial in some
- More extensive cases … (similar to PV)
  - ○ Systemic **corticosteroids** – 60–100 mg PO every morning or more often as required to abort acantholysis; alternatively, 0.5–2 mg/kg/day PO; taper as condition improves; single morning dose is safer for long-term use, but

divided doses have more anti-inflammatory effect
○ **Azathioprine** – 100–200 mg PO qd in combination with prednisone; alternatively, 1 mg/kg/day PO for 6–8 week; increase by 0.5 mg/kg q 4 week until response or dose reaches 2.5 mg/kg/day
○ **Mycophenolate mofetil** – start 1.5–2 g/day and increase by 500 mg every month until reach benefit or 3 g/day maximum. Once stable, may decrease dose by 500 mg/day every month
○ **Cyclophosphamide** – 50–100 mg IV qd in combination with prednisone; 2.5–3 mg/kg/day PO divided qid
○ **Cyclosporine** – 2–5 mg/kg/day
○ **IVig** – 2 g/kg q 4 weeks
○ **Rituximab** reported to be helpful – [*Dermatology*. 2007;214(4):310–8]
○ **Plasmapheresis** is another therapeutic option (recalcitrant disease)
  ■ May decrease autoantibody titers in some patients and favorably influence the clinical outcome
  ■ Often used in conjunction with cytostatic agents, such as cyclophosphamide or azathioprine, to reduce a predictable rebound increase in autoantibody synthesis
  ■ Potential complications, including the need for maintaining venous access, a bleeding tendency, electrolyte shifts, pulmonary edema, fever, chills, hypotension, and septicemia, should be considered

Pearls and Pitfalls

– UV protection is important (can cause flares)
– Monitor pemphigus foliaceus (PF) patients for other autoimmune disorders, particularly thymoma and myasthenia gravis

Pemphigoid Gestationis

Etiology and Pathogenesis

- AKA – herpes gestationis (term not favored because misleading)
- Appears to be caused by an anti-basement membrane "serum factor" – called the "herpes gestationis (HG) factor" that induces C3 deposition along the dermal–epidermal junction
- Majority have antibodies to BPAG2 (collagen XVII)
    - Anti-BPAG2 antibodies belong to the IgG1 subclass
- Exclusively a disease in pregnancy and the immediate postpartum period
- Has been reported in association with hydatidiform moles and choriocarcinomas

Clinical Presentation

- Abrupt onset of intensely pruritic urticarial lesions which occur during late pregnancy
- Lesions commonly start on the trunk and rapidly progress to a generalized eruption sparing only the face, mucous membranes, palms, and soles
    - In 50% of patients, lesions begin on the abdomen often within or adjacent to the umbilicus. The other 50% have an atypical presentation (palms, soles, extremities)
    - Flares occur with delivery in approximately 75% and may be dramatic and within hours
    - Up to 25% present during the immediate postpartum period
    - Most disease remits spontanetously over weeks to months but can have protracted disease
    - Clinical picture can vary from fairly mild to severe
- Recurrences associated with menstruation, oral/hormonal contraceptives in at least 25%
- Can skip pregnancies in about 5%
- **Newborns** – affected up to 10% of time, but disease is mild and self-limited. Increased risk of prematurity and small babies. No increased risk in morbidity or mortality. No evidence that systemic corticosteroids in the mother alters the risk of prematurity

Labs – routine labs are normal

DDx – PUPPP, allergic contact dermatitis, drug eruption

Histology

- H&E – subepidermal vesicle, perivascular infiltrate of lymphocytes and eosinophils. Eosinophils may be lined up along the dermal–epidermal junction and typically fill the vesicular space
- DIF – Essential component is the finding of C3, +/– IgG, in a linear band along the basement membrane zone of perilesional skin
- Complement added indirect immunofluroescence – reveals the circulating HG factor in the majority of patients. Indirect IF only occasionally shows IgG deposition
- Salt-split skin – staining remains with epidermal fragment as it does with bullous pemphigoid
- ELISA – a BP180 NC 16A enzyme-linked immunosorbent assay is now commercially available, and when a cut-off value of 10 ELISA units was employed, this condition could be distinguished from PUPPP with a specificity and sensitivity of 90%

Fig. 16 Where to biopsy SKIN lesions of pemphigoid gestationis for DIF

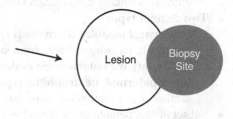

Treatment (No randomized controlled clinical trials)

- Topical corticosteroids (with the possible exception of Class I)
- Antihistamines
- Systemic corticosteroids are cornerstone of therapy – SE include placental calcifications, lower birthweight infants. Most respond to 0.5 mg/kg prednisone daily
  - Maintenance therapy, usually at a lower dose, may or may not be required during remainder of pregnancy
- Many will experience spontaneous disease regression during the third trimester, only to experience a flare during parturition
- No maternal risk other than discomfort from the lesions, which can be severe. Critical to weigh risks of therapy against the severity of symptoms

Pearls and Pitfalls

- Patients with pemphigoid gestationis appear to be at increased risk for developing Graves disease
- Increased incidence of antithyroid antibodies in these patients

Pemphigus, IgA type

Etiology and Pathogenesis

- *In vivo* bound and circulating IgA autoantibodies directed against the cell surface of keratinocytes, but with no IgG autoantibodies

Clinical Presentation and Types

- Vesiculobullous eruption usually occuring in middle-aged or elderly patients
  - Both types have flaccid vesicles or pustules on either erythematous or normal skin
  - Both types – pustules tend to form annular or circinate pattern with crusts in the center of the lesion
  - Distribution – axilla and groin most common, but trunk and proximal extremities may be involved. Mucous membrane involvement is rare
  - Pruritus is usually a significant symptom
- **Two distinct types**
  - **Subcorneal pustular dermatosis type – (Desmocollin 1)** Clinically and histologically indistinguishable from subcorneal pustular dermatosis (Sneddon–Wilkinson), but immunologic evaluation will distinguish the two diseases
  - **Intraepidermal neutrophilic type – (target remains to be identified)** sunflower-like configuration is characteristic
- Subset of IgA pemphigus patients have IgA antibodies directed against DSG1 or DSG3

Labs

- TB skin test (or quantiFERON gold test), CXR, CBC + diff, complete metabolic profile prior to starting immunosuppressives
- Bacterial cultures
- Viral cultures

DDx – bullous pemphigoid, dermatitis herpetiformis, erythema multiforme, Hailey–Hailey, linear IgA dermatosis, pemphigus erythematosus, pemphigus foliaceos, pemphigus herpetiformis, drug-induced pemphigus, IgA pemphigus, paraneoplastic pemphigus, erythema multiforme, aphthous ulcers, herpetic stomatitis, bullous lichen planus

Histology

- DIF → IgA deposition on cell surfaces of epidermal keratinocytes is present in all cases
- IIF → many patients have detectable circulating IgA autoantibodies
  - SPD type – IgA autoantibodies react against upper epidermal surfaces
  - IEN type – IgA autoantibodies found throughout the entire epidermis

Treatment

- Treatment similar to pemphigus vulgaris

Pearls and Pitfalls

- Be diligent about looking for secondary infections (bacterial, viral, fungal)
- Once clinical remission is obtained, changes in the titer of circulating autoantibodies, as determined by indirect IF or ELISA, are helpful in gauging the dose of prednisone

Pemphigus Vulgaris (PV)

Etiology and Pathogenesis

- Pemphigus vulgaris (oral lesions only) – Antibodies to desmoglein 3
- Pemphigus vulgaris (oral and skin lesions) – Antibodies to desmoglein 3 and 1

Clinical Presentation

- Flaccid blisters that may appear on skin and mucosa
- All patients develop painful erosions on the oral mucosa (especially buccal and palatine mucosa). Intact blisters are rare as they are fragile and break easily. Lesions may extend out onto vermilion lip and lead to thick fissured hemorrhagic crusts
  - Involvement of throat may lead to hoarseness and difficulty swallowing
- Conjunctivae, nasal mucosa, vagina, penis, anus, and labia can develop lesions as well
- Some patients have both oral erosions and cutaneous erosions
- Nikolsky sign +
- Without treatment, pemphigus vulgaris can be fatal if large body surface area involved as skin loses its barrier function and prone to secondary infection
- Mean age of onset is approximately 50–60 years
- **Drug-induced PV**: Drugs reported most significantly in association with PV include penicillamine, captopril, and other thiol-containing compounds. Rifampin also reported

Labs

- TB skin test (or quantiFERON gold test), CXR, CBC + diff, complete metabolic profile prior to starting immunosuppressives
- Bacterial cultures
- Viral cultures

DDx – bullous pemphigoid, dermatitis herpetiformis, erythema multiforme, Hailey–Hailey, linear IgA dermatosis, pemphigus erythematosus, pemphigus foliaceos, pemphigus herpetiformis, drug-induced pemphigus, IgA pemphigus, paraneoplastic pemphigus, , aphthous ulcers, herpetic stomatitis, bullous lichen planus

Histology

- Intraepidermal blister formation due to loss of cell–cell adhesion of keratinocytes (acantholysis) without keratinocyte necrosis. Acantholytic keratinocytes seen in blister cavity
- Although basal cells lose lateral desmosomal contact, they maintain their attachment to the basement membrane via hemidesmosomes, thus giving the appearance of a "row of tombstones"
- Acantholysis may involve hair follicles
- Usually maintain appearance of dermal papillae
- Blister cavity may contain inflammatory cells, especially eosinophils
- Rarely, earliest findings may be eosinophilic spongiosis
- DIF (normal perilesional skin) – IgG and often C3
  - ○ Mucosal PV – IgG binds to DSG3 (near base of epidermis)
  - ○ Cutaneous PV – chicken wire appearance – DSG3 and DSG1
- Autoantibodies (IgG) detected by IIF or ELISA. Titer usually correlates with disease activity

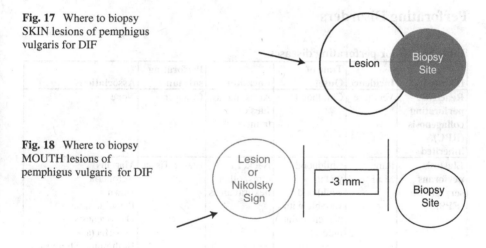

Fig. 17 Where to biopsy SKIN lesions of pemphigus vulgaris for DIF

Fig. 18 Where to biopsy MOUTH lesions of pemphigus vulgaris for DIF

Treatment

- Corticosteroids
  - ○ Bone density q 6 months, eye exam q 6 months, CXR/PPD at baseline and at regular intervals
  - ○ Follow blood glucose and triglycerides
  - ○ Avoid live vaccinations (intranasal flu, polio, yellow fever, typhoid)
- Start steroid-sparing agents early in course
  - ○ Mycophenolate mofetil and azathioprine are the usual first-line agents
  - ○ Azathioprine (Imuran) – 1 mg/kg/day qd/bid (empiric) or based on TPMT level; increase dose by 0.5 mg/kg/day after 6–8 week if necessary; increase q 4 week; 2 mg/kg/day maximum dose for most dermatologic purposes

- ○ **Rituximab** and **intravenous immunoglobulin (IVig)** have also proved useful alone or in combination
  - **IVIG** – 2 g/kg q 3–4 weeks until clear. Then taper off steroids and other immunosuppressants, then start decreasing IVIG. Average time to clearing is 4.5 months. More helpful in milder disease
  - ○ Cyclophosphamide is used for refractory disease
- Consultants – ophthamology, dental
- Patients with oral disease may benefit from avoiding foods, such as spicy foods, tomatoes, orange juice, and hard foods that may traumatize the oral epithelium mechanically, such as nuts, chips, and hard vegetables and fruit
- Advise patients to minimize activities that traumatize the skin and that may precipitate blistering, such as contact sports. Nontraumatic exercises, such as swimming, may be helpful
- Dental plates, dental bridges, or contact lenses may precipitate or exacerbate mucosal disease
- Oral care – see *Lichen Planus*

Perforating Disorders

Table 88 Major perforating diseases

Disease	Incidence	Time of Onset	Location	Perforating substance	Associations
Reactive perforating collagenosis (RPC), inherited	Very rare	Childhood	Arms, hands, sites of trauma	Collagen	None
Elastosis perforans serpiginosa (EPS)	Rare, M > F	Childhood, young adulthood; variable with penicillamine-induced	Neck, face, arms, other flexural areas	Elastic Tissue	**M**arfans **A**crogeria **D**own's **P**enicillamine **O**steogenesis imperfecta **R**othmund–Thompson **E**hlers–Danlos **S**cleroderma
Perforating folliculitis	Common	Young adulthood	Trunk, extremities	Necrotic material	May simply be ordinary folliculitis with follicular rupture, i.e., not a specific entity

Disease	Incidence	Time of Onset	Location	Perforating substance	Associations
Acquired perforating dermatosis – includes RPC, Kyrle's* and occasion-ally, EPS	Common (10% of dialysis patients)	Adulthood	Legs or generalized	Necrotic material, collagen or, uncommonly, elastic tissue	Diabetes, renal disease, pruritus, rarely liver disease; may be end stage of perforating folliculitis
Perforating periumbilical calcific elastosis	Very rare, more common in black women	Adulthood	Abdomen, periumbilical	Calcified elastic tissue	Multiparity

In the opinion of some authors.
Reference: Used with permission from Elsevier. Rapini RP. Perforating Diseases. In: Dermatology. Eds: Bolognia JL, Jorizzo JL, Rapini RP. 2nd ed, 2008. Mosby: New York; 1461

- Treatment
  - Retinoids – systemic and topical
  - Salicylic acid
  - Corticosteroids (topical, intralesional)
  - Menthol-containing lotions – sarna and antihistamines
  - Imiquimod
  - Cryotherapy
  - Light therapy – nbUVB, PUVA
  - Excision

Periodic Fever Syndromes

Table 89   Characteristics of the periodic fever syndromes

Disease	Inheritance	Gene	Characteristics
Familial Mediterranean Fever(FMF)	AR	MEVF gene (pyrin)	• Jewish, Turkish, Armenian, Arab, Italian heritage • 90% have initial episode before age 20 – fever of short duration (6–72 h), **erysipelas-like lesions** of lower extremities (symmetric or unilateral, well-demarcated), monoarticular arthritis, severe abdominal pain, pleurisy • Pericarditis in 1%, scrotal swelling • Vasculitides such as HSP, PAN more frequent • AA amyloidosis is severe complication – usually in untreated disease • May be asymptomatic b/n attacks but biochemical evidence of inflammation • Histology of erysipelas lesions → dermal infiltrate of predominantly neutrophils and nuclear dust • Tx – **Colchicine** (75% respond), azathioprine, anti-TNF, anakinra
Cryopyrin Associated Periodic Syndrome (The Cryopyrinopathies, IL-1 pathways) → FCAS, Muckle Wells, NOMID			
Familial Cold Auto-inflammatory Syndrome (FCAS)	AD	CIAS1/NALP3 gene (cryopyrin)	• Urticarial rash, arthralgias, bouts of fever induced by cold • Rash lasts 12 h • Headache, nausea, sweating, drowsiness, extreme thirst, conjunctivitis, blurred vision, ocular pain • Histology → neutrophilic infiltrate with vascular changes, including swelling and narrowing of lumen • Tx – **Canakinumab (Ilaris).** Avoid cold exposure, NSAIDs for arthralgias, corticosteroids, anakinra

Table 89 (continued)

Disease	Inheritance	Gene	Characteristics
Muckle Wells Syndrome	AD	CIAS1/NALP3 gene (cryopyrin)	• Fever, urticarial rash, limb pain with eventual sensorineural deafness (50–75%). Nephropathy and amyloidosis in 25% • Rash has "circadian rhythm" – don't see in the AM, comes after • lunch. Not pruritic, but "tightness or warmth". Usually on trunk, unusual on face. Can get conjunctivitis • Most have onset at birth, arthralgias, infertility in some • Progressive flu-like symptoms throughout day • Conjunctivitis 3–4x/week • Histology → looks like neutrophilic urticaria • Labs – CRP, UA (look for proteinuria) • Tx – Anakinra (massive rebound after stopping), **Canakinumab (Ilaris)**. Modest benefit -steroids, cyclosporine, cellcept
NOMID/ CINCA Syndrome	Sporadic in most	CIAS1/NALP3 gene (cryopyrin)	• Triad – disabling arthropathy, skin eruption and CNS inflamm • 2/3 have "urticaria-like" eruption at birth. Most develop it within 6 months of life. Rash lasts throughout life • Neurologic – headaches, macrocephaly, cerebral atrophy, chronic aseptic meningitis, high-freq hearing loss, developmental delay • Eye – may get anterior uveitis • 50% have severe arthropathy before age 1 • Labs – ↑ ESR, thrombocytosis, leukocytosis, eosinophilia, hyperglobulinemia • Histology → Sup/deep perivascular infiltrate of lymphs, neuts, occ eosinophils. No mast cells • Tx – high-dose steroids for pain and inflammation but don't help other manifestations. May add MTX. Anakinra very helpful
Other			

(continued)

Table 89 (continued)

Disease	Inheritance	Gene	Characteristics
Blau Syndrome	AD	NOD2 (CARD15) – *often mutated in Crohns dz but different loci*	• Looks like juvenile sarcoid but no pulmonary involvement; some describe this as a type of early onset sarcoidosis. May be misdiagnosed as JRA, unless histology is performed • Usually present by age 4 • Get granulomatous arthritis, uveitis, and dermatitis • Histologically → same as sarcoid, but clinically different • Skin lesions most commonly show scaly maculopapules with tapioca-like appearance and are described as the lichenoid-type, which are rarely seen among sarcoidosis in adults. Erythema nodosum also occurs
Tumor Necrosis Factor Assoc Receptor Syndromes (TRAPS)	AD	TNFRSF1A	• Protracted periods of fever, inflammation – lasts between 7 and 21 days. Fever tends to vary in duration/severity b/n pts • Age of onset → 2 weeks–50 years • >80% with abdominal pain, GI symptoms • Headaches in 68%, arthralgias in 52% • Conjunctival problems – pain, redness, edema (44%) • Pleuritic chest pain (40%) • Skin – generalized reticulated and serpiginous lesions or red macules/patches. Edematous plaques in some. Skin often assoc with underlying myalgias – migrate distally (may limit its movement). Skin lesions may resolve, leaving ecchymoses. • AA amyloidosis in 10% → renal/hepatic failure • Path – infiltrate of CD68+, CD3+, CD4+ and CD8+ T cells. IF of lesional skin – IgM and C3 at DEJ, diffuse IgA, IgG and C3 deposition and fibrinogen in the upper dermis • Tx – High-dose steroids. **No response to colchicine.** Etanercept, anakinra may help

Disease	Inheritance	Gene	Characteristics
Pyogenic Arthritis, Pyoderma Gangrenosum and Acne Syndrome (PAPA)	AD	CD2BP1	• CD2BP1 interacts with pyrin. PAPA-assoc mutations lead to ↑binding to pyrin resulting in CD2BP1 sequestering pyrin. Reduces pyrin's inhibitory role in regulation of IL-1β pathway • Skin – typically get cystic acne, sterile abscesses, cutaneous ulcers (including pyoderma gangrenosum-like lesions). May develop sterile abscesses at injection sites • Histology – sup and deep perivascular, interstitial, periadnexal infiltrate of lymphocytes and neutrophils • Skeletal – develop severe, sterile, pyogenic, destructive arthritis that affects the nonaxial skeleton at a young age • Irritable bowel syndrome and fever have been described in association with PAPA • Tx – Corticosteroids. Etanercept and infliximab reportedly helpful. Anakinra can also be helpful for arthritis
Deficiency of the interleu-kin-1-receptor antagonist (DIRA)	AR	IL1RN	• Within 3 weeks of life → fetal distress, joint swelling, oral mucosal lesions and painful movement • Skin – severe pustulosis and psoriasis-like changes • Histology – epidermal and dermal infiltrate of neuts, especially along hair follicles. Acanthosis and hyperkeratosis • Bone – widening of anterior rib ends and periosteal elevation along long bones • ↑ inflammatory markers (ESR, CRP) • Tx – anakinra

Disease	Inheritance	Gene	Characteristics
Hyper-IgD Syndrome	AR	MVK gene	• MVK=enzyme that catalyzes mevalonic acid to 5-phosphomevalonic acid in sterol biosynthesis pathway. HIDS-assoc mutation causes reduction in this enzyme • Only during febrile periods do pts have ↑ concentrations of mevalonic acid in urine • European descent, especially Dutch (50%) • Presents usually in childhood; most first attacks before age 1 • Typical attack is 3–7 days long with 4- to 8-week asymptomatic period • Attack=fever, cervical LN, abdominal pain, skin lesions. 50% with splenomegaly • Skin – during febrile periods → red macules, papules, nodules or urticarial lesions. Less common – aphthous oral or vaginal ulcers • Very rare to get AA amyloidosis or arthritis • Labs – IgD levels > 100 mg/L (document twice). Need this with clinical to make diagnosis. **NOTE – ↑ serum IgD levels not unique or specific to HIDS. Seen in 10–15% of TRAPS, FMF** • Tx – IVIG, cyclosporine, steroids. Simvastatin, etanercept, anakinra may help
Schnitzler Syndrome	NA	NA	• Acquired autoinflammatory syndrome • Periodic fever, non-pruritic urticarial rash, arthralgia or arthritis, bone pain, and IgM gammopathy. Fatigue, weight loss common • Workup should include SPEP/UPEP or serum/urine IFE • Tx – anakinra

Perioral Dermatitis (POD)

Etiology and Pathogenesis

- Etiology unknown but some possibilities...
  - *Drugs*: abuse of topical steroid preparations. No clear correlation exists between the risk of POD and strength of the steroid or the duration of the abuse
  - *Cosmetics*: Fluorinated toothpaste; skin care ointments and creams, especially those with a petrolatum or paraffin base, and the vehicle isopropyl myristate are suggested to be causative factors
  - *Physical factors*: UV light, heat, and wind worsen POD
  - *Microbiologic factors*: Fusiform spirilla bacteria, *Candida* species, and other fungi have been cultured from lesions. Their presence has no clear clinical relevance. In addition, candidiasis is suggested to provoke POD
  - *Miscellaneous factors*: Hormonal factors are suspected because of an observed premenstrual deterioration. Oral contraceptives may be a factor. Gastrointestinal disturbances, such as malabsorption, have been considered as well

Clinical Presentation

- Mostly occurs in women, although a distinct papular variant occurs in children
- Erythematous papulopustules irregularly grouped and symmetric. Lesions increase in number with central confluence and satellites. Some areas may appear eczematous. No comedones
- Distribution – initially perioral with rim of sparing around vermilion border of lips. May involve periorbital areas and occasionally is on glabella/forehead

Labs – bacterial culture to rule out staph infections

DDx – rosacea, acne vulgaris, irritant dermatitis, allergic contact dermatitis, lupus miliaris disseminatus faciei, demodex folliculitis, Haber syndrome, granuloma faciale, granulomatous rosacea, steroid acne

Histology – perifollicular granulomatous infiltrate (not diagnostic)

Treatment

- Metronidazole or erythromycin in a non-greasy base (lotion, gel, cream)
- PO ABX – tetracycline, doxycycline, minocycline, metronidazole

- Topical retinoids such as adapalene have been useful
- Azaleic acid
- Pimecrolimus cream
- Consider isotretinoin in severe cases
- Avoid ointments on the face
- Zero-therapy – ceasing use of all topical medications and cosmetics (for compliant patients). This is often a limited option because of the patient's tendency to overtreat themselves
- If over-using topical steroids, wean them off by going to lower potency (hydrocortisone 1–2.5%)
- Consider avoidance of fluorinated products (such as toothpaste)

Pearls and Pitfalls

- Blepharitis or conjunctivitis may be seen
- Can occur around any orifice and is rarely a generalized eruption

Pigmented Purpuric Dermatoses

Etiology and Pathogenesis

- Etiology unknown but believed to be cell-mediated immune injury with subsequent vascular injury and erythrocyte extravasation
- Other etiologies include: pressure, trauma, medications
  - Medications implicated → acetaminophen, ampicillin, diuretics, NSAIDs, zomepirac sodium, glipizide, topical 5-FU

Clinical Presentation and Types

- AKA – Capillaritis
- Variants:
  - **Schamberg's disease** (progressive pigmentary dermatosis)
    - Can occur during childhood, but most frequently seen in middle-aged and older men. Lesions consist of oval to irregular patches
    - Yellow-brown in color with superimposed "cayenne-pepper" appearance
    - Favors lower legs and ankles, but can occur on thighs, buttocks, trunk, arms. Usually bilateral
  - **Purpura annularis telangiectodes of Majocchi**
    - Seen most often in adolescents or young adults, especially women. Annular plaques usually 1–3 cm in diameter with punctate telangiectasias and cayenne pepper petechiae. Usually asymptomatic
  - **Lichen aureus**
    - Uncommon. Usually see solitary lesion on lower extremity (often over a perforator vein). Chronic patches or plaques or often rust-colored to purple-brown but may be golden. Usually asymptomatic
  - **Eczematid-like purpura of Doucas and Kapetanakis**
    - Usually affects middle-aged men and older. Presents with scaly petechial or purpuric macules, papules and patches
    - Lesions favor lower extremities and are typically pruritic
  - **Lichenoid purpura of Gougerot and Blum**
    - Usually seen in middle-aged men. Lichenoid papules, plaques and macules in association with lesions of Schamberg's disease

Labs – CBC to exclude thrombocytopenia, and coagulation screening to exclude other causes of purpura

DDx – early CTCL, purpuric clothing dermatitis, stasis, scurvy, LCV, purpuric generalized lichen nitidus, regressing Kaposi's sarcoma, and drug hypersensitivity reactions (e.g., allergy to rituximab, carbamazepine, meprobamate, chlordiazepox-ide, furosemide, nitroglycerin, or vitamin B-1)

Histology

- Red cell extravasation, endothelial cell swelling, perivascular lymphocytic infil-trate, and hemosiderin-containing macrophages
- Lichen aureus and Gougerot–Blum variants → lichenoid infiltrate and epidermal spongiosis
- Gougerot–Blum and Eczematoid-like purpura of Doucas and Kapetanakis → patchy parakeratosis

Treatment

- Pruritus – topical corticosteroids and antihistamines
- Associated venous stasis should be treated by compression stockings
- Prolonged leg dependency should be avoided
- Ascorbic acid 500 mg PO BID
- Rutoside 50 mg PO BID (a flavonoid)
- Pentoxifylline 400 mg PO TID
- PUVA or NbUVB for severe cases
- Systemic tetracycline or minocycline

Pearls and Pitfalls

– Biopsy if clinically unclear. Can clinically resemble a vasculitis in some cases.

Pitted Keratolysis

Etiology and Pathogenesis

- Infection with *Micrococcus sedentarius* (now renamed to *Kytococcus sedentarius,*) *Dermatophilus congolensis,* or species of *Corynebacterium* and *Actinomyces*
  - Under appropriate conditions (i.e., prolonged occlusion, hyperhidrosis, increased skin surface pH), these bacteria proliferate and produce proteinases that destroy the stratum corneum, creating pits
- Malodor associated is presumed to be from the production of sulfur-compound by-products, such as thiols, sulfides, and thioesters

Clinical Presentation

- Crateriform pitting that primarily affects the pressure-bearing aspects of the plantar surface of the feet and, occasionally, the palms of the hand as collarettes of scale
- Prominent malodor

DDx – plantar warts, tinea pedis, palmoplantar punctate keratoderma, pits of nevoid basal cell carcinoma syndrome, palmar or plantar hypokeratosis

Histology – Biopsy usually not needed

- Well-defined erosions of stratum corneum with filamentous organisms confined entirely to area of erosion. Pits extend about 2/3 of way into stratum corneum
- Bacteria best seen with Grocott–Gomori methenamine silver stain

Treatment

- Avoid occlusive footwear and reduce foot friction with properly fitting footwear
- Absorbent cotton socks must be changed frequently to prevent excessive foot moisture. Wool socks tend to whisk moisture away from the skin and may be helpful
- Reduce associated hyperhidrosis with the application of 20% aluminum chloride soln (Drysol)
- Clindamycin or erythromycin (soln or gel) BID may be sufficient
- PO Erythromycin

- ○ 250 mg erythromycin stearate/base (or 400 mg ethylsuccinate) PO q 6 h, or 500 mg q 12 h (1 h ac or 2 h pc); alternatively, 333 mg PO q 8 h; increase to 4 g/day depending on severity of infection
- Topical mupirocin (Bactroban), econazole, tetracycline have been effective
- For cases resistant to topical antibiotic treatments and/or associated with hyperhidrosis, the use of botulinum toxin injections has been effective
- Effective treatment of pitted keratolysis clears both the lesions and odor in 3–4 weeks

Pearls and Pitfalls

– May be misdiagnosed as warts by the non-dermatologist

Pityriasis Lichenoides

Etiology and Pathogenesis

- Etiology unclear, but the most commonly reported associated pathogens are Epstein–Barr virus (EBV), *Toxoplasma gondii,* and human immunodeficiency virus (HIV)

Clinical Presentation and Types

- Encompasses spectrum of clinical presentations ranging from acute papular lesions that rapidly evolve into pseudovesicles and central necrosis (pityriasis lichenoides et varioliformis acuta or **PLEVA**) to small, scaling, benign-appearing papules (pityriasis lichenoides chronica or **PLC**)
- **Pityriasis lichenoides et varioliformis acuta (PLEVA)**
  - Presents with abrupt appearance of multiple papules on the trunk, buttocks, and proximal extremities. Papules rapidly progress to vesicles with necrotic centers and hemorrhagic crusts
  - Minor constitutional symptoms may be present
  - A patient with febrile ulceronecrotic PLEVA presents with acute constitutional symptoms such as high fever, malaise, and myalgias – can cause scarring
  - Lesions may be associated with burning and pruritus
- **Pityriasis lichenoides chronica (PLC)**
  - At the subacute end of the spectrum, PLC may develop over days
  - PLC also is distributed over the trunk, buttocks, and proximal extremities
  - Papules are erythematous to red-brown and scaly. Pursue a more indolent course
  - PLEVA and PLC are not distinct diseases, but rather, they are different manifestations of the same process, although the process is accelerated in PLEVA

Labs to Consider – Antistreptolysin O titers, EBV IgM/IgG, Hep B surf Ag, Hep B surf Ab and anticore IgM, Hep C Ab, HIV screening, Monospot or heterophil antibody test, RPR, throat cultures, *Toxoplasma* Sabin–Feldman dye test, enzyme-linked immunoassay, and indirect immunofluorescence/hemagglutination

DDx – chickenpox, Gianotti–Crosti syndrome, lichen planus, pityriasis rosea, psoriasis (guttate), secondary syphilis, arthropod bite, disseminated herpes zoster, drug eruption, primary HIV infection, vasculitis, viral exanthem

Histology

- **PLEVA** – focal parakeratosis often with scale crust. Dense wedge-shaped infiltrate in dermis with prominent lymphocytic exocytosis into the epidermis. Necrotic keratinocytes common. Sometimes see spongiosis and intraepidermal vesiculation. Basal layer degeneration and extravasation of erythrocytes, often in the epidermis
- **PLC** – histologically similar to PLEVA but less acute, more chronic form. See less scale, fewer neutrophils, less spongiosis, fewer vesicles, and fewer necrotic keratinocytes

Treatment

- **Topical corticosteroids**
- Topical coal tar products
- **Oral erythromycin**
- **Oral tetracycline**
- Phototherapy – UVB, PUVA
- Methotrexate (MTX)
- Other – sulfonamides, dapsone, chloroquine, streptomycin, INH, penicillin, pentoxifylline

Pearls and Pitfalls

- A diagnosis of lymphomatoid papulosis should not be missed because of the theoretical possibility of subsequent development of a myeloproliferative disorder. Biopsies should be obtained to confirm a diagnosis of PLEVA
- Erythromycin (EES) in solution form has been difficult to obtain recently. Can crush pills into food for kids with PLEVA
- Aggressively treat and follow kids with PLEVA as significant scarring can occur

Pityriasis Rosea (PR)

Etiology and Pathogenesis

- Etiology unknown but viral etiology proposed. May be the result of HHV-6 or -7
- Some drugs can cause a PR-like drug eruption – ACE inhibitors, Flagyl, Gold, NSAIDs, metronidazole, isotretinoin, arsenic, beta-blockers, barbiturates, sulfasalazine, bismuth, clonidine, imatinib, organic mecurials, methoxypromazine, D-penicillamine, tripelennamine, ketotifen, salvarsan

Clinical Presentation

- Initial lesion is the "herald patch" (2–4 cm) which is common on the neck, trunk or proximal extremities. Lesion is a skin-colored to pink- to salmon-colored patch or plaque with a slightly raised advancing margin. Margin has a more obvious trailing collarette of scale with free edge pointing inward
- 5% experience a mild prodrome of headache, fever, arthralgias, or general malaise
- Within next couple of days, numerous lesions appear on trunk and extremities
- In darker skin types, lesions tend to be more papular and hyperpigmented
- Lesions on the trunk are distributed in "Christmas tree" pattern
- Minute pustules may be seen during the initial phase of PR
- Eruption usually last 6–8 weeks
- Oral lesions uncommon
- Pruritus may be intense and is seen in > 75% of cases
- Atypical variants – inverse pattern, urticarial lesions, EM-like lesions, vesicular, pustular, and purpuric

Labs – usually none are performed, but consider …

- RPR
- Blood profiles are normal; however, leukocytosis, neutrophilia, basophilia, and lymphocytosis have been seen
- Minimal increases in the erythrocyte sedimentation rate (ESR), total protein, albumin, alpha1-globulin, and alpha2-globulin have been noted
- Test findings for rheumatoid factor (RF), cold agglutinins, and cryoglobulins have been normal

DDx – erythema multiforme, secondary syphilis, CTCL, psoriasis, pityriasis alba, tinea, PR-like drug eruption, nummular eczema, seborrheic dermatitis, erythema dyschromicum perstans, lichen planus, lichenoid reaction, Kaposi's sarcoma, pityriasis lichenoides

Histology

- See focal parakeratosis and sometimes mild acanthosis
- Spongiosis present and rarely see spongiotic vesicles
- Perivascular lymphocytes and rarely eosinophils
- Sometimes – Extravasated erythrocytes and dyskeratosis

Treatment

- **Topical** or Oral corticosteroids – especially if the disease is severe or widespread (vesicular)
- Pruritus
  - PO hydroxyzine, cetirizine, loratidine, fexofenadine
- Ultraviolet radiation therapy (NbUVB) has been demonstrated to be effective for PR but may leave postinflammatory pigmentation at the site of the PR lesion
- Azithromycin does not seem to help
- Erythromycin may be helpful in children older than 2 (not all studies show this)
  - 250 mg erythromycin stearate/base (or 400 mg ethylsuccinate) PO 1 h ac q 6 h, or 500 mg q 12 h
  - Alternatively, 333 mg PO q 8 h; increase to 4 g/day depending on severity of infection
  - Pediatric dose: 30–50 mg/kg/day (15–25 mg/lb/day) PO divided q 6–8 h; double dose for severe infection
- Acyclovir has been shown in one study to hasten resolution, especially if given within 1 week of rash but this was a non-randomized, non-blinded trial
  - 800 mg PO five times daily for 5 days
  - Pediatric Dose 10–20 mg/kg PO q 6 h for 5–10 day

Pearls and Pitfalls

- Have a low threshold to rule out syphilis
- There is no reason to exclude children from school for PR

Pityriasis Rubra Pilaris (PRP)

Etiology and Pathogenesis

- No clear etiology. The therapeutic success of systemic retinoids has suggested a possible dysfunction in keratinization or vitamin A metabolism, but not proven. Various minor traumas to the skin, UV exposure, and infections have been reported to precede onset of PRP. May be an autoimmune process

Clinical Presentation and Types

- Reddish-orange scaly plaques, orange-red waxy palmoplantar keratoderma (PPK), and keratotic follicular papules. Disease may progress to erythroderma with distinct areas of uninvolved skin, the "islands of sparing". Nail involvement is characterized by a thickened plate, yellow-brown discoloration, and subungual debris. Mucous membranes are rarely involved, but may resemble lichen planus
- Six categories:
  - **Type I is classic adult PRP** – Most common form of PRP (**>50% of all cases**), best prognosis
    - Acute onset, features are classic (w/erythroderma, islands of sparing), PPK, and follicular hyperkeratosis
    - Reportedly, about 80% of patients have remission in an average of 3 years
  - **Type II is atypical adult PRP – 5%** of all cases
    - Characterized by ichthyosiform lesions, areas of eczematous change, alopecia, and long duration (often 20 years or more)
  - **Type III is classic juvenile PRP – 10%** of all cases of PRP
    - Very similar to type I but onset is within the first 2 years of life
    - Remission can occur sooner than with type I, within an average of 1 year
  - **Type IV is circumscribed juvenile PRP – 25%** of all cases of PRP
    - Occurs in prepubertal children, characterized by sharply demarcated areas of follicular hyperkeratosis and erythema of the knees and the elbows
    - Long-term outcome is unclear, with some reports of improvement in the late teenaged years. This form of PRP rarely progresses
  - **Type V is atypical juvenile PRP – 5%** of all cases of PRP
    - Most cases of familial PRP belong to this group; early onset, runs chronic course
    - Characterized by prominent follicular hyperkeratosis, scleroderma-like changes on the palms and the soles, and infrequent erythema
  - **Type VI is HIV-associated PRP**

- ■ May have nodulocystic and pustular acneiform lesions
- ■ Elongated follicular plugs or lichen spinulosus-type lesions also been reported
- ■ Tend to be resistant to standard treatments, but may respond to HAART

DDx – Seb derm, CTCL, atopic dermatitis, allergic contact dermatitis, psoriasis, dermatomyositis, drug reaction, ichthyosis, GVHD

Histology

- Psoriasiform dermatitis with irregular hyperkeratosis and alternating vertical and horizontal ortho- and parakeratosis ("checkerboard pattern") is distinctive
- Hair follicles are dilated and filled with a keratinous plug while the shoulder of the stratum corneum at the edge of these follicles frequently show parakeratosis
- Interfollicular epidermis often has hypergranulosis and thick, shortened rete ridges
- Sparse lymphohistiocytic perivascular infiltrate
- Acantholysis within the epidermis has been described

Treatment

- (Emollients, dry skin care)
- Topical corticosteroids
- **Acitretin**
- **Isotretinoin** – 1–1.5 mg/kg/day. May go up to 2 mg/kg/day
- Calcipotriol may help
- Azathioprine – 1 mg/kg/day PO for 6–8 week; increase by 0.5 mg/kg q 4 week until response; not to exceed 2.5 mg/kg/day
- Methotrexate – 10–25 mg PO q week
- Cyclosporine
- Infliximab
- Extracorporeal photochemotherapy

Pearls and Pitfalls

- If PRP appears in older pt or if seems atypical, the pt should be evaluated for possible underlying malignancy (such as renal cell carcinoma, lung carcinoma, hepatocellular carcinoma, etc.)
- There are reports of PRP in association with myasthenia gravis, celiac disease, myositis, inflammatory arthritis, and hypothyroidism
- Both photoaggravated and phototriggered forms of PRP can occur

Polymorphous Light Eruption (PMLE)

Etiology and Pathogenesis

- Appears to be a delayed-type hypersensitivity response to undefined, endogenous, cutaneous photo-induced antigen(s)
- Susceptibility appears to be genetic

Clinical Presentation

- Appearance is most common in the spring and early summer and follows minutes to hours (sometimes days) of being in the sun
- Outbreaks may occur in the winter months with snow-reflected sunlight
- Eruption last for one to several days or occasionally weeks (especially with continued sun exposure)
- Tendency for the eruption to diminish or cease as summer progresses → "hardening"
- Distribution → face, neck, outer arms, dorsal hands, and other sun-exposed surfaces
- Morphology – most common is grouped, pinhead-sized papules in sun-exposed areas. Can see vesicles, bullae, papulovesicles, confluent edematous swelling
- General malaise, headache, fever, nausea, and other symptoms rarely occur
- Variant – **Juvenile Spring Eruption**
  - Dull-red edematous papules which may become vesicular and crusted. These lesions usually confined to the helix of the ears. Lesions may occur on hands and trunk
  - More common in boys and appears in the spring/early summer
  - Considered subset of PMLE, but eruption cannot be reproduced with UV light exposure
  - Topical steroids helpful, but sunscreens do not appear to prevent recurrences

Labs to Consider

- ANA
- SSA, SSB
- Urine, stool, blood porphyrin levels
- MEDs are normal in PMLE (lowered/abnormal in chronic actinic dermatitis)
- Photopatch testing to rule out photoallergic or airborne contact dermatitis

DDx – allergic contact dermatitis, SCLE, tumid lupus, actinic prurigo, chronic actinic dermatitis, solar urticaria, porphyrias, photodrug eruption, airborne allergic contact dermatitis

Histology

- Variable epidermal spongiosis and a superficial and deep perivascular and periappendageal lymphohistiocytic dermal infiltrate. Eosinophils and neutrophils often present. May be difficult to differentiate from lupus if there are significant interface changes

Treatment

- Sun-protective measures
- Sunscreen with high SPF are not protective against UVA-induced PMLE. Use zinc- or titanium-based sunscreens
- Antioxidants may be helpful (Vitamin E 400 IU/day, Beta-carotene 30–300 mg QD)
- PUVA → oral prednisone may be useful initially in conjunction with phototherapy to avoid eruption during therapy
- NBUVB
- Antimalarials sometimes helpful
- Nicotinamide 3 g/day orally → rationale for its use based on its blockade of kynurenic acid formation, a photosensitizer that may play a role in PMLE
- Azathioprine 0.8–2.5 mg/kg/day for 3 months
- Thalidomide

Pearls and Pitfalls

- Rule out porphyrias in unusual cases

Porokeratoses

Etiology and Pathogenesis

- Thought to be a disorder of keratinization, but definitive pathogenesis unknown. Lesions may represent expanding mutant clone of keratinocytes in genetic predisposed individuals.

Clinical Presentation and Types

- Clonal disorder of keratinization characterized by one or more atrophic patches surrounded by a clinically and histologically distinctive ridgelike border called the cornoid lamella
- Formation of SCCs or BCCs – reported in all forms of porokeratoses except in punctate form
- **Risk factors** – genetic inheritance (AD has been established for familial cases of all forms of porokeratosis), ultraviolet radiation, immunosuppression (HIV, lymphoma, iatrogenic causes), electron beam therapy, radiation therapy
- **Five clinical variants of porokeratosis are recognized**:
  - ○ **Classic porokeratosis of Mibelli (PM)** 2x more common in men
    - ▪ Small, asymptomatic, or slightly pruritic lesion develops; expands over years
    - ▪ Occasionally, patients have a history of an antecedent trauma, such as a burn wound
    - ▪ PM circumferentially involving the digits may induce pseudoainhum
  - ○ **Disseminated superficial actinic porokeratosis (DSAP)**
    - ▪ Usually third to fourth decade; 3x more common in women
    - ▪ Multiple, brown, annular, keratotic lesions that develop predominantly on the extensor surfaces of the legs and the arms
  - ○ **Porokeratosis palmaris et plantaris disseminata (PPPD)**
    - ▪ Any age; 2x more common in men
    - ▪ Small, relatively uniform lesions are first seen on the palms and the soles, and, then, they develop in a generalized distribution, including mucosal membranes
    - ▪ Lesions may itch or sting, but they are usually asymptomatic
  - ○ **Linear porokeratosis**
    - ▪ May develop at any age but common in infancy or childhood
    - ▪ Unilateral, linear array of papules develop which follow lines of Blaschko
    - ▪ Most common on extremities
  - ○ **Punctate porokeratosis**
    - ▪ Multiple, asymptomatic, tiny, hyperkeratotic papules with thin, raised margins develop on the palms and the soles during adulthood

DDx

- Linear porokeratosis – inflammatory linear epidermal nevus, incontinentia pigmenti, lichen striatus, linear lichen planus
- Punctate porokeratosis – May resemble punctate keratoderma, Darier disease, Cowden disease, arsenical keratoses
- Actinic keratoses

Histology – Cornoid lamella is the histopathologic hallmark of all forms of porokeratosis – take biopsy from hyperkeratotic edge. This is characterized by a thin column of tightly packed parakeratotic cells extending from an invagination of the epidermis through the adjacent stratum corneum, often protruding above the surface of adjacent skin. Looks like smoke from a train.

Treatment

- Cryotherapy
- Topical 5-fluorouracil (5-FU)
  - Enhancement of penetration, which heightens the response, may be achieved by occlusion or the addition of topical tretinoin. Concurrent use of topical steroids may ease discomfort without reducing long-term improvement
- Topical vitamin D-3 analogue – calcipotriol
- Topical imiquimod 5% cream – shown effective for PM
- Oral retinoids (isotretinoin and acitretin): The use of oral retinoids in patients who are immunosuppressed, who are at higher risk for malignant degeneration, may reduce the risk of carcinoma in porokeratotic lesions
  - Oral isotretinoin at 20 mg daily combined with topical 5-fluorouracil is reported to be effective for DSAP and PPPD
- Excision – for both porokeratosis (if size permits) and for malignant degeneration
- ED & C
- Laser therapy – 585 nm, frequency-doubled Nd:YAG, CO_2 laser ablation – helpful for some
- Photodynamic therapy
- Dermabrasion

Pearls and Pitfalls

- DSAP has lowest risk of malignant change
- Porokeratosis is sometimes inherited as an autosomal dominant condition
- Thread-like raised hyperkeratotic border is characteristic

Porphyria Cutanea Tarda (PCT)

Etiology and Pathogenesis

- Excess iron enhances the formation of toxic oxygen species and increases oxidative stress and apparently facilitates porphyrinogenesis by catalyzing the formation of oxidation products that inhibit UROD. Reduction of UROD activity to approximately 25% of normal leads to clinical expression of the disease
  - Uroporphyrinogen decarboxylase (UROD) – inherited or acquired
    - Familial types with *UROD* gene mutations
    - Acquired types that may occur in individuals with a genetic predisposition (sporadic PCT)
- When hepatic UROD activity falls below a critical threshold, porphyrin by-products of the heme biosynthetic pathway with 4–8 carboxyl group substituents are overproduced
- These porphyrins accumulate in the liver and disseminate to other organs
- Porphyrins with high carboxyl group numbers are water soluble; excreted primarily by kidneys
  - The porphyrin with 8 carboxyl groups is termed uroporphyrin
  - 4-carboxyl porphyrins include coproporphyrin, isocoproporphyrin – chiefly excreted in feces
- Porphyrins are photoactive molecules that efficiently absorb energy in the visible violet spectrum. Photoexcited porphyrins in the skin mediate oxidative damage to biomolecular targets, causing cutaneous lesions

Clinical Presentation

- Characterized by increased mechanical fragility after sun exposure
  - Typically on hands and arms; occasionally on the face, feet
- Erosions, blisters form painful indolent sores – heal with milia, dyspigmentation, scarring
- Hypertrichosis, scleroderma-like plaques that may develop dystrophic calcification
- Photo-onycholysis and scarring alopecia may occur in severe cases
- Excretion of discolored urine – resembles port wine or tea due to porphyrin pigments
- **Aggravating factors** – ethanol, estrogen, hepatitis and HIV, hemochromatosis (HFE gene), hepatic tumors

Labs and Workup

- 24 h urine porphyrin level; consider stool porphyrins
- CBC+diff, LFTs, serum ferritin level and screening for hepatitis viruses and HIV

- Consider checking for HFE gene if Hgb/Hct high – often see concomitant hemochromatosis
- Urine – the excess porphyrin pigment is often grossly evident in visible light and yields a pink fluorescence under Wood lamp; false negatives up to 50%
- Alpha-fetoprotein presence in serum is useful to screen for hepatocellular carcinoma
- Ascorbic acid (vitamin C) serum levels are deficient in some patients with PCT
- Pseudoporphyria – urine porphyrins are negative; commonly caused by NSAIDs

DDx – Pseudoporphyria, EBA, variegate porphyria, hereditary coproporphyria, bullous lupus, Hydroa Vacciniforme

Histology

- Subepidermal bullae with minimal dermal inflammatory infiltrate and dermal papillae protruding upward into the blister cavity (festooning)
- Thickened upper dermal capillary walls and DE basement membrane zone – accentuated with the periodic acid-Schiff stain. Elastosis, sclerosis of dermal collagen, and hyaline deposits may be seen in the dermis. Linear, eosinophilic, PAS–positive globules composed of basement membrane material and degenerating keratinocytes ("caterpillar bodies") may be observed in the blister roof
- **DIF** – deposition of immunoglobulins and complement in and around the dermal blood vessels and at the basement membrane zone

Treatment

- **Phlebotomy** – 1 unit q 2–4 weeks until serum ferritin levels are at lower limit of reference range
  - Chelation with desferrioxamine is an alternative means of iron mobilization when venesections are not practical

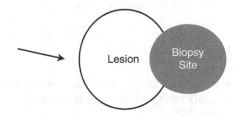

Fig. 19 Where to biopsy lesions suspicious for porphyria for DIF

- Sunlight avoidance is main defense for photosensitivity until clinical remission induced
  - Use sunscreens with zinc oxide and titanium dioxide or Mexoryl → every day!
- Avoid alcohol, estrogens
- Plaquenil 200–400 mg, **2–3 times per week**; larger doses can cause severe hepatotoxicity
- For patients with PCT who are anemic due to other chronic diseases (e.g., renal failure, human immunodeficiency viral infection), human recombinant erythropoietin can be used to stimulate erythropoiesis (50–100 U/kg IV/SC three times/week)
  - Mobilizes tissue iron and may increase circulating erythrocyte mass to a degree that permits therapeutic phlebotomies to be performed at judicious volumes and intervals

Pearls and Pitfalls

- The estrogen-receptor antagonist tamoxifen has been associated with the development of PCT in a few women treated with this agent for breast carcinoma
- Iron-rich foods should be consumed in moderation; strict avoidance not usually necessary
- The risks of PCT patients using plant-derived, estrogen-like compounds are not well established, but these agents probably should be avoided
- UROD enzyme activity assay is commercially available in at least one laboratory in the United States – may help determine patterns of inheritance in familial PCT and confirm the diagnosis in cases with confusing biochemical data
- **Differentiate from Variegate Porphyria** – VP can have identical cutaneous findings, but with VP can also get seizures, colicky abdominal pain, N/V/C, peripheral neuropathy. NPO can be dangerous and acute attacks can leave residual neurologic damage
  - Check ratio of URO to COPRO in the urine
    - PCT 8:1 (URO > COPRO), VP 1:1 (or COPRO > URO)

Progressive Macular Hypomelanosis

Etiology and Pathogenesis

- *Propionibacterium acnes* residing in hair follicles may play a role

Clinical Presentation

- Seen in darker-skinned individuals. Characterized by poorly defined, nummular, non-scaly hypopigmented macules and patches on the trunk and rarely on proximal extremities, head, and neck
- Confluence of lesions may occur centrally
- Occasionally – large circular lesions
- No associated pruritus or preceding inflammation

Labs – Consider KOH if tinea versicolor is a consideration (negative in PMH)

DDx – tinea versicolor, seborrheic dermatitis, pityriasis alba, hypopigmented mycosis fungoides, tuberculoid or borderline tuberculoid leprosy, post-inflammatory hypopigmentation

Histology

- Decreased pigment in the epidermis and a normal appearing dermis
- Electron microscopy demonstrates a shift from large melanosomes in uninvolved skin to small aggregated membrane-bound melanosomes in hypopigmented skin

Treatment

- Topical 1% clindamycin and 5% benzoyl peroxide
- Oral minocycline + topical 1% clindamycin and 5% benzoyl peroxide
- Oral doxycycline + topical 1% clindamycin and 5% benzoyl peroxide
- NbUVB 3x/weeK (usually in combination with topicals)
- UVA 3x/week (usually in combination with topicals)

Pearls and Pitfalls

– Patients have usually failed topical steroids and antifungals
– May recur when treatment is discontinued

Reference:

Relyveld GN, et al. Progressive macular hypomelanosis: an overview. Am J Clin Dermatol. 2007;
8(1):13–9.

Prurigo of Pregnancy

Etiology and Pathogenesis

- Etiology unknown. Theories include:
  - May simply have atopic dermatitis as some patients have elevated IgE levels
  - Other patients have been reported to have cholestasis suggesting an overlap with cholestasis of pregnancy

Clinical Presentation

- Patients report onset of lesions during the second or third trimester with discrete, excoriated papules, mostly on extensor surfaces
- Lesions may or may not be follicular and are typically 0.5–1 cm
- May or may not have a central crust
- Pustules or follicular pustules may be seen, but blisters are not
- Disease may last for week to months postpartum
- Recurrence in subsequent pregnancies is variable

Labs – LFTs are normal (by definition)

DDx – cholestasis of pregnancy, bacterial folliculitis

Histology – Nonspecific.

- Direct IF – negative
- Indirect IF – negative

Treatment – May respond to:

- Topical corticosteroids
- Benzoyl peroxide
- UVB
- Proper skin care
- No maternal or fetal risk with this condition

Pruritic Urticarial Papules and Plaques of Pregnancy (PUPPP)

Etiology and Pathogenesis

- Etiology unknown. Theories include:
  - Some speculate that increased maternal weight gain may play a role as it is more frequent with multiple gestation pregnancies (tenfold higher)
  - Increased levels of progesterone in association with multiple gestations and peripheral chimerism (deposition of fetal DNA) that favors skin with increased vascularity and damaged collagen

Clinical Presentation

- Pruritic urticarial papules usually begin in the abdominal striae, typically with umbilical sparing
- Onset is usually in third trimester or immediately postpartum
- Eruption typically spread over a matter of days, but generally spares the face, palms, soles
- Microvesiculation may occur but bullae formation not present
- Less commonly, can see target or annular and polycyclic lesions
- No fetal or maternal morbidities associated with this condition

Labs – LFTs normal, cortisol levels normal

DDx – allergic contact dermatitis, pemphigoid gestationis, urticaria, viral exanthem, drug eruption

Histology – Skin biopsy findings are nonspecific

- **H&E**
  - Epidermis may show spongiosis, parakeratosis, or eosinophilic spongiosis
  - Dermis shows a nonspecific perivascular lymphocytic infiltrate with variable degree of edema
  - There may be neutrophils or eosinophils within infiltrate but the number of eosinophils is far fewer than that seen in pemphigoid gestationis
- **DIF** – no relevant findings
- **IIF** – negative

Treatment

- Majority benefit from potent topical corticosteroids
- Oral antihistamines
- Occasionally, women may require systemic corticosteroids
- Proper skin care and emollients helpful
- Resolution typically occurs within 7–10 days of delivery

Pruritus

Etiology and Pathogenesis

- Generalized pruritus may be classified into the following categories:
  - Renal pruritus, cholestatic pruritus, hematologic pruritus, endocrine pruritus, pruritus related to malignancy, and idiopathic generalized pruritus
- **Renal pruritus** occurs in patients with CRF, most often those receiving hemodialysis
  - Exact cause not known, although toxic substances retained during HD, histamine, opioids, and neural proliferation have been postulated as potential causes
- **Cholestatic pruritus**
  - Particularly common with cholestasis caused by primary biliary cirrhosis, primary sclerosing cholangitis, chronic hepatitis C, choledocholithiasis, obstructive carcinoma of the pancreas/biliary system, cholestasis of pregnancy, and end-stage liver disease of any cause
  - Drug-induced cholestasis may be caused by chlorpropamide, tolbutamide, phenothiazines, erythromycin, anabolic steroids, and oral contraceptives
- **Hematologic pruritus** may be seen in association with the following conditions:
  - Iron deficiency
  - Polycythemia rubra vera
  - Hypereosinophilic syndrome
  - Essential thrombocythemia
  - Myelodysplastic syndrome
- **Endocrine pruritus** may be seen in association with the following disorders:
  - Hyperthyroidism
  - Hypothyroidism
  - Diabetes mellitus
  - Hyperparathyroidism
  - Hypoparathyroidism
- The following **malignancies** are known to have the potential to cause itching:
  - Hodgkin disease
  - Non-Hodgkin lymphoma
  - Leukemias
  - Paraproteinemias and myeloma
  - Carcinoid syndrome
  - Sipple syndrome (multiple endocrine neoplasia)
  - Solid tumors, including GI malignancies, CNS tumors, and lung cancer
- **Other causes**
  - Drug-induced pruritus without a rash, mastocytosis, HIV infection and AIDS, sarcoidosis, eosinophilia-myalgia syndrome, dermatomyositis, scleroderma, SLE, Sjögren syndrome, neurofibromatosis, hemochromatosis, multiple

sclerosis, brain abscess, parasitic infections, parvoviral infection, leptospirosis, chemical intoxication with mercury or diamino diphenylmethane, primary cutaneous amyloidosis, starvation, fibromyalgia, chronic fatigue syndrome, dumping syndrome, notalgia paresthetica

Clinical Presentation

- Secondary excoriations and erosions but no primary lesion
- May develop prurigo nodules and/or lichen simplex chronicus
- Skin is often very dry, which complicates and precipitates itching

Labs and Imaging to Consider

- CBC+diff
- Cr, BUN, GFR
- TSH, free T4
- Fasting glucose
- Occult blood in stool (three samples)
- HIV if risk factors
- SPEP, UPEP
- Stool for ova and parasites (three samples)
- Urine for 5-HIAA and mast cell metabolites
- Chest x-ray
- Consider liver ultrasound or CT scan
- Scabies prep – if papules, vesicles and burrows on hands, wrists, feet, genital area

DDx – Scabies, xerosis

Treatment

- **Renal Pruritus**
    - ○ Systemic
        - nbUVB – 3x/week is treatment of choice
        - Activated charcoal (cholestyramine is not as effective and is associated with more side effects such as acidosis)
            - □ Charcodote 6 g PO QD
        - Thalidomide
        - PO opioid antagonists – naltrexone (start at 12.5 mg PO QD – cut pill)
        - Nicergoline and free fatty acids (e.g., those in primrose oil)
        - Gabapentin (worsens cholestatic pruritus)

- Butorphanol, an opioid that displays mu antagonism and kappa agonism
  - Topicals
    - Capsaicin cream 0.025%. Can apply EMLA prior to applying capsaicin to reduce burning sensation of capsaicin
    - Tacrolimus ointment (Protopic)
  - Low protein diet may help in chronic renal failure
- **Cholestatic Pruritus**
  - Cholestyramine – first-line treatment
    - 4–16 g PO qd in divided doses (4 g before or after meals to coincide with gall bladder contraction); further increases may be given before midday and evening meals; not to exceed 16 g/day
  - Rifampin – be aware of drug interactions
  - Opioid antagonists – oral naltrexone
  - Ursodeoxycholic acid (Actigall, Urso 250, Urso Forte) and S-adenosyl-L-methionine have both been reported to decrease pruritus in women with cholestasis of pregnancy
  - Extracorporeal albumin dialysis – consider when severe pruritus is refractory
  - Ondansetron – affects opioid pathway
  - Removal of the offending agent should be initiated in patients with drug-induced cholestasis
  - Thalidomide
  - Other – infused propofol, SSRIs (such as sertraline), UV-B, phenobarbital, dronabinol, Remeron
- **Hematologic and Endocrine Pruritus**
  - Treat underlying problems such as anemia, thyroid abnormalities
  - Polycythemia vera – aspirin
  - UV-B light therapy, cholestyramine, naloxone, and activated charcoal
  - Paroxetine (Paxil) relieves itch in patients with advanced cancer; however, the effect usually lasts only 4–6 weeks
- **Other General Treatments**
  - Atarax 25 mg PO q 6 h
  - Doxepin 25–50 mg QHS
  - Non-sedating
    - Allegra
    - Claritin
    - Clarinex
    - Zyrtec (nonsedating in most)
    - Xyzal
  - Neurontin
  - Lyrica
  - Pramoxine
  - Capsaicin

- ○ Pimecrolimus (Elidel® Cream 1) and tacrolimus (Protopic 0.1% oint)
- ○ Cutaneous field stimulation (CFS)
  - ▪ Electrically stimulates thin afferent fibers, including nocireceptive C-fibers, was reported to inhibit histamine-induced itching. The reduction in itching is accompanied by degeneration of the epidermal nerve fibers
- ○ Reflex therapy, acupuncture, and hydrotherapy are three treatments that may be beneficial as adjunctive therapy, however further research is needed. There is little research available regarding the effectiveness of reflex therapy and hydrotherapy. These options may be considered in difficult-to-treat patients where traditional approaches have been unsuccessful

Pearls and Pitfalls

- – Some treatments have a rare risk of tardive dyskinesia (Remeron). Always discuss and warn patient about this potential side effect
- – Paroxetine has been labeled "pack it on" as it does cause significant weight gain in many patients. This can be helpful in cancer patients who are losing weight and struggling with pruritus
- – Always review good dry skin care with the patient

Pseudofolliculitis Barbae (PFB)

Etiology and Pathogenesis

- Mechanism: (1) extrafollicular penetration occurs when a curly hair reenters the skin, and (2) transfollicular penetration occurs when the sharp tip of a growing hair pierces the follicle wall
- Once the hair penetrates the dermis, a foreign body inflammatory reaction occurs

Clinical Presentation

- Inflammatory papules and pustules in the beard area and on the anterolateral neck. Hyperpigmentation and firm papules form. Keloids and hypertrophic scars can also form and be somewhat disfiguring
- Mostly seen in men who shave and more common in African-Americans. Can also affect white men and hirsute women
- Pseudofolliculitis pubis is a similar condition occurring after pubic hair is shaved

DDx – facial acne, sarcoidosis, dermatophyte folliculitis

Histology

- Perifollicular or intrafollicular mixed infiltrate of lymphocytes, histiocytes, or plasma cells
- Often see ruptured follicle surrounded by neutrophils and multinucleated giant cells
- Perifollicular fibrosis in older lesions

Treatment

- Chemical depilatories
  - Barium sulfide powder depilatories (2% strength) can be made into a paste with water and applied to the beard area. Paste is removed after 3–5 min
  - Calcium thioglycolate preparations come as powder, lotions, creams, and pastes
    - The mercaptan odor is often masked with fragrance. In rare cases, this fragrance can cause an allergic reaction
    - This depilatory takes longer to work and is left on 10–15 min; chemical burns result if left on too long

- ○ Chemical depilatories should not be used every day – cause skin irritation. Every second or third day is an acceptable regimen
  - ■ Irritation can be countered by using hydrocortisone cream. A lower pH or concentration, or a different brand, may also prove less irritating
  - ■ Trying a different product is encouraged if one depilatory unacceptable
- Topical retinoid QHS – relieves hyperkeratosis
- Topical combination cream (tretinoin 0.05%, fluocinolone acetonide 0.01%, and hydroquinone 4%) (Triluma) – some benefit by targeting the hyperkeratosis (tretinoin), inflammation (fluocinolone), and post-inflammatory hyperpigmentation (hydroquinone)
- Mild topical corticosteroid creams reduce inflammation of papular lesions (IL Kenalog to very large lesions)
- If pustules and abscesses → topical and PO ABX (similar to acne regimens)
- Vaniqa cream (13.9%) cream – decreases the rate of hair growth. In addition, the treated hair may become finer and lighter
- Laser hair removal

Pearls and Pitfalls

- Give handout with shaving tips, including topics such as:
  - ○ Using needles or toothpicks to dislodge stubborn tips is controversial. It usually is not recommended because overly aggressive digging with sharp objects can cause further damage to the skin
  - ○ Shave only on moist skin
  - ○ **Razor type** – single-edged, foil-guarded, safety razors are recommended. Double- or triple-bladed razors shave too closely and may not be tolerated well by some, although some men find these to be MORE tolerated
  - ○ **Electric razor** – use three-headed rotary electric razor and keep the heads slightly off the surface of the skin. Shave in a slow, circular motion. Do not press the electric razor close to the skin or pull the skin taut because this results in too close of a shave
  - ○ Avoid shaving all-together, if possible

Psoriasis

Etiology and Pathogenesis

- Thought to be a T-cell driven disease. Some have regarded psoriasis as an auto-immune disease, but to date no true autoantigen has been definitively identified
  - Dogma up until the early–mid 1990s was that this was considered a disease of keratinocytes
- Factors/Triggers associated with Psoriasis – genetics, infections (Strept), HIV, endocrine factors (hypocalcemia), psychogenic stress, medications (lithium, IFN, beta-blockers, anti-malarials, rapid steroid tapers), alcohol consumption, smoking, and obesity
  - Psoriasis associated with various HLA types → HLA-B13, HLA-B17, HLA-B37, HLA-Bw16, HLA-Cw6, HLA-DR7
  - Pustulor psoriasis and acrodermatitis continua of Hallopeau (but not in pustulosis of palms and soles)→ increased prevalence of HLA-B27
  - Guttate psoriasis in children and in erythroderma → HLA-B13, HLA-B17

Clinical Presentation and Types

- **Chronic Plaque Psoriasis** – relatively symmetrical distribution. Lesions are erythematous, micaceous plaques, and typically involved elbows, knees, scalp, presacrum, and sometimes hands and feet
- **Guttate Psoriasis** – small erythematous patches, often diffusely located on body. In over 50%, an elevated antistreptolysin O, anti-DNase B, or streptozyme titer is found. Often seen in children after strept throat. In adults, guttate lesions can become chronic
- **Erythrodermic Psoriasis** – diffuse erythema and scaling covering most of body. Clues include classic locations, nail changes
- **Pustular Variants**
  - **Generalized pustular psoriasis** – erythema and pustules predominate the picture. Triggers include rapid taper of systemic steroids, pregnancy, hypocalcemia, infections. Four distinct patterns – von Zumbusch, annular, exanthematic, localized (within existing psoriatic plaques)
  - **Pustulosis of the palms and soles** – deep-seated, multiple, sterile pustules admixed with yellow-brown macules. Minority of patients also have chronic plaque psoriasis lesions elsewhere. Focal infections, stress can trigger this. Smoking can aggravate. This is one of the entities most commonly associated with sterile inflammatory bone lesions
  - **Acrodermatitis continua of Hallopeau** – pustules at the distal portions of the fingers and sometimes the toes. Pustulation often followed by scaling and crust formation. Pustules may also form in the nail bed (beneath the nail plate) and there may be shedding of the nail plates. Can transition into other forms of psoriasis

- **Inverse Psoriasis** – Shiny, pink to red, sharply demarcated plaques. Much less scale seen than in other areas. Central fissuring common. Typical sites = axillae, inguinal creases, intergluteal cleft, inframammary region, and retroauricular folds
- **Nail Psoriasis** – Reported in 10–80% of psoriatic patients. Fingernails > Toenails. Findings including "oil spots", distal onycholysis, splinter hemorrhages, subungual hyperkeratosis, leukonychia
- Disorders related to psoriasis – inflammatory linear verrucous epidermal nevus (ILVEN), reactive arthritis, Sneddon–Wilkinson disease (subcorneal pustular dermatosis)

Labs – TB skin test or quanitFERON gold, and CXR prior to starting biologics, immunosuppressives

DDx – seborrheic dermatitis, SCC in situ (if only 1–2 lesions), mycosis fungoides, hypertrophic lichen planus (especially if on shins), keratotic eczema, PRP, drug reactions, tinea capitis (with scalp involvement). If guttate psoriasis pattern, DDx includes small plaque parapsoriasis, PLC, secondary syphilis, PR. For inverse psoriasis, consider extramammary Paget's, contact dermatitis, necrolytic migratory erythema.

Histology

- Confluent parakeratosis, hyperkeratosis
- Neutrophils in stratum corneum (Munro microabscesses) and in spinous layer (spongiform pustules of Kogoj)
- Hypogranulosis and suprapapillary thinning of epidermis
- Regular acanthosis, often with clubbed rete ridges
- Dilated capillaries in dermal papillae (cause of Auspitz sign)
- Perivascular lymphocytes

Treatment – *See following tables and see drug monitoring section*

Pearls and Pitfalls

- Patients with psoriasis have an increased risk of cardiac disease
- Many patients with psoriasis are obese. Encourage weight loss
  - ○ Obese patients may not respond to systemic treatment as well as many of the medications are not weight-based
  - ○ Many of these patients have fatty liver prior to starting medications, but it can

   complicate treatment (e.g., with methotrexate)
- Encourage cessation of smoking as this may aggravate psoriasis. Additionally, these patients already have an increased risk of heart disease and stroke
- Crohn's disease, ulcerative colitis, and psoriasis share an important association with sacroiliitis, and HLA-B27 positivity
- Always screen for joint pain, psoriatic arthritis. This may significantly change the management of disease
- Get a sense as to how much the disease bothers patient and consider this when deciding how aggressive you will be in your treatment plan
- Avoid systemic steroids in psoriasis, as a pustular or erythrodermic flare may occur in some patients (which can require hospitalization)

Psoriasis

Table 90 Topical treatments commonly used in psoriasis

Body Site	Treatment options	Directions	Comments
Scalp Rx	Steroids	**Oluxfoam** (clobetasol) **Olux-E** – ethanol free form **Luxiq foam**(betamethasone) **Diprolenesoln or lotion** (betamethasone) **Temovate soln**(clobetasol) **Dermasmoothe FSoil** (fluocinolone) – use w/ shower cap overnight	
	Anthralin	**Dritho-Scalp**0.5% cream: apply QD × 5–10 min, increase to 20–30 min if tolerated. Shampoo out. **Anthralin 0.1%, 0.25%, 0.5%, 0.1% cream or oint**: start at low strength and can titrate up every 3 weeks until improvement	May stain (purple/brown) shower, bath, hair, nails, fabric Local irritation common
	Vitamin D analogue	**Dovonexscalp soln** 0.005%	Apply to scalp BID
	Shampoo	**Clobexshampoo** (clobetasol), T-gel shampoo, T-sal shampoo **Carmol Scalp Treatment Kit** – contains medicated shampoo and sulfacetamide lotion	
Body Rx	Palmoplantar	10% LCD + 2–8% salicylic acid in Lidex ointment (or ultravate, etc). Disp: 4 oz (equivalent to 120 g)	Dr. Elewski's formula
	Vitamin D analogue	Dovonex cream BID M-F and Ultravate BID Sat and Sun	Minimizes risk of atrophy from topical steroids. Dovonex ointment discontinued but cream, scalp soln available
	Topical steroids	Medium to high potency BID	
	Topical retinoid	Tazorac gel (0.05%, 0.1%) – Apply QHS	Reduces scaling and plaque thickness
	Vit D + steroid	Taclonex – Apply to lesions QD	Combination of betamethasone + calcipotriene
	6% Salicylic acid + 6% lactic acid in propylene glycol	Apply BID	Useful to remove excess scale
	NB UVB	3x per week. Start at 50% MED and increase by 5% per treatment protocol as tolerated	
	Topical PUVA	Rx: 0.1% oxsoralen solution in Aquaphor	Apply immediately prior to treatment
	Goekerman treatment	Goeckerman protocol is UVB and tar treatments May modify by adding the following: 1) Valisone wraps: valisone under occlusion for 4–6 h; helps to thin plaques 2) Scalp/face regimen: D/S/K/N 3) Antihistamines – for pruritus	D/S/K/N = Dermasmoothe FS Oil Sebulex shampoo Kenalog lotion Nizoral 2% cream

Psoriasis

Table 91 Systemic treatments commonly used in psoriasis (excluding the biologics)

Systemicmedications: Generic name	Trade name	Treatment regimen	Monitoring	Comments
Acitretin 10 mg capsule 25 mg	Soriatane	Start at 0.3–0.5 mg/kg/day and increase to 0.75 mg/k/day over 3–4 weeks Take with food	Fasting lipids, Chem, LFTs, BUN/ Cr, βHcG at baseline and q 1–2 week (except βHcG) until stable does	Effective in pustular psoriasis; start at 1 mg/kg and taper after clinical improvement to 0.5 mg/kg SE – **Category X**, not for women of childbearing potential, no pregnancy for 3 yrs after last dose. Palmar/plantar desquamation, hair loss, sticky palms
Methotrexate 2.5 mg tablet	Trexall Rheumatrex dose pack	Test dose of 5–7 mg after baseline labs ok Usual dose varies from 5 to 15 mg PO **q week** on average	Baseline LFTs, CBC, Chem, BUN/Cr	Liver toxicity – avoid in patients with history of liver dz or ETOH abuse. Liver biopsy recommended every 1.5 g of cumulative treatment. **Category X** SE – nausea, diarrhea, ulcerative stomatitis, ↓ plts, ↓ WBC, ↓ Hgb, pulm fibrosis, pneumonitis, radiation recall
Cyclosporine 25 mg capsule 100 mg	Neoral	3–5 mg/kg/day	Baseline BUN/Cr, BP, Mg, uric acid, K+, UA, βHcG	Most effective in erythroderma, pustular and severe chronic plaque psoriasis SE – renal toxicity, hypertension, hyperkalemia, ↓ plts, ↓ WBC, hirsutism, headache, N/V/D, gingival hyperplasia, tremor, fatigue
PUVA Oxsoralen ultra 10 mg tablets	–	Oxsoralen Ultra – 0.4–0.6 mg/kg; 30 mg for 70 kg patient PUVA 3x/week – start at ¼ or ½ J and increase by ½ J per Rx as tolerated		Patient to take dose 1.5 h prior to UVA exposure. Important to take at same time before tx to ensure consistent systemic levels at time of light exposure

Preventative Measures:
 (1) Avoid oral steroids – may cause significant rebound flare with steroid taper
 (2) Daily moisturizers; emollients to wet skin BID
 (3) Patients may flare with streptococcus infection (pharyngitis)

Psoriasis – Biologics (Dosing)

Table 92 Biologics commonly used in the treatment of psoriasis

Generic name	Trade name	Treatment regimen	Monitoring	Comments
Alefacept	Amevive	15 mg IM q week×12 weeks	CD4 at baseline and q 2 weeks	May repeat course 12 weeks after end of last course in normal CD4+
Etanercept	Enbrel	(1) 50 mg SC 2x/ week×3 months, then decrease to maintain dose of 50 mg SC weekly (2) 50 mg SC 2x/ week×3 months, then 25 mg SC 2x/week	PPD at baseline	Psoriatic arthritis dosing is 25 mg SC 2x/week
Adalimumab	Humira	40 mg SC q 2 week	PPD at baseline	**Black box warning** re: TB, invasive fungal infections, opportunistic infections
Efalizumab	Raptiva	Start 0.7 mg/kg SC (max 200 mg/dose)×1, then 1 mg/kg SC q week	Monitor plts q months initially, then q 3 months	The only biologic that is weight-based. May potentially cause flare in arthritic symptoms. **(Removed from US market in April 2009 for increased risk of PML)**
Infliximab	Remicade	Start 5 mg/kg IV×1 on weeks 0, 2, 6 then 5 mg/kg IV q 8 weeks	PPD at baseline	Psoriatic arthritis dosing is the same **Black box warning** re: TB, invasive fungal infections, opportunistic infections
Ustekinumab	Stelara	<100 kg 45 mg SC at week 0, week 4, q 12 weeks >100 kg 90 mg SC at week 0, week 4, q 12 weeks	PPD at baseline	Approved for psoriasis, but not for psoriatic arthritis

Workup prior to starting biologic:	Rule of Nines(Body surface area):
1) History of CHF? 2) History of multiple sclerosis? 3) History of any malignancy (except NMSC)? 4) Family history of multiple sclerosis? 5) History of tuberculosis? 6) History of chronic infections? 7) History of IV Antibiotics in past year? 8) History of hepatitis? 9) PPD +/– Chest x-ray 10) CBC+diff, LFTs, CMP 11) Document body surface area (BSA)	**Arm+Hand (each)** ------- **9%** **Leg+Foot (each)** --------- **18%** **Front Torso** ----------------- **18%** **Back Torso+Buttocks** --- **18%** **Head+Neck** ---------------- **9%** **Genital Area (perineum) – 1%**

Purpura

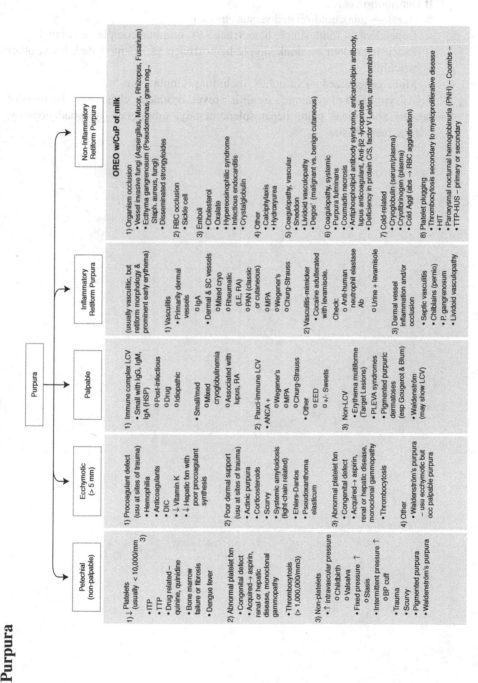
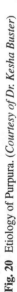

Fig. 20 Etiology of Purpura. (*Courtesy of Dr. Kesha Buster*)

Pearls and Pitfalls

- If Distribution is ….
    o Acral → think cold-related versus embolic
    o Dependent → think simple hemorrhage vs. immune complex mediated
    o Pauci or random → think simple hemorrhage vs. IC-mediated, PAN, other vasculitis
    o Multi-generalized → vasculitis, including lymphocytic
- Signs/symptoms of systemic vasculitis = fever, headache, chest pain, shortness of breath, abdominal pain, hepatosplenomegaly, athralgias, lymphadenopathy, edema, paresthesias

Pyoderma Gangrenosum (PG)

Etiology and Pathogenesis

- Disease is idiopathic in 25–50% and an underlying immunologic abnormality is favored given its frequent association with other autoimmune diseases
- Pathergy is seen in 20–30%

Clinical Presentation and Types

- Lesion begins as a tender papulopustule with surrounding erythematous or violaceous induration, an erythematous nodule, or a bulla. Lesion undergoes necrosis leading to a central ulcer. Loss of tissue can expose underlying tendons and muscles
- Border described as "irregular, undermined with an overhanging gun-metal gray border". Expands centrifugally. Ulcers heal with atrophic cribiform pigmented scars
- The primary variants of PG
    o **Ulcerative** – usually observed on the legs. May occur around stoma
    o **Vesiculobullous** – also known as atypical or bullous PG. Occurs most commonly in setting of AML, myelodysplasia, and myeloproliferative disorders such as CML. Eruption favors face and upper extremities (especially dorsal hands). Clinical appearance overlaps Sweet's syndrome and neutrophilic dermatosis of the dorsal hands
    o **Pustular** – characterized by multiple small pustules in patients with inflammatory bowel disease with or without PG. Lesions usually regress without scarring, but can evolve into PG. Similar eruption seen in Behçet's or bowel-associated dermatosis-arthritis syndrome
    o **Superficial granulomatous** – characterized by superficial vegetative or ulcerative lesion which usually follows trauma such as surgery. Predilection for the trunk and responds more easily to treatment
    o **Vulvar or penile PG** – must be differentiated from sexually transmitted diseases
    o **Pyostomatitis vegetans** – assoc with inflammatory bowel disease and characterized by chronic vegetative sterile pyoderma of the labial and buccal mucosa
- Associated with systemic diseases in at least 50% of patients
    o Common – inflammatory bowel disease (either ulcerative colitis or Crohn disease), polyarthritis that is usually symmetric and may be either seronegative or seropositive, hematologic diseases/disorders, such as leukemia or preleukemic states, predominantly myelocytic in nature or monoclonal gammopathies (primarily immunoglobulin A [IgA]).

- ○ Less common – other forms of arthritis (such as psoriatic arthritis, osteoar-thritis, or spondyloarthropathy), hepatic diseases (hepatitis and primary biliary cirrhosis), myelomas (IgA type predominantly), and immunologic diseases (lupus, Sjögren synd)
- Involvement of other organs may occur
  - ○ Involvement of other organ systems commonly manifests as sterile neutro-philic abscesses (as in Sweet's syndrome)
  - ○ Culture-negative pulmonary infiltrates are most common extracutaneous manifestation. Other organs systems that may be involved – heart, CNS, GI tract, eyes, liver, spleen, bones, and lymph nodes

Labs and Imaging to Consider

- CBC, CMP, LFTs, urinalysis
- Hepatitis profile to rule out hepatitis
- SPEP (to eval for IgA monoclonal gammopathy), UPEP, peripheral smear, bone marrow aspiration – if concern for hematologic malignancy
- ANCAs, PTT, and antiphospholipid antibody test to rule out Wegener granulo-matosis, vasculitis, and antiphospholipid antibody syndrome
- Cultures of the ulcer/erosion – bacteria, fungi, atypical mycobacteria, and viruses
- CXR
- Colonoscopy or other tests to exclude inflammatory bowel disease
- Angiography or doppler studies may be performed in patients suspected of having arterial or venous insufficiency

DDx – Sweet's, aphthous stomatitis, Behçet's disease, chancroid, Churg–Strauss, Ecthyma, Ecthyma gangrenosum, herpes simplex, LCV, impetigo, arthropod assault, sporotrichosis, SCC, venous insufficiency, verrucous carcinoma, Wegener's, anthrax, arterial insufficiency, factitial disease, traumatic ulceration, tuberculosis gumma

Histology – Can be nonspecific.

- Early → there is a neutrophilic vascular reaction, which can be folliculocentric. Neutrophilic infiltrates, often with leukocytoclasia, are seen in untreated expand-ing lesions
- Developed ulcers → marked tissue necrosis with surrounding mononuclear cell infiltrates

Treatment

- **Treatment of Pyoderma Gangrenosum**
  - ○ Topical therapies
    - Local wound care and dressings
    - Superpotent topical corticosteroids
    - Cromolyn sodium 2% solution
    - Nitrogen mustard
    - 5-aminosalicylic acid
    - Tacrolimus and pimecrolimus may have some benefit in certain patients
  - ○ Systemic therapies
    - **Corticosteroids** → Prednisone 0.5–2 mg/kg/day PO; taper as condition improves; single morning dose is safer for long-term use, but divided doses have more anti-inflammatory effect
    - Cyclosporine → 3–5 mg/kg/day PO/IV, sometimes initial loading therapy at 10–12 mg/kg/day is useful for first 3–5 days
    - Mycophenolate mofetil → 1–2 g/day PO
    - Azathioprine → 1–2 mg/kg/day (50–200 mg) PO
    - Dapsone
    - Tacrolimus → 0.05 mg/kg/day IV or 0.15–0.30 mg/kg/day PO divided bid
    - Cyclophosphamide → 1–2 mg/kg/day PO
    - Chlorambucil (Leukeran) → 4–6 mg/day PO
    - Tumor necrosis factor-alpha (TNF-alpha) inhibitors
      - □ Etanercept (Enbrel) → 50–100 mg SC q week
      - □ Adalimumab(Humira) → 40 mg SC q week or every other week
      - □ Thalidomide → 50–300 mg/day PO qd with water, preferably QHS and at least 1 h pc; 50–200 mg usually yields results
    - Clofazimine (Lamprene) → 200–400 mg/day PO qd
  - ○ Intravenous therapies
    - Pulsed methylprednisolone
    - Pulsed cyclophosphamide
    - Infliximab → 3–5 mg/kg IV infusion over 2–4 h
      - □ Initial induction dose then repeat at week 2, then week 6, then q 6–8 week
      - □ May increase to 10 mg/kg IV q 8 week for patients who respond, then lose their response; d/c treatment in those who do not response by week 14
    - Intravenous immune globulin → 2 g/kg IV over 2–5 days
  - ○ Other therapy includes hyperbaric oxygen
  - ○ **Avoid surgery** – can result in enlargement, worsening of the area due to pathergy. If surgery is required (for grafting, etc), patient should be on appropriate treatment first (but still a risk)
  - ○ Some patients with ulcerative colitis have responded to total colectomy; however, in others, the disease is peristomal and occurs following bowel resection

Pearls and Pitfalls

- Keep the surgeons away
- In children, the clinical appearance is similar but lesions tend to more frequently involve the head and genital and perianal areas
- **Consultations to consider**
  - ○ Gastroenterologist or GI surgeon, proctorectal surgeon, or general surgeon in patients with inflammatory bowel disease
  - ○ Rheumatologist for patients with arthritis
  - ○ Ophthalmologist if ocular disease is present
  - ○ Hematologist/oncologist when preleukemia, leukemia, monoclonal gammopathy, or other neoplasm is associated
  - ○ Plastic surgeon or general surgeon when debridement or grafting is deemed necessary

Reactive Arthritis *(formerly Reiter's Syndrome)*

Etiology and Pathogenesis

- HLA-B27 association. Reactive arthritis is triggered following enteric or urogenital infections
  - Bacteria associated – are generally enteric or venereal and include:
    - *Shigella flexneri, Salmonella typhimurium, Salmonella enteritidis, Streptococcus viridans, Mycoplasma pneumonia, Cyclospora, Chlamydia trachomatis, Yersinia enterocolitica,* and *Yersinia pseudotuberculosis*
    - Bacteria or their components (RNA, DNA) have been identified in synovial fluid

Clinical Presentation

- Triad of arthritis, nongonococcal urethritis, conjunctivitis → **"Can't see, can't pee, can't climb a tree"**
- In category of seronegative spondyloarthropathies, which includes ankylosing spondylitis, psoriatic arthritis, the arthropathy of associated inflammatory bowel disease, juvenile-onset ankylosing spondylitis, and juvenile chronic arthritis
- Scoring system – **Two or more of the following points establishes diagnosis (one of which must pertain to the musculoskeletal system):**
  - Musculoskeletal
    - **Asymmetric oligoarthritis** affecting mainly lower legs with low-grade inflammation. Knee may become markedly edematous
    - Distinctive arthropathy of reactive arthritis includes local enthesopathy, which is **inflammation at the tendinous insertion into bone**, rather than synovium (common in insertions into calcaneus, talus, and subtalar joints)
    - **Sausage finger or toe** is caused by uniform inflammation
  - Urogenital
    - Meatal edema and erythema and clear mucoid discharge
    - Prostatic tenderness (up to 80%) and vulvovaginitis
    - Genital ulceration or urethritis
    - Cervicitis
  - Dermatologic
    - **Balanitis circinata** – Shallow painless ulcers at meatus and glans penis; moist on uncircumcised patients; may harden and crust causing pain and scarring
    - **Keratoderma blennorrhagica** – Hyperkeratotic skin, which begins as clear vesicles on erythematous bases and progresses to macules, papules, and nodules (found on soles of feet, toes, palms, scrotum, trunk, and scalp)
    - Nail thickening and ridging and superficial oral ulcers

○ Ophthalmologic signs – Conjunctivitis (most common), with mucopurulent discharge, chemosis, lid edema, and iritis
○ Cardiac signs – Aortic regurgitation caused by inflammation of aortic wall and valve
○ GI – acute diarrhea within 1 month of the arthritis

Labs and Imaging to Consider

- Document bacterial infection
  ○ Cervical or urethral swab may be performed. Look for *Chlamydia* in every case of reactive arthritis, preferably by DFA, enzyme immunoassay, or DNA probe for ribosomal RNA. Culture techniques unreliable but serology may be useful
  ○ Obtain stool cultures even when bowel symptoms are in apparent or mild
  ○ Arthrocentesis and fluid analysis often are needed to rule out an infectious process, especially in monoarticular arthritis with constitutional symptoms
- Acute cases
  ○ Neutrophilic leukocytosis
  ○ Elevated CRP or C3 and C4 (nonspecific)
  ○ ESR – Usually elevated during acute phase of disease
- Chronic cases – Mild normocytic anemia
- RF and ANA are negative
- Consider HIV testing – if risk factors or if sudden explosive onset
- Plain radiography → May show no abnormalities early in the disease

DDx – other seronegative spondyloarthropathies, and various diseases affecting the joints such as gout, gonococcal arthritis, septic arthritis, rheumatoid arthritis, and psoriatic arthritis. Skin manifestations can resemble pustular psoriasis, atopic dermatitis, Behçet's disease, and contact dermatitis. Keratoderma, uveitis, and balanitis may be syphilis mimicking reactive arthritis. Children → consider Kawasaki's

Histology – psoriasiform dermatitis identical to psoriasis but often see more pustules, more massive hyperkeratosis in keratoderma blenorrhagicum

Treatment

- Mainstays of therapy for joint symptoms are **NSAIDs**
- **Sulfasalazine** 1,000 mg enteric-coated PO BID → may be used for patients who do not respond to NSAIDs or who have contraindications to NSAIDs
- COX-2 inhibitors – for patients who don't tolerate NSAIDs (no published data)
- Intra-articular injection of steroid to joints
- Short course of systemic corticosteroids may be helpful in severe or prolonged

disease
- Acitretin may be useful in reducing the amount of NSAIDs required by patient for joint symptoms
- Systemic steroid-sparing immunosuppressants (HIV testing beforehand recommended)
  - Methotrexate
  - Azathioprine
  - Cyclosporine
- Reactive arthritis in patients with HIV/AIDS is more recalcitrant to therapy and requires careful management → acitretin can improve skin and joints
- ABX use → No consensus about the use of antibiotics in reactive arthritis. Some suggest that treatment with antibiotics should be prescribed pending culture results; however, its effect on the severity and duration of Reiter's syndrome is not clear

Pearls and Pitfalls

- Variable course – It usually has a duration of 3–12 months, and may resolve spontaneously or progress to chronic illness
- Check for HIV in explosive cases

Reference:

(1) Wu IB and Schwartz RA. Reiter's syndrome: the classic triad and more. JAAD 2008; 59(1): 113–21.

Relapsing Polychondritis

Etiology and Pathogenesis

- Circulating antibodies to cartilage-specific collagen types II, IX, and XI present in 30–70% of patients
- Antibodies to type II collagen are present during acute episodes and levels correlate with severity
- Association with HLA-DR4, while extent of organ involvement negatively assoc with HLA-DR6

Clinical Presentation

- Severe, episodic, and progressive inflammatory condition involving cartilaginous structures, predominantly those of the ears, nose, and laryngotracheobronchial tree. Other affected structures may include the eyes, cardiovascular system, peripheral joints, skin, middle and inner ear, and CNS
- Most common in fifth decade, but can occur at any age
- **Skin Findings**
  - Ear – pain, swelling, redness, sparing the lobules (85–95% develop auricular chondritis)
  - Nasal chondritis – onset is acute, painful, and accompanied by feeling of fullness over the nasal bridge (48–72%)
  - Aphthous ulcers, LCV, urticarial vasculitis, PAN, panniculitis, Sweet's syndrome
  - Isolated reports of – hyperpigmentation, pustular psoriasis, macular purpura of palms/soles/lower limbs/buttocks, purpura, actinic granulomas, alopecia universalis, urticaria, angioedema, livedo reticularis, erythema nodosum, erythema multiforme, limb ulceration, ulcerating abscesses
- **Diagnosis**
  - **McAdam et al. criteria (three of six clinical features are present)**
    - Bilateral auricular chondritis
    - Nonerosive, seronegative inflammatory polyarthritis
    - Nasal chondritis
    - Ocular inflammation
    - Respiratory tract chondritis
    - Audiovestibular damage
  - **Damiani and Levine criteria (one of three conditions is met)**
    - Three McAdam et al. criteria
    - One McAdam et al. criterion plus positive histology
    - Two McAdam et al. criteria plus therapeutic response to corticosteroid or dapsone administration

○ **Michet et al. criteria (one of two conditions is met)**
  ▪ Proven inflammation in 2 of 3 of the auricular, nasal, laryngotracheal cartilages
  ▪ Proven inflammation in 1 of 3 of the auricular, nasal, or laryngotracheal cartilages plus two other signs including ocular inflammation, vestibular dysfunction, seronegative inflammatory arthritis, and hearing loss

Labs and Imaging to Consider – No specific labs available to make diagnosis
- Cultures to rule out infection
- Nonspecific elevation in inflammatory markers – ESR, CRP
- Mild leukocytosis may be present
- ANA, RF, antiphospholipid antibody syndrome – to eval for other autoimmune diseases
- Vasculitis workup – CBC+diff, CMP (including renal, LFTs), urinalysis and microscopic eval of sediment, cryoglobulins, hepatitis panel, ANCA tests (c-ANCA, p-ANCA, antimyeloperoxidase and antiproteinase 3 antibody titers)
- CXR – may see tracheal stenosis, calcification of cartilaginous structures, pulm parenchymal infiltrates may suggest vasculitis
- CT, MRI, bone scans, PFTs, EKG, Echo

DDx – cellulitis, CNH, reactive arthritis, Wegener's, rheumatoid arthritis, polyarteritis nodosa, Cogan syndrome, infectious perichondritis, MAGIC syndrome (RP plus Behçet disease), trauma, congenital syphilis, chronic external otitis, auricular calcification (secondary to trauma, Addison dz, diabetes, hyperthyroidism)

Histology

- Loss of basophilic staining and breakdown of normal lacunar structure of the cartilage, with neutrophilic infiltrates initially and later lymphocytes or plasma cells. CD4>CD8 T cells
- Late → replacement of cartilgage with granulation tissue and fibrosis
- DIF → nonspecific

Treatment and Management

- Complete workup to exclude involvement of other organ systems
- Systemic corticosteroids – Prednisone (20–60 mg/day) – mainstay of treatment
  ○ Administered in acute phase and tapered to 5–25 mg/day for maintenance
  ○ Severe flares may require 80–100 mg/day. Most patients require low-dose maintenance
  ○ Treatment of choice during pregnancy

- Dapsone (25–200 mg/day) – may not be as useful as MTX
- Methotrexate (MTX) – 7.5–22.5 mg/week → decreases steroid requirements
- Other – Cyclophosphamide, cyclosporine, azathioprine, infliximab, etanercept, anakinra

Pearls and Pitfalls

- NSAIDs are **NOT** effective in the treatment
- Elapsed time from patient presentation for medical care for a related symptom to diagnosis was reported to be 2.9 years
  - 1/3 of patients have seen five or more physicians before diagnosis is made
- **Morbidity**
  - Five-year survival rate reported to be 66–74% (45% if RP occurs with systemic vasculitis) with a 10 year survival rate of 55%
  - Most frequent causes of death include infection secondary to corticosteroid treatment or respiratory compromise (10–50% of deaths result from airway complications), systemic vasculitis, and malignancy unrelated to RP
  - Complications – vertigo, tinnitus, voice hoarseness, joint deformity, epiglottitis, scleritis, conjunctivitis, iritis, need for permanent tracheotomy (severe cases), severe pulmonary infection, blindness, frail chest wall, respiratory failure, aortic regurgitation, mitral regurgitation, aortic dissection, and glomerulonephritis-associated renal failure

Rosacea

Etiology and Pathogenesis

- Etiology likely multifactorial, but clearly related to vascular hyperreactivity. Medications and foods that induce facial vasodilation seem to accelerate the development of rosacea, but why this happens is unclear
  - Theoies to etiology – *H. pylori, Demodex folliculorum, Propionibacterium acnes*
- Patients also tend to have sensitive skin
- Can be induced by mid- to high-potency topical corticosteroids

Clinical Presentation and Types

- Four major types of rosacea
  - **Erythematotelangiectatic (vascular)** – flushing and persistent facial erythema with or without telangiectasias
  - **Papulopustular** – persistent central facial erythema with transient papules and/or pustules
  - **Phymatous** – thickening of the skin, irregular surface nodularities, and enlargement. May occur on the nose, chin, forehead, cheeks, or ears
  - **Ocular** – Foreign body sensation in the eye, burning or stinging, dryness, itching, ocular sensitivity, blurred vision, telangiectasia of the sclera or other parts of the eye, or periorbital edema. May get recurrent styes (especially in children). Can be seen in conjunction with other types of rosacea
    - Epithelium-derived protease activity, especially matrix metalloproteinase (MMP)-9 is elevated in ocular rosacea tear fluid and doxycycline reduces this
    - Ocular rosacea may precede skin involvement
- Variants of Rosacea
  - **Granulomatous Rosacea** – large granulomatous nodules may occur. Some patients present with more persistent, discrete, red to red-brown paules. Occasionally see extra-facial lesions
  - **Periorificial dermatitis** – *see perioral derm section*
  - **Pyoderma faciale (Rosacea fulminans)** – Eruptions of inflamed papules and yellow pustules in the centrofacial region. Papules and pustules can coalesce into very large plaques. Patients are typically younger and tend to be female. Often misdiagnosed as having chronic skin infections and have not responded to antibiotics or antifungals. Often have low-grade fever, myalgias, elevated WBC, and ESR
  - **Steroid Rosacea** – Clue is the presence of red papules on the upper lip and around the nasal alae. Fluorinated another other potent topical steroids cause problems more quickly but any topical or inhaled steroid can induce this. Herbal creams have been known to contain corticosteroids

- Complications
  - ○ Rosacea keratitis and keratoconjunctivitis sicca
  - ○ Scarring generally does not occur

Labs – Consider labs for flushing *(see flushing section)*

DDx – acute lupus erythematosus, perioral dermatitis, sarcoidosis, seborrheic dermatitis, photodermatoses, carcinoid syndrome, pheochromocytoma, mitral valve incompetence, acne, pustular folliculitis, erythromelanosis faciei and keratosis pilaris rubra, lupus miliaris disseminatus faciei, Haber syndrome, demodex folliculitis

Histology – vascular ectasia and mild edema. With advancing disease, see perivascular and perifollicular lymphohistiocytic inflammation. Sebaceous hyperplasia may be prominent in some and elastolysis can occur. No comedones. Severe disease can show non-caseating granulomas

Treatment

- **General measures**
  - ○ Identify triggers and avoid
  - ○ Sunscreen and gentle cleansers
  - ○ Avoid astringents, toners, menthols, camphor, products containing sodium lauryl sulfate, waterproof cosmetics requiring solvents to be removed
- **Rosacea fulminans** – prednisolone 30–60 mg/day followed by PO isotretinoin
- **Telangiectasias and Erythema** – Lasers (pulsed dye, potassium-titanyl-phosphate, diode, IPL, etc)
- **Rhinophyma** – Mechanical dermabrasion, carbon dioxide laser, surgical shave techniques
- **Flushing** – beta-blockers, clonidine, naloxone, ondansetron, SSRIs
- **Papulopustular type** – antibiotics helpful – tetracycline, **doxycycline, minocycline**. Occasionally, azithromycin, erythromycin, **metronidazole (topical)**, clindamycin, fusidic acid
- **Oral contraceptives** can be helpful in females who flare with hormonal cycle
- **Acne products** – Benzoyl peroxide, azelaic acid (Azelex 20% cream, **Finacea 15% gel**), sodium sulfacetamide, and **sulfur (Plexion, Clenia, Rosula, Rosac**)
- Immunosuppressants – Tacrolimus (Protopic), pimecrolimus
- Tretinoin→ may be helpful for recalcitrant disease. Long-term, low-dose may be suitable for selected patients

- **Ocular rosacea**
  - Lid hygiene → hot compresses to eyelid margins can help liquefy thick meibomian gland secretions and thus facilitate their expression. Light pressure can aid in gland expression. Use a nonirritating cleaning solution (like baby shampoo)
  - Artificial tears → use liberally
  - Lubricating ointment QHS (may contain antibiotic)
  - Antibiotics – TCNs (tetracycline, doxycycline, minocycline), erythromycin, clarithromycin, metronidazole (do not take with EToH → disulfiram reaction)
  - Topical steroids (prescribed by ophthamology)

Pearls and Pitfalls

- Symptoms of ocular rosacea are often present and these symptoms are often blamed on contact lenses, allergies, etc. Always ask about symptoms as oral antibiotics are quite helpful
- Severity of ocular rosacea does not correlate with skin disease
- Be careful about certain topicals as they can cause irritation – tretinoin, benzoyl peroxide. Although not commonly used in practice for rosacea, they can be useful in some patients. Use every other day or 3x/week to begin
- Topical erythromycin, clindamycin seem to have little effect on rosacea
- Hydrocortisone 1% cream can be compounded with 0.5–1% precipitated sulfur and applied twice daily to treat mild rosacea
- Severe forms require isotretinoin

Rosacea Diet *(from Dr. Boni Elewski)*

1. Foods to Avoid

Raisins	All cheeses – except cottage cheese
Herring	Yogurt, sour cream
Chocolate	Coffee, tea
Bananas	Vinegar – except white vinegar
Soy sauce	Anything fermented, pickled, marinated, or smoked
Yeast extract	Citrus fruits
Vanilla	Nuts
Figs	Pods of broad beans such as: Lima, Navy, Pea pods
Liver	

2. Liquor to Avoid

   Beer

   Dry Red Burgandy

   All Bourbons

   Gin

   Vodka

   Champagne

3. Avoid very hot beverages and solid foods, both thermal and chemical irritants (spices)

Sarcoid

Etiology and Pathogenesis

- Multisystem granulomatous disease characterized by hyperactivity of the cell-mediated immune system. Upregulation of CD4 T cells of the T_H1 subtype occurs following antigen presentation by monocytes with MHC class II molecules
- Unclear what starts the cascade of events leading to granuloma formation – autoimmune? Infectious?
- Associated with HLA-B8, HLA-A1, HLA-DR3
- Polymorphisms in the gene encoding angiotension-converting enzyme (ACE) have been identified in sarcoid patients

Clinical Presentation and Types

- Cutaneous – papules and plaques, often red-brown in color. Papules may be flat-topped in appearance and may have an "apple jelly" appearance
  - Less common presentations – hypopigmentation, subcutaneous nodules, ichthyosis, alopecia, and ulcerations. Erythroderma and erythema multiforme are rare manifestations
  - Erythema nodosum associated with sarcoid in some cases
  - Classic – lesions tend to develop at sites of previous trauma or within scars, tattoos
  - **Angiolupoid sarcoidosis** – individual plaques develop central clearing leading to an annular configuration or they can contain prominent telangiectasias
  - **Lupus pernio,** especially involving nasal rim, is associated with involvement of the upper respiratory tract (50%) and lungs (75%). Treat this cutaneous process more aggressively as it can scar. Cystic lesions in bones, distal phalanges seen more common
  - Nail changes can be seen – clubbing, subungual hyperkeratosis, onycholysis
- Distribution – skin lesions favor face, lips, neck, upper trunk, and extremities and tend to be symmetrical
- May affect any organ – skin, lungs, heart, CNS, eyes, kidneys, pituitary, bone, liver, etc
- In US, 10–17 times more common in African-Americans than in Whites

Table 93 Sarcoid syndromes

Mikulicz	Bilateral sarcoidal involvement of the parotid gland, submandibular, sublingual, and lacrimal glands
Löfgren's	• Erythema nodosum • Bilateral hilar lymphadenopathy +/– pulmonary fibrosis • Migratory polyarthritis, fever, iritis, acute sarcoid Excellent prognosis, typically resolving spontaneously in 6–8 weeks
Heerfordt's	Fever, parotid enlargement, anterior uveitis, **facial nerve palsy**
Darier–Roussy (Subcutaneous nodular sarcoid)	Painless, non-tender nodules on trunk and extremities. Patients often have non-severe systemic sarcoid
Blau (AD)	On Differential of Sarcoid, but actually a familial disorder • Arthritis • Uveitis • Skin lesions • **Lack of pulmonary involvement**

Labs to Consider

- CBC+diff – leukopenia, thrombocytopenia common. May see eosinophilia, anemia
- Serum calcium – increased calcium due to increased intestinal absorption resulting from increased vitamin D metabolite by pulmonary macrophages
- 24-h urine for calcium – Hypercalciuria in 49%
- Serum angiotensin-converting enzyme (ACE) – elevated in 60% (not sensitive in diagnosing sarcoid). May help in monitoring response to treatment and disease activity. Reflects granuloma load
- ALT, AST, Alk phos
- BUN, Cr, GFR
- ESR – may be elevated
- ANA – elevated in 30%
- **Kveim Test**
  - Intradermal injection of tissue from spleen or lymph node of a patient with sarcoidosis. Biopsy obtained 4–6 weeks after injection and histologically examined for non-caseating granulomas. If found – test is positive
  - Not commonly done for fear of transmitting infection

Imaging to Consider

- CXR (pulmonary involvement occurs in 90% of cases)
  - Stage I disease – bilateral hilar lymphadenopathy
  - Stage II disease – BHL plus pulmonary infiltrates
  - Stage III disease – pulmonary infiltrates without BHL
  - Stage IV disease – pulmonary fibrosis

- CT of thorax
- **Bronchoalveolar lavage** with CD4/CD8 ratio: a CD4/CD8 ratio of more than 3.5 has a specificity of 94% for sarcoidosis
- **EKG** – rule out arrhythmias (anomalies in 10%)
- Whole body gallium Ga^{67} screening – lambda and panda patterns common
  - **Lambda Sign** – uptake of right paratracheal and BHL lymph nodes
  - **Panda Sign**– symmetric uptake by lacrimal and parotid glands

DDx – cutaneous tuberculosis, drug eruption, granuloma annulare, granuloma faciale, lamellar ichthyosis, leprosy, lichen planus, DLE, SCLE, lymphocytoma cutis, NL, plaque psoriasis, syphilis, tinea corporis, lichen planopilaris, B-cell lymphoma, foreign body reaction

Histology

- Superficial and deep dermal epithelioid cell granulomas with minimal or absent associated inflammation ("naked granulomas"). Central casseation usually absent
- Multinucleated giant cells usually of the Langhans type. Giant cells may contain eosinophilic stellate inclusions known as Schaumann bodies (likely represent degenerating lysosomes).
- Asteroid bodies represent engulfed collagen
- Darier–Roussy sarcoidosis → characteristic tubercles with little surrounding lymphocytic infiltration and these extend into the fat

Treatment

- PO steroids – prednisone 30–40 mg for 2–3 months. Gradual taper over 1 year to 10–20 mg QOD
- **Topical and/or Intralesional steroids**
- **Methotrexate** – 7.5–25 mg PO q week
- **Azathioprine** – 1–3 mg/kg/day PO; 1 mg/kg/day PO for 6–8 week; increase by 0.5 mg/kg q 4 week until response or dose reaches 2.5 mg/kg/day
- **Hydroxychloroquine** – 200–400 PO mg/day
- TNF-α inhibitors
  - Infliximab – dose not established but extrapolation from other uses: 3 or 5 mg/kg IV over 2 h on weeks 0, 2, and 6 and then q 8 week (TNF-α inhibitor)
  - Etanercept, adalimumab
  - Thalidomide – 50–300 mg/day PO qd with water, preferably hs and at least 1 h pc
  - <50 kg (110 lb): Start at low end of dose regimen
- Other – Chloroquine, cyclosporine, chlorambucil, isotretinoin, allopurinol,

minocycline, doxycycline, PUVA, leflunomide, pentoxyfylline, melatonin, radiation, pulsed-dye laser. Experimental – Golimumab, ustekinumab (clinical trials)

Pearls and Pitfalls

- Counsel patients about fact that hydroxychloroquine is not as effective in smokers
- JAAD CME 2001 → Testicular cancer is common with sarcoid
- 2/3 of patients have cutaneous anergy to tuberculin skin test; consider quantiF-ERON gold test
- Most common neurologic presentation → **CN VII palsy**
- Radiographic involvement seen in almost 90% of patients
- **Childhood sarcoidosis**
  - Rare, but usually presents with triad of arthritis, uveitis, cutaneous lesions along with constitutional symptoms
  - Peripheral lymphadenopathy common
  - Pulmonary involvement less common
  - Consider this diagnosis in kids with joint pain and especially with ocular symptoms

Scabies

Etiology and Pathogenesis

- Intensely pruritic skin infestation caused by the host-specific mite, *Sarcoptes scabiei* var *hominis* usually transmitted through direct contact with an infested individual
  - Mites can survive up to 3 days away from human skin, so fomites such as infested bedding or clothing are an alternate but infrequent source of transmission
- Entire life cycle of the mite lasts 30 days and is spent within the human epidermis
  - After copulation, the male mite dies and the female mite burrows into the superficial skin layers and lays a total of 60–90 eggs
  - The ova require 10 days to progress through larval/nymph stages to become mature adult mites. Less than 10% of the eggs laid result in mature mites
  - Mites move through the top layers of skin by secreting proteases that degrade the stratum corneum. They feed on dissolved tissue but do not ingest blood. Scybala (feces) are left behind as they travel through the epidermis, creating linear lesions clinically recognized as burrows

Clinical Presentation

- Common, extremely pruritic eruption consisting of papules, pustules, vesicles, and linear burrows
- Distribution – wrists, fingerweb spaces, toewebs, umbilicus, genital area, breast (women), axillae. May involve the face and scalp in infants
- Nodular scabies more common in children
- Prevalence rates are higher in children and sexually active individuals than in other persons
- Norwegian crusted variant is more common in …
  - Poor sensory perception due to entities such as leprosy , cerebral palsy, paraplegics
  - Immunocompromised patients – s/p transplantation, HIV disease, and old age

Labs

- Light microscopic (LM) identification of mites, larvae, ova, or scybala (fecal pellets) in skin scrapings
  - Place drop of mineral oil on a glass slide, touch a No. 15 blade to the oil, and scrape infested skin sites (preferably 1° lesions – vesicles, juicy papules, and burrows)
  - Skin scrapings placed on glass slide, cover slip, examine under LM at 40X mag

- o Multiple scrapings may be required to identify mites or their products
- o **Crusted scabies**: Add 10% KOH to the skin scraping – dissolves excess keratin and permits adequate microscopic examination
- Elevated IgE titers and eosinophilia may be demonstrated in some patients with scabies

DDx – acropustulosis of infancy, AD, bedbug bites, chickenpox, ACD, ICD, dermatitis artefacta, DH, dyshidrotic eczema, eosinophilic folliculitis, folliculitis, Gianotti–Crosti syndrome, Id reaction, insect bites, Kyrle disease, lice, lichen planus, neurotic excoriations, papular urticaria, prurigo nodularis, guttate psoriasis, pustular psoriasis, seabather's eruption, syphilis, fiberglass dermatitis, urticaria, delusions of parasitosis, urticaria pigmentosa (in young child with nodular scabies). Crusted scabies – psoriasis, seb derm, Langerhans cell histiocytosis

Histology – In rare cases, mites are identified in biopsy specimens obtained to r/o other dermatoses

- Eggs or mites or scybala (feces) are present in the subcorneal zone
- Sometimes see spongiosis or epidermal hyperplasia
- Perivascular or moderately diffuse dermal lymphocytes and eosinophils

Treatment

- **Home**
  - o All family members and close contacts must be evaluated and treated, even if they do not have symptoms
  - o Pets do not require treatment
  - o All carpets and upholstered furniture should be vacuumed and vacuum bags immediately discarded
  - o Instruct patients to launder clothing, bed linens, and towels used within last week in hot water the day after treatment is initiated and again in 1 week. Items that cannot be washed may be professionally dry cleaned or sealed in plastic bags for 1 week
  - o Affected individuals should avoid skin-to-skin contact with others
  - o Decontamination of clothing, bed linens, personal items must coincide with medical tx
  - o Patients with typical scabies may return to school/work 24 h after the first treatment

- **Medical Treatment** – Application of topical antiscabietic agents (see table below); repeat in 7–10 days
  - Pruritus
    - Antihistamines , menthol (Sarna), and pramoxine (Prax)
    - More severe sx may require short course of topical or oral steroids
  - **Crusted Scabies** (can mimic eczema)
    - Patients with crusted scabies or their caregivers should be instructed to remove excess scale to allow penetration of the topical scabicidal agent and decrease the burden of infestation
    - Achieved with warm water soaks followed by application of a keratolytic agent such as 5% salicylic acid in petrolatum, Lac-Hydrin cream, or urea cream. (Salicylic acid should be avoided if large body surface areas are involved because of the potential risk of salicylate poisoning)
    - The scales are then mechanically debrided with a tongue depressor or similar non-sharp device
    - Assessment of immune function may be indicated in individuals presenting with crusted scabies

Table 94 Topical and oral treatment for scabies

Topical	Adult dosage	Peds dosage
Permethrin 5% cream (Preg Cat B)	Apply from chin to toes and under fingernails and toenails; rinse off in shower 12 h later; repeat in 1 week	>2 months: Apply as in as adults but include head and neck in children <5 years; repeat in 1 week
Lindane 1% lotion or cream	Apply thin layer from chin to toes; use on dry skin and shower off 10 h later; repeat in 1 week	Apply thin film topically over entire body, including hairline, neck, scalp, temple, and forehead; leave on 6–8 h before washing off with water; may repeat in 1 week if necessary; – not to exceed 30 g per application – not for neonates or infants (risk of neurotoxicity)
Precipitated 6% sulfur in petrolatum (Preg Cat B)	Applied to entire body below head on three successive nights; bathe 24 h after each application	Administer as in adults, including head and neck
Crotamiton (Eurax) 10% cream or lotion	Apply a thin layer onto skin of entire body from neck to toes; repeat application in 24 h; take cleansing bath 48 h after last application	Not FDA approved
Oral	Adult dosage	Peds dosage
Ivermectin (3, 6 mg tabs) Dose of 0.2 mg/kg given at diagnosis; repeat in 7–14 days	<120 lb: 12 mg 200 lb: 18 mg 200 lb: 24 mg	<5 years or <15 kg: Not estab >5 years: Administer as in adults
Ivermectin – Crusted scabies may require three or more doses given at 1- to 2-week intervals – An ideal agent in cases for where topical tx is difficult or impractical, such as in widespread institutional infestations and bedridden patients – Not for pregnant or breastfeeding patients		

Pearls and Pitfalls

- Failure to repeat the treatment in 7–10 days is a common reason for relapse
- Failure to treat close contacts (even those without symptoms) is a common reason for relapse
- Resistance to permethrin is emerging
- Treat any secondary infections
- Scabies nodules can be treated symptomatically with topical steroids

Seborrheic Dermatitis

Etiology and Pathogenesis

- Seborrheic dermatitis is associated with normal levels of *Malassezia* but an abnormal immune response. Helper T cells, phytohemagglutinin and concanavalin stimulation, and antibody titers are depressed compared with those of control subjects. The contribution of *Malassezia* may come from its lipase activity – releasing inflammatory free fatty acids – and from its ability to activate the alternative complement pathway.

Clinical Presentation

- Papulosquamous disorder patterned on the sebum-rich areas
  - Distribution – scalp, eyebrows, around nose, central chest
- Commonly aggravated by changes in humidity, changes in seasons, trauma (e.g., scratching), or emotional stress
- The severity varies from mild dandruff to exfoliative erythroderma (erythroderma more often occurs in association with AIDS, congestive heart failure, Parkinson disease, and immunosuppression in premature infants)
- Seborrheic dermatitis may worsen in Parkinson disease, neurologic disorders, and in AIDS
- **Infantile form** – usually begins 1 week after birth and can persists for several months. Initially, see greasy scales that adhere to crown, but may extend to cover entire scalp, face, retroauricular folds, neck, trunk, and proximal extremities. May get infected with candida

Labs

- Rule out tinea infection
- Rule out immunodeficiency such as HIV-1 or -2 in severe cases that are recalcitrant to therapy

DDx – asteatotic eczema, atopic dermatitis, cutaneous candidiasis, ACD, irritant dermatitis, dermatomyositis, discoid lupus, drug eruption, drug-induced photosensitivity, erythrasma, extramammary paget's, glucagonoma syndrome, impetigo, Darier's disease, Grover's disease, pemphigus foliaceus, intertrigo, LSC, acute lupus erythematosus, perioral dermatitis, pityriasis alba, pityriasis rosea, rosacea, tinea capitis, tinea corporis, tinea cruris, tinea versicolor, sebopsoriasis, pityriasis amiantacea, Letterer–Siwe disease, pityrosporum folliculitis

Histology – spongiosis with a superficial perivascular and perifollicular lymphocytic infiltrate. Older lesions have acanthosis and focal parakeratosis. Unlike psoriasis, does NOT have Munro's microabscesses, confluent parakeratoic horny layers

Treatment

- Ketoconazole based
  - Xolegel 2%
  - Ketoconazole cream
  - Extina foam – ketoconazole 2%
- Shampoos
  - Capex Shampoo – fluocinolone acetonide
  - DHS (tar)
  - Head and shoulders
  - Ionil: 2% salicylic acid shampoo
  - Ionil-T: 1% coal tar
  - Ionil-T Plus: 2% coal tar shampoo
  - Ketoconazole shampoo 2% three times a week
  - Loprox shampoo
  - Selseb (selenium sulfide) 2.25% shampoo
  - Selsun blue (selenium sulfide)
  - Sebulex shampoo (2% salicylic acid + 2% urea)
  - T-gel (tar)
  - T-sal (contains salicylic acid)
- Topical corticosteroids (useful in very inflammatory cases) –
  - Hydrocortisone 2.5% (cream, lotion)
  - Desonide (cream, lotion)
  - Synalar (cream, soln) – **not to face**
  - Kenalog lotion (0.1% or 0.025% triamcinolone)
  - Apply 15–20 gtts (drops) to scalp qAM – **not to face**
  - Dermasmoothe FS oil (fluocinolone acetonide 0.01% in peanut/mineral oil) – **not to face**
    - Apply to scalp QHS × 2 weeks and then prn; cover scalp with shower cap
  - Olux foam to scalp – **not to face**
  - Luxiq foam to scalp – **not to face**
- Selenium sulfide based (other than shampoos)
  - Tersi Foam – selenium sulfide 2.25%
- Sodium sulfacetamide (helpful for facial seb derm)
  - Ovace – comes in 10% cream, gel, foam, wash
  - Plexion – cleanser, cleansing cloths, topical suspension
  - Rosanil cleanser – 10% sulfacetamide and 5% sulfur wash

○ Rosula – sodium sulfacetamide–sulfur–urea → cleanser and gel, medicated pads, wash
- Keratolytics
  ○ Coal tar – DHS Tar, MG217, Theraplex T, Psoriasin
  ○ Thick scalp involvement – Carmol scalp solution
- Immunosuppressives
  ○ Tacrolimus (Protopic) ointment 0.03% and 0.1%
  ○ Pimecrolimus (Elidel cream 1%)
- Severe cases
  ○ Consider PO ketoconazole, fluconazole, or itraconazole
- Seborrheic blepharitis
  ○ Wash eyelashes with baby shampoo

Pearls and Pitfalls

- Can mimic psoriasis and vice versa. Look for other signs of psoriasis
- Check for HIV-1 and -2 for severe cases that are recalcitrant to therapy

"Signs" in Dermatology

Table 95 "Signs" in dermatology

Name of sign	Description	Disease associations
Albright's sign	Dimple on 4th MCP Extension of	Gorlin's Syndrome
Asboe Hansen sign	Blister with direct pressure	Pemphigus
Auspitz sign	Pinpoint bleeding upon scale removal	Psoriasis
Beighton's sign	Thumb touches arm	EDS
Berliner's sign	Palpebral edema seen in exanthema subitum	Exanthema subitum
Crowe's sign	Axillary freckling	NF
Darier's sign	Whealing with skin striking	Urticaria pigmentosa
Deck–Chair Sign	Skinfold sparing	Papuloerythroderma of Ofuji
Dimple Sign	Pushing edges of lesion together produces central dimpling	Dermatofibroma
Dory flop sign	When the foreskin is retracted, mucosal surface chancres flip briskly	Seen in syphilis
Forscheimer's Sign	Enanthem of soft palate and uvula	Rubella
Gorlin's Sign	Ability to touch tip of tongue to nose	Marfan syndrome
Gottron's sign	Eruption occurs on knuckles, knees, and elbows	Dermatomyositis
Groove sign	Groove appears on extremity	Eosinophilic fasciitis, lymphogranuloma venereum
Headlight sign	Perinasal and periorbital pallor	Atopic dermatitis
Hertoghe's sign	Thinning of the lateral eyebrows	Atopic dermatitis
Higouménaki's sign	Unilateral thickening of inner 1/3 of clavicle	Syphilis
Higoumenaki's sign	Unilateral, irregular enlargement of the clavicle at site of sternocleidomastoid attachment, secondary to periostitis	Seen in syphilis
Hutchinson's sign	Nasal tip zoster	Seen in Herpes Zoster – warns of ophthalmic involvement of nasociliary branch
Hutchinson's sign	Pigmentation over nail fold	Indicator of melanoma
Nikolsky sign	Extension of blister with lateral pressure	Toxic epidermal necrolysis, pemphigus vulgaris, staphylococcal scalded skin syndrome, acute generalized exanthematous pustulosis
Ollendorf's sign	Exquisitely tender papule to blunt probe	Secondary syphilis
Ollendorf's sign	Papules tender to palpation	Seen in syphilis
Osler's sign	Pigmentation of sclerae	Alkaptonuria
Rumpel–Leede sign	Distal shower of petechiae that occurs immediately after release of pressure from tourniquet or sphygmomanometer	
Russel's sign	Excoriations on knuckles	Anorexia nervosa
Shoulder pad sign	Prominent deltoid muscle	Primary systemic amyloidosis

(continued)

Table 95 (continued)

Name of sign	Description	Disease associations
Sign of Leser-Trelat	Sudden occurrence of seborrheic keratoses	Associated with underlying malignancy
Tent sign	Surface of the tumor appears to be angulated or has several facets	Pilomatricoma
Trousseau's sign	Migratory thrombophlebitis	Associated with underlying malignancy
Winterbottom's sign	Posterior cervical lymphadenopathy	African trypanosomiasis
Wimberger's (cat-bite) sign	A radiographic "saw tooth" appearance at medial aspect of proximal tibial metaphysis	Seen in syphilis

Sjögren's Syndrome

Etiology and Pathogenesis

- Autoimmune disease that primarily affects the secretory glands (especially the lacrimal and salivary glands)
- Antibodies often present to anti-fodrin, anti-SSA (Ro), and anti-SSB (La)

Clinical Presentation

- Classic triad = xerostomia (dry mouth), keratoconjunctivitis sicca (dry eyes), and arthritis
- Can occur as primary disease of exocrine gland dysfunction or in association with several other autoimmune diseases (e.g., SLE, rheumatoid arthritis, scleroderma, systemic sclerosis, cryoglobulinemia, polyarteritis nodosa)
  - These primary and secondary types occur with similar frequency, but the sicca complex seems to cause more severe symptoms in the primary form
- Virtually all organs may be involved. Commonly affects eyes, mouth, parotid gland, lungs, kidneys, skin, and nervous system
- **Morbidity**
  - Eyes – Chronic keratoconjunctivitis, corneal ulcers
  - Oral dryness leads to caries, fissures, candidal infections, and difficulty speaking and swallowing food, altered sense of taste, higher incidence of dental caries, and periodontal disease
  - Dyspareunia
- American-European Consensus criteria
  - Diagnosis of primary SS requires four of six of the below criteria; in addition, either criterion number five or criterion number six must be included. Diagnosis of SS can be made in patients who have no sicca symptoms if three of four objective criteria are fulfilled. The criteria are as follows:
  - (1) Ocular symptoms
    - Dry eyes for more than 3 months
    - Foreign-body sensation
    - Tear substitutes are used more than three times per day
  - (2) Oral symptoms
    - Feeling of dry mouth
    - Recurrently swollen salivary glands
    - Liquids are frequently used to aid swallowing
  - (3) Ocular signs
    - Schirmer test performed without anesthesia (<5 mm in 5 min)
    - Positive vital dye staining results
  - (4) Oral signs
    - Abnormal salivary scintigraphy findings
    - Abnormal parotid sialography findings

■ Abnormal sialometry findings (unstimulated salivary flow <0.1 mL/min)
○ (5) Positive lip biopsy findings
○ (6) Positive anti-SS-A or anti-SS-B antibody results

Labs

- Schirmer test
  ○ A test strip of number 41 Whatman filter paper placed near lower conjunctival sac to measure tear formation. Healthy persons wet 15 mm or more after 5 min. A positive test occurs when less than 5 mm is wet after 5 min
  ○ This test can be useful to help exclude or confirm significant dryness of the eyes, but it is not disease specific. False-positive results occur
- ESR is elevated in 80% of patients
- Rheumatoid factor is present in 52% of cases of 1° Sjögren's and in 98% of 2° Sjögren's
- CBC – mild anemia is present in 50% of patients, leukopenia occurs in up to 42% of patients. Pernicious anemia can occur (B12)
  ○ Check for SLE especially if leukopenia or thrombocytopenia
- SSA and SSB
  ○ Anti-SSA found in approx 50%
  ○ Anti-SSB found in approx 40–50%
  ○ Absence does not exclude disease
- ANA (speckled and homogeneous) present in most cases of 1° Sjögren syndrome
- Creatinine clearance may be diminished in up to 50% of patients
- SPEP/UPEP – many have polyclonal gammopathy
- Patients with primary SS may have positive test results for lupus anticoagulant and/or anticardiolipin antibodies
- May have increased freq of autoimmune thyroid disease with hypothyroidism (10–15%)

DDx – dry mouth/dry eyes from hepatitis C, HIV, amyloidosis

Histology – Biopsy of the minor salivary glands is often performed. Presence of two or more aggregates of lymphocytes (50+) in 4 mm^2 of salivary gland tissue is required for diagnosis. Biopsy of the parotid gland can have diagnostic changes at an earlier stage than a minor salivary gland biopsy

Treatment

- Dry Eyes
  ○ Artificial tears – liberally; patients may need more if they enter an environ-

ment with low humidity (e.g., air conditioning, airplanes). Examples: Celluvisc, Murine, Refresh, Tears Naturale

- Artificial tears with hydroxymethylcellulose or dextran are more viscous and can last longer before reapplication is needed; encourage patients to try various products
- If artificial tears burn when they are instilled, the preservative in the artificial tears is likely irritating the eye
- If patients wake up in the morning with severe matting in the eyes, then they should use a more viscous preparation, such as Lacri-Lube, at night

o Patients should avoid medications with anticholinergic and antihistamine effects
o The use of humidifiers may help – distilled water is best

- Dry Mouth
  o Sip frequently (q 2 h); add lemon slices or lemon juice to water – stimulates saliva
  o **Sugar-free** lemon drops prn to stimulate salivary secretion
  o Artificial saliva can be used as needed, although patient tolerance is variable
    - Preparations include Salivart, Saliment, Saliva Substitute, MouthKote, and Xero-Lube
  o Patients should be **seen regularly by a dentist**, who might advise fluoride treatments
    - Toothpaste without detergents can reduce mouth irritation in patients with SS. Brands include Biotene toothpaste, Biotene mouth rinse, Dental Care toothpaste, and Oral Balance gel
  o **Avoid antihistamines and anticholinergics**
  o Avoid eating dry, rough, or irritating foods – crackers, cereals, steaks, chips, salt, salad dressings, spicy food
  o Rinse mouth with water or saline water after each meal
  o **Minimize tobacco** use
  o Watch for and treat oral candidiasis and angular cheilitis with topical antifungal agents, such as nystatin troches. PO fluconazole may be needed occasionally. Patients also need to be sure to disinfect their dentures
  o Sinusitis and sinus blockade should be treated because these problems may contribute to mouth breathing
- Skin and vaginal dryness
  o Patients should use skin creams to help with dry skin
  o Patients should use vaginal lubricants, such as Replens, for vaginal dryness. Vaginal estrogen creams can be considered in postmenopausal women. Evaluate for and treat vaginal yeast infections
- Arthralgias and arthritis
  o Acetaminophen or NSAIDs can be taken for arthralgias
  o Consider Plaquenil if NSAIDs are not sufficient for the synovitis occasionally associated with primary SS. Does not relieve sicca symptoms
  o Patients with RA associated with SS likely require other disease-modifying agents

- Other
  - In patients with major organ involvement (i.e., lymphocytic interstitial lung dz, consider tx with steroids and immunosuppressive agents, such as cyclophosphamide)
  - While cyclophosphamide and similar agents may be helpful to treat serious manifestations of SS or disorders associated with SS, clinicians should understand that these agents are also associated with the development of lymphomas
  - Long-term anticoagulation may be needed in those patients with vascular thrombosis related to antiphospholipid antibody syndrome
  - During surgery – anesthesiologist should use as little anticholinergic meds as possible and use humidified oxygen to help avoid inspissation of pulmonary secretions. Good postop resp therapy should also be provided. Patients at higher risk for corneal abrasions, so ocular lubricants should be considered
  - Cholinergic parasympathomimetic agents can ↑salivary secretion
    - **Pilocarpine (Salagen)** – 5 mg PO tid/qid
    - **Cevimeline (Evoxac)** – 30 mg PO tid

Pearls and Pitfalls

- Patients with hepatitis C, HIV can get a "Sjögren's-like" xerostomia
- Unlikely to have SSB + but SSA– → if present, also consider primary biliary cirrhosis and autoimmune hepatitis
- **Avoid Mycelex lozenges** – contain a lot of sugar and can cause dental caries
- Encourage smoking cessation
- Patients may find the newsletter *Moisture Seekers,* published by the Sjögren's Syndrome Foundation, useful

Squamous Cell Carcinoma (SCC)

Etiology and Pathogenesis

- SCC is a malignant tumor of epidermal keratinocytes associated with p53 mutations from UV-induced DNA damage

Clinical Presentation and Types

- Second most common form of skin cancer and frequently arises on the sun-exposed skin of middle-aged and elderly individuals
- Some cases of SCC occur de novo (i.e., in the absence of a precursor lesion); however, some SCCs arise from sun-induced precancerous lesions known as actinic keratoses (AKs) and patients with multiple AKs are at increased risk for developing SCC
- SCC is capable of locally infiltrative growth, spread to regional lymph nodes, and distant metastasis, most often to the lungs
- Clinical Variants
    - **SCC *in situ* (Bowen's disease)** – red, scaly patch that arises in sun-exposed areas or in genital area (HPV-16 or -18 typically)
    - **Invasive SCC** – Erythematous, keratotic papule or nodule arising on background of sun-damaged skin. Often tender and may enlarge rapidly
    - **Periungual SCC** – can look like a wart
    - **Marjolin ulcer** – subtype of SCC appears as a new area of induration, elevation, or ulceration at the site of a preexisting scar or ulcer
    - **Keratoacanthoma** – rapidly enlarging crateriform nodule which develops over a few weeks. Common on the head or extremities
        - **Types = solitary KA**, multiple, grouped, giant, subungual, intraoral, multiple spontaneously regressing (Ferguson–Smith), multiple non-regressing generalized eruptive (Grzybowski), keratoacanthoma centrifugum marginatum, KAs associated with Muir–Torre syndrome and KAs assoc with immunosuppression
    - **Perioral SCC**
    - **Anogenital SCC**
    - **Verrucous carcinoma** – locally destructive, but rarely metastasizes
- Risk Factors
    - age > 50, male sex, fair skin, geography (closer to equator), Hx of prior NMSC, exposure to UV light (high cumulative dose), exposure to chemical carcinogens (arsenic, tar), exposure to ionizing radiation, chronic immunosuppression, chronic scarring condition, genodermatoses, HPV infection (specific subtypes)

Labs and Imaging to Consider

- Imaging may be necessary in patients with → those with symptoms suspicious for perineural invasion, lymphadenopathy, those with significant local destruction. No formal guidelines for imaging, however

DDx – superficial basal cell carcinoma, verruca vulgaris, actinic keratosis, condyloma accuminata in genital area, neuroendocrine carcinoma, amelanotic melanoma, adnexal tumors, prurigo nodule, irritated seborrheic keratose, atypical fibroxanthoma.

Histology

Table 96 Histologic and clinical variants of squamous cell carcinoma

Tumor	Histologic characteristics	Clinical characteristics
SCC	Invasion of dermis by atypical keratino-cytes. Squamous eddies or keratin pearls. Variable infiltrate. Perineural invasion in some aggressive forms	Keratotic nodule on sun-damaged skin
Keratoacanthoma	Keratin-filled crater Well-differentiated (mild atypia) Neutrophil microabscesses Eosinophils in dermal infiltrate	Solitary nodule Central craterlike depression Rapid growth May spontaneously involute
Spindle-cell SCC	Atypical spindle cells Foci of squamous differentiation May resemble other spindle cell tumors (e.g., atypical fibroxanthoma)	Resembles typical SCC May be clinically aggressive
Acantholytic (adenoid) SCC	Glandlike differentiation Acantholysis May resemble adenocarcinoma or sweat gland carcinoma	Arises on sun-damaged skin Elderly patients Resembles typical SCC Clinically aggressive
Verrucous carcinoma	Well-differentiated (minimal atypia) Resembles verruca Bulbous downward proliferation "Bulldozing" invasion	Oral, genital, or plantar foot Indolent growth Locally destructive Rarely metastasizes

Treatment

- **SCC in situ** – Surgical excision, Mohs, Imiquimod, 5-Fluorouracil cream (5-FU), photodynamic therapy, cryotherapy
- **SCC** – Surgical excision (4 mm margins), Mohs, Radiation – for select patients
  - Consider radiation if multiple involved nodes or extensive extracapsular extension is present or inoperable disease (latter +/– chemotherapy with cisplatin)

○ Patients in high-risk groups may develop lesions in short periods of time and thus ED&C may be a preferred treatment for clinically low-risk tumors because of the ability to treat numerous lesions at one visit. F/u on pathology, however, to make sure no high-risk features that would require more aggressive intervention

- **Risk Factors for recurrence**
  ○ Large size
    ■ ≥20 mm on trunk/extremities
    ■ ≥10 mm on cheeks, forehead, scalp, neck
    ■ ≥6 mm on "mask areas of face", genitals, hands, or feet
  ○ Poorly defined borders, history of recurrence, immunosuppression present, site of prior radiation therapy, rapidly growing tumor, neurologic symptoms, perineural invasion, Clark's level IV or V
  ○ Moderately or poorly differentiated on pathology)
  ○ Path variants – adenoid (acantholytic), adenosquamous (with mucin production), or desmoplastic types
- **Staging of SCC– TNM system** (*www.cancer.gov*)
  ○ The primary tumor (T) is classified according to the following categories:
    ■ TX: The primary tumor cannot be assessed
    ■ T0: There is no evidence of primary tumor
    ■ T1: Tumor is 2 cm or less in greatest dimension
    ■ T2: Tumor is more than 2 cm, but less than 5 cm in greatest dimension
    ■ T3: Tumor is more than 5 cm in greatest dimension
    ■ T4: Tumor invades the deep, extradermal structures (cartilage, bone, or muscle)
  ○ The regional lymph nodes (N) are clinically divided into the following categories:
    ■ NX: Regional (nearby) lymph nodes cannot be assessed
    ■ N0: There is no regional lymph node metastasis
    ■ N1: Regional lymph node metastasis is present
  ○ The state of metastasis (M) is defined as follows:
    ■ MX: Distant metastasis cannot be assessed
    ■ M0: There is no distant metastasis
    ■ M1: Distant metastasis is present
  ○ There are four basic stage groupings within the TNM system, as well as a "Stage 0" classification, which refers to carcinoma in situ:
    ■ Stage 0: Tis, N0, M0
    ■ Stage 1: T1, N0, M0
    ■ Stage 2: T2, N0, M0; or T3, N0, M0
    ■ Stage 3: T4, N0, M0; or T(any), N1, M0
    ■ Stage 4: T(any), N(any), M1

Pearls and Pitfalls

- The National Comprehensive Cancer Network (NCCN) has established guidelines for care of non-melanoma skin cancers (www.nccn.org), which is a useful resource
- Always do a lymph node examination
- If a large aggressive tumor is present, send to ENT for possible head/neck dissection
- Patients with chronic lymphocytic leukemia (CLL) tend to get aggressive SCC's which can be life-threatening. Follow these patients very closely. Mohs surgery may be difficult as the inflammation can obscure tumor, but this is still the treatment with the highest cure rate.

Subacute Cutaneous Lupus Erythematosus (SCLE)

Etiology and Pathogenesis

- May occur in patients with SLE, Sjögren's syndrome, and deficiency of C2d. May be drug-related
  - **Medications associated with SCLE** – ACE-inhibitors, aldactone, azathioprine, calcium-channel blockers, cimetidine, glyburide, griseofulvin, leflunomide, NSAIDs, penicillin, penicillamine, piroxicam, sulfonylureas, terbinafine, TNF-α inhibitors

Clinical Presentation

- Skin lesions have an annular configuration, with raised red borders and central clearing. May have a papulosquamous appearance
- Post-inflammatory pigmentary alteration may occur after lesions resolve, but do not scar
- More common in whites (85%), M < F (1:4)
- Photosensitivity common

Labs

- **SSA (Anti-Ro)** positive in high proportion
- SSB (Anti-La) positive frequently but less than SSA
- Anti-dsDNA usually reflects SLE but may occur in SCLE
- Anemia, leukopenia, thrombocytopenia may be present
- ↑ ESR in some
- RF may be positive
- Complement levels may be ↓
- Get urinalysis initially and periodically

DDx – Dermatomyositis, erythema annulare centrifugum, erythema gyratum repens, erythema multiforme, granuloma annulare, Henoch–Schönlein purpura, hypersensitivity vasculitis, lichen planus, acute lupus erythematosus, DLE, PMLE, plaque psoriasis, sarcoid, tinea corporis

Histology – Findings similar to that seen in acute cutaneous lupus erythematosus

- Keratinocyte damage and epidermal atrophy common. Basal cell layer may have degeneration. Perivascular and interface lymphohistiocytic infiltrate in upper dermis

- Have little or no hyperkeratosis, basement membrane thickening, perifollicular infiltrate, follicular plugging, deep dermal infiltrate, or scarring

Treatment

- **General** – good sun-protective measures, broad-spectrum sunscreen
- Steroids (topical, IL)
- Antimalarials
- Immunosuppressive – MTX, azathioprine, mycophenolate mofetil, IFN-α
- Dapsone
- Retinoids (PO)
- Other – thalidomide, IFN, clofazimine, auranofin (gold)

Pearls and Pitfalls

- Always rule out drug-induced SCLE (see medication monitoring chapter for list)
- Long-term prognosis is not entirely known, but approximately 10–15% develop systemic disease such as nephritis. Long-term follow-up recommended

Sweet's Syndrome (Acute Febrile Neutrophilic Dermatosis)

Etiology and Pathogenesis

- Exact pathogenesis unknown but associated with infections, autoimmunity, inflammatory bowel disease, medications, and malignancies. Up to 50% have idiopathic disease
- **Malignancy** (15–20%) – *most are hematologic malignancies*
  - Hematologic malignancy – AML, CML
  - Non-myeloid hematologic malignancies – CTCL, multiple myeloma, hairy cell leukemia, Hodgkin disease, non-Hodgkin lymphoma
  - Non-hematologic malignancy – rates of genitourinary, breast, and gastrointestinal cancers appear to be slightly increased in this group. Rarely reported associations include osteosarcoma, oral cancer/tonsil cancer, ovarian cancer, thyroid cancer, lung cancer, pheochromocytoma, and rectal carcinoma
  - Some authors recommend a directed systemic evaluation in all patients with Sweet's
- **Infections**
  - Infections often involve the upper respiratory tract – especially Streptococcal pneumonia
  - *Salmonella* or *Staphylococcus* species, *Yersinia enterocolitica* (may improve with ABX), *Entamoeba coli, Helicobacter pylori, Borrelia burgdorferi,* non-tuberculous organisms, (atypical), and *Tuberculous mycobacteria*
  - Sweets may be a presenting feature of coccidiomycosis
  - HIV, cytomegalovirus (CMV), hepatitis A, and hepatitis B have been implicated
- **Medications**
  - Note: Some of these reactions have been noted in patients with underlying malignancy; therefore, the validity of these possible associations is unclear
  - G-CSF, trimethoprim-sulfamethoxazole (Bactrim), all-*trans* retinoic acid, and minocycline
  - Anecdotal or limited reports include lithium, furosemide, hydralazine, carbamazepine, OCPs, the Mirena intrauterine device, COX-2 inhibitors, doxycycline, diazepam, diclofenac, nitrofurantoin, propylthiouracil, lenalidomide, bortezomib, abacavir, imitinib, and vaccinations (e.g., for bacille Calmette–Guérin, smallpox, pneumococcal organisms)
- **Systemic Disorders**
  - Crohn disease, ulcerative colitis – especially with bullous or ulcerative lesions (can get these skin lesions with malignancy, too)
  - Sjögren's, Behçet's, lupus, rheumatoid arthritis, and other connective tissue disease

- **Miscellaneous**
  - Spinal surgery, sarcoidosis, erythema nodosum, relapsing polychondritis, or thyroiditis
  - A few cases have been observed during pregnancy
    - Can occur during pregnancy and may recur in subsequent pregnancies
    - Presently, it is believed that disease is not associated with fetal harm
  - Several cases have occurred with polycythemia vera

Clinical Presentation

- Reactive process characterized by abrupt onset of tender, red-to-purple papules, and nodules that coalesce to form plaques. Bullous or vesicular lesions may be present (frequently associated with myelogenous leukemia)
- Distribution – Plaques usually occur on upper extremities, face, or neck and are typically accompanied by fever and peripheral neutrophilia. Oral lesions uncommon. Leg involvement may mimic erythema nodosum
- Constitutional symptoms 1–3 weeks prior to onset of rash (fevers, arthralgias, myalgias, malaise, …)
- **Diagnostic Criteria** – The presence of two major and two minor clinical findings have been proposed as criteria for diagnosis, as suggested by Su and Liu and revised by von den Driesch
  - Major criteria
    - Abrupt onset of tender or painful erythematous plaques or nodules, occasionally with vesicles, pustules, or bullae
    - Predominantly neutrophilic infiltration in dermis without LCV
  - Minor criteria
    - Preceding nonspecific respiratory or gastrointestinal tract infection or vaccination or associated with inflammatory disease, hemoproliferative disorders, solid malignant tumors, or pregnancy
    - Periods of general malaise and fever (body temperature >38°C)
    - Laboratory values during onset showing a erythrocyte sedimentation rate >20 mm, positive C-reactive protein (CRP) result, segmented nuclear neutrophils, bands >70% in peripheral blood smears, and leukocytosis (count >8,000/μL) (meeting three of four of these values is necessary)
    - Excellent response to tx with systemic corticosteroids or potassium iodide

Labs and Imaging to Consider

- CBC+diff and peripheral blood smear – rule out underlying hematologic malignancy
  - Neutrophilia is typically present, but the absence of neutrophilia in a patient who is neutropenic does not rule out Sweet syndrome
  - Anemia and ↓plts are common in patients with underlying malignancy
  - Abnormalities in CBC should prompt consideration of bone marrow biopsy

- ESR, CRP – nonspecific markers of inflammation; ESR elevated in >90%
- Urinalysis – may show proteinuria or hematuria
- LFTs – may be nonspecifically elevated
- ANCAs have been described, but not consistently found, in patients with Sweet syndrome
- Lesions should be sent for tissue culture to rule out infection (fungal, AFB, bacterial)
- CXR – to rule out pulmonary involvement
- Bone marrow biopsy is indicated if abnormal CBC, and should be considered in all cases of atypical bullous or ulcerative Sweet syndrome
- Imaging such as ultrasonography, CT, PET, or MRI may be helpful in identifying underlying malignancies

DDx – Behçet disease, drug eruption, erythema multiforme, erythema nodosum, herpes simplex, pyoderma gangrenosum, bowel-associated dermatitis-arthritis syndrome, neutrophilic rheumatoid dermatitis, LCV, acral erythema, leukemia cutis, acute hemorrhagic edema of childhood, infection (AFB, fungal, bacterial)

Histology

- Epidermal changes variable. Sometimes see epidermal necrosis
- Often see superficial dermal edema and occasionally subepidermal blister
- Diffuse dermal infiltrate consisting mostly of neutrophils, but also lymphocytes, histiocytes, and a few eosinophils
- No true vasculitis (no vessel wall necrosis)
- Extravasated erythrocytes – sometimes
- Stains for infectious organisms negative

Treatment

- Attempt to identify and treat an underlying cause
- In most cases, **prednisone** is extremely and rapidly effective → 0.5–1 mg/kg/day
  - Prompt relief typical
  - May need prolonged low-dose prednisone for 2–3 months to prevent recurrence
  - Pulmonary infiltrates also respond to prednisone
- High-potency **topical corticosteroids** or intralesionals may be used for localized lesions
- Topical calcineurin inhibitors

- For long-term management, numerous drugs may be helpful. Many of the medications work by inhibiting neutrophil chemotaxis
  - Potassium iodide (SSKI) – 900 mg/day
  - Dapsone 100–200 mg/day
  - Colchicine 0.6–1.5 mg/day
- Other medications which may be helpful – NSAIDS, cyclosporine, thalidomide, IFN-α, clofazamine, isotretinoin, methotrexate, cyclophosphamide, TNF-α inhibitors

Pearls and Pitfalls

- Pulmonary involvement can occur and may look like anything on imaging (can mimic other lung diseases)
- Rule out malignancy, infection prior to starting immunosuppressive therapy
- Consider injectable medication or infusion in patients with poor GI absorption (inflammatory bowel, hx of bowel bypass)
- Always exclude cutaneous infection
- **Pediatric population**
  - Sweet's is rare, but presentation similar to adults. May or may not be able to find a cause, but always look for one. Treatment in this population is with systemic corticosteroids (1–2 mg/kg/day) and taper over 2–3 months to prevent recurrent. Colchicine and dapsone have also been recommended

Syphilis

Etiology and Pathogenesis

- Etiology: *Treponema pallidum* – spirochete
- **Transmission**
  - Intimate contact with infectious lesions (most common)
  - Blood transfusions (blood collected during early syphilis)
  - Transplacentally from an infected mother to her fetus

Clinical Presentation and Types *(also see table)*

- **Types of Syphilis**
  - **Primary** syphilis occurs within 3 weeks of contact with infected individual. Usually present with solitary red papule that rapidly forms painless non-bleeding ulcer or chancre. Chancre usually heals within 4–8 weeks, with or without therapy
  - **Secondary** syphilis usually presents with cutaneous eruption within 2–10 weeks after primary chancre and is most florid 3–4 months after infection. Eruption may be subtle; 25% of patients unaware of skin changes. Commonly see red-violaceous scaly patches on trunk, extremities, palms, and soles. May mimic pityriasis rosea
    - Mild constitutional symptoms
    - Small % develop acute syphilitic meningitis and present with headache, neck stiffness, facial numbness or weakness, and deafness
  - The lesions of benign **tertiary** syphilis usually develop within 3–10 years of infection. Typical lesion is a gumma, and patient complaints usually are secondary to bone pain, which is described as a deep boring pain characteristically worse at night. Trauma may predispose a specific site to gumma involvement
    - CNS involvement may occur, w/ presenting sx representative of area affected
    - Some patients may present up to 20 years after infection with behavioral changes and other signs of dementia, which is indicative of **neurosyphilis**
  - A small percentage of infants infected in utero may have a latent form of infection that becomes apparent during childhood and, in some cases, during adult life
    - Prior to age 2 years is rhinitis (snuffles), followed by cutaneous lesions
    - After age 2 years, parents may see problems with child's hearing and language development and with vision. Facial and dental abnormalities may be noted

Labs

- In suspected acquired syphilis, perform nontreponemal serology screening using VDRL, RPR
  - Then, test sera yielding a positive or equivocal reaction by the FTA-ABS, quantitative VDRL/RPR, and microhemagglutination assay *Treponema pallidum* (MHA-TP) tests
  - For evaluation of infants with suspected congenital syphilis, the 19 S immunoglobulin M FTA-ABS serology test or the Captia Syphilis-M test currently is recommended

DDx

- Primary syphilis – HSV, chancroid, granuloma inguinale, fixed drug eruption, trauma
- Secondary syphilis – pityriasis rosea, guttate psoriasis, viral exanthem, drug eruption, lichen planus, pityriasis lichenoides chronica, acute HIV infection, nummular eczema, folliculitis. If mucous membranes involved – lichen planus, apthae, herpangioma, perleche. Condyloma lata may mimic condyloma accuminata
- Tertiary syphilis – lupus vulgaris, chromoblastomycosis, deep fungal infections, leishmaniasis, lupus erythematosus, mycosis fungoides, sarcoidosis, venous ulcer, tumor

Histology – Regardless of the stage of disease and location of lesions, two histopathologic hallmarks of syphilis have been noted, including obliterative endarteritis and plasma cell-rich mononuclear infiltrates. Spirochetes may be seen with **Warthin–Starry stain**

Treatment and Management → *Also See Table*

- Follow-Up
  - Patients with treated primary or secondary syphilis
    - Perform quantitative VDRL testing at 1, 3, 6, and 12 months following tx
    - If VDRL titer of 1:8 or more fails to fall at least fourfold within 12 months or if the titer starts to rise, consider more intensive retreatment, and examine the CSF
    - If all clinical and serologic examinations remain satisfactory for 2 years following treatment, the patient can be reassured that cure is complete, and no further follow-up care is needed

- o Patients with latent syphilis
  - Perform quantitative reagin testing for up to 2 years
  - Schedule annual follow-up visits for an indefinite period of time for patients with persistently positive serologic tests
  - Patients with benign tertiary or cardiovascular syphilis: Patients should be observed by the physician for the rest of their lives to monitor for complications
- o Patients with neurosyphilis (both symptomatic and asymptomatic): Examine the CSF (cell count, protein, reagin titer) q 3–6 months for 3 years or until CSF findings return to normal
- o For patients who are pregnant and have early syphilis, it is likely that the mother will deliver a child not infected by syphilis (assuming the mother was treated appropriately)

Pearls and Pitfalls

- HIV patients (especially with low CD4 counts) may have negative RPR, VDRL – consider biopsying any lesions. Labs will usually convert in a couple of months
- **Lues Maligna** type of syphilis is more common in HIV. Anyone presenting with this type should be checked for HIV-1 and -2
- Always ask about and look for eye involvement. If any signs/symptoms, send for eye exam. Spirochetes frequently seen on eye exams
  - o If they have eye involvement, they have neurosyphilis and need to be treated accordingly
- Pregnant women – need Penicillin G. If allergic, desensitize. This is the only reliable treatment in this population
- **Prozone effect** – The lack of agglutination at high concentrations of antibodies is called the prozone effect and can result in a negative RPR. Lack of agglutination in the prozone is due to antibody excess resulting in very small complexes that do not clump to form visible agglutination
  - o Can call the lab and have them dilute the sample if there is high clinical suspicion

Table 97   Syphilology: manifestations and treatment of *T. pallidum* infection

Stage	Manifestations		Treatment	
Congenital (Prenatal)	*Placenta*	*Fetus*	*Primary*	*Secondary* (f/u mandatory)
	Langerhan's cell layer Placentitis: • Acute chorioamnionitis • Chronic villitis • Hydrops placentalis • Necrotizing funisitis	• Hydrops fetalis • Intrauterine growth retardation • Premature delivery • Stillbirth	**Aqueous crystalline PCN G** 100,000–150,000 µg/kg/day administered as 50,000 µg/kg/dose IV q 12 h × first 7 days of life, then q 8 h × 7–21 days	**Procaine PCN G** 50,000 u/kg/dose QD IM × 10 days Pregnancy and syphilis: skin test for PCN allergy. Desensitize if necessary. Parenteral **PCN G** is only tx with documented efficacy
Congenital (Postnatal)	*Early* • Chorioretinitis ("Salt and Pepper" fundus) • Dactylitis • Epiphysitis • Hepatomegaly, hepatitis • **Parrot's pseudoparalysis** • **Pneumonia alba** • **Snuffles** • **Syphilitic pemphigus** • **Rhagades** • **Wimberger's sign**	*Late* • **Clutton's joints** • Frontal bossing • **Higoumenaki's sign** • Interstitial keratitis • **"Mulberry" molars** • Neurosyphilis • Protruding mandible • **Saber shins** • **Saddle nose** • Short maxillae	*Pregnancy and syphilis*: same as for non-pregnant. Some recommend second dose (2.4 mill U) **benzathine PCN G** 1 week after initial dose especially in third trimester or with 2° syphilis	
Primary	*Cutaneous*: **balanitis of Follman, chancre rédux, "dory flop" sign**, primary chancre (genital area or head/neck), **syphilis d'emblee** *Other*: Regional lymphadenopathy		Primary, secondary or early latent (<1 year): **Benzathine PCN G** – 2.4 mill U IM in single dose *Use of benzathine procaine PCN is inappropriate*	**Doxycycline** 100 mg BID PO × 14 days or **Tetracycline** 500 mg QID PO × 14 days or **Ceftriaxone** 1 g IM/IV QD × 8–10 days **Doxycycline** 100 mg PO BID PO × 28 days or **Tetracycline** 500 mg QID PO × 28 days

Table 97 (continued)

Stage	Manifestations	Treatment	
Secondary	*Cutaneous*: **Biette's collarette, condyloma lata,** "corona veneris", **corymbiform, "frambesiform syphilid", leukoderma colli** (collar of Venus), **lues maligna** (ulceronodular, "la grand verole"), moth-eaten alopecia, **mucous patches (plaques fauchées en prairie). Ollendorf sign,** "raw ham" papules, **ringed** (annular) plaques, **rupial plaques, split papule** *Other*: Acute meningitis, acute nephritic syndrome, GI involvement, granulomatous iritis, pharyngitis, retrobulbar optic neuritis, syphilitic hepatitis	*Late latent (>1 year) or syphilis of indeterminate duration, late benign*: **Benzathine PCN G** 2.4 mill U IM q week×3 weeks *Neurosyphilis, including ocular syphilis*: **(all need CSF exam) Aqueous crystalline PCN G**, 3–4 mill U IV q 4 h×10–14 days	**Procaine PCN G** 2.4 mill U QD IM plus **Probenecid** 500 mg QID PO, both×10–14 days
Latent	**Asymptomatic**		
Tertiary (Late)	*Cutaneous*: Gummas, **pseudochancre redux** *Neurosyphilis*: Asymptomatic, Gummas, meningeal, Meningovascular, Parenchymatous (paresis, **tabes dorsalis, Argyll Robertson pupil**) *Rheum*: **bilateral bursitis of Verneuil, Charcot joints** *Vascular*: Aortitis, aortic aneurysm, coronary ostial stenosis *Lumbar Puncture if*: neuro sx, tx failure, titer≥1:32, HIV +, non-PCN rx, evid of other active syphilis		

HIV patients– Treatment same as uninfected patients, but with closer follow-up. LP on all HIV-infected patients with late syphilis and serum RPR≥1:32 (neurosyphilis risk 19-fold in this group and CSF changes less likely to normalize) Treat neurosyphilis for 10–14 days regardless of CD4 count

Table 98 Syphilology: glossary of terms

Argyll Robertson pupil	Pupil accommodates, but does not react to light
Balanitis of Follman	Chancres may be atypical [multiple, painful, purulent, and destructive]
Biette's collarette	Thin, white ring of scales on surface of the papules
Chancre rédux	(**Monorecidive chancre**) the reappearance of a chancre after partial healing as a result of insufficient treatment
Charcot joint	Enlarged, painless, uninflammed joints, +/– deformity, in the extremities and spine
Clutton's joints	Synovitis with effusions of the knees and elbows
Corona veneris	Macules and/or papules along the hairline
Corymbose (bomb shell)	A large central papule surrounded by satellite raised pustules
Condyloma lata	Skin-colored or hypopigmented, moist, oozing papules located perianally and on the genitalia. They become flattened and macerated. These are teeming with treponemes, and thus are extremely infectious
Frambesiform syphilid	Condyloma lata in intertriginous areas may proliferate forming nodular lesions that resemble raspberries
Gummas	Rubbery tumors with predilection for skin or long bones, may also develop in the eyes, mucous membranes, throat, liver, or stomach lining
Hutchinson's teeth	Centrally notched, widely spaced, peg-shaped upper incisors
Hutchinson's triad	Hutchinson's teeth, CN VIII deafness, and corneal opacities (2° to interstitial keratitis)
Langerhan's cell layer	Layer of the cytotrophoblast of the placenta: a controversial protective placental barrier until 20 week gestation. Recently – evidence that treponemas cross placenta in early preg
Leukoderma colli	(Syphilitic leukoderma/collar of pearls/**collar of Venus**/venereal collar), round or oval, ill-defined, depigmented macules with hyperpigmented borders occurring on the anteriolateral neck and chest
Lues maligna	Areas of ulcerated and necrotic tissue – in 2° syphilis (more likely in patients with HIV)
Mulberry molars	(**Moon's or Fournier's molar**) sixth-year molars, is seen in the first lower molar
Mucous patches	Painless, shallow, rounded gray macerated erosions, located on the oral, genital and anal mucosa. These are teeming with treponemes
Parrot's pseudoparalysis	Reduced movement of the extremities due to pain
Pneumonia alba	Yellowish-white, heavy firm, and grossly enlarged lungs (pneumonitis)
Pseudochancre redux	A solitary gumma of the penis
Rhagades (Parrot's lines)	Perioral fissures. Depressed linear scars radiating from mouth
Rupial lesion	Ulcerative lesions with a heaped-up crust, oyster-shell-like
Saber shins	Anterior tibial bowing
Snuffles	Bloody or purulent mucinous nasal discharge
Split papule	Lesions at the angle of the mouth or corner of the nose which have central linear erosion

Table 98 (continued)

Syphilitis d'emblee	Syphilis occurring without an initial sore
Syphilitic pemphigus	Vesiculobullous eruption
Tabes dorsalis	Presents with signs of demyelination of the posterior columns, dorsal roots, and dorsal root ganglia (e.g., ataxic wide-based gait and foot slap, areflexia and loss of position, deep pain and temperature sensations)

References: – Berman SM. Maternal syphilis: pathophysiology and treatment. Bull World Heath Organ. 2004 June; 82(6):433–8.
– Czelusta A, Yen-Moore A, Van der Straten M, Carrasco D, Tyring SK. An overview of sexually transmitted diseases. Part III. Sexually transmitted diseases in HIV-infected patients. J Am Acad Dermatol. 2000 Sep; 43(3):409–32.
– Gilbert DN, Moellering RC Jr, Eliopoulos GM, Chambers HF, Saag MS, editors. The Sanford guide to antimicrobial therapy 2010. 40th ed. USA: Antimicrobial Therapy Inc.; 2010.
– Singh AE, Romanowski B. Syphilis: review with emphasis on clinical, epidermiologic, and some biologic features. Clin Microbiol Rev. 1999 Apr; 12(2): 187–209.

Systemic Lupus Erythematosus (SLE)

- Diagnosis (**requires 4 of 11** criteria for diagnosis)
  - Malar erythema (tends to spare nasolabial folds)
  - Discoid lupus erythematosus
  - Photosensitivity (patient history or examination)
  - Oral ulcers (oral/nasopharyngeal ulceration; usually painless)
  - Arthritis (nonerosive) involving >2 peripheral joints. Characterized by ten-derness, swelling, or effusion
  - Serositis (pericarditis or pleuritis)
  - Nephropathy
    - Persistent proteinuria >0.5 g/day or 3+ (or)
    - Cellular casts (red cell, hemoglobin, granular, tubular, mixed)
  - **Neurologic disorder** (seizures/psychosis in absence of drugs or metabolic derangements)
  - **Hematologic disorder**
    - Hemolytic anemia with reticulocytosis OR
    - Leukopenia <4,000/mm3 on two occasions OR
    - Lymphopenia <1,500/mm3 on two occasions OR
    - Thrombocytopenia <100,000/mm^3
  - **Immunologic disorder** (+LE-prep; anti-DNA Ab or Sm Ag or false + for syphilis known to be + for ≥6 months)
  - **Antinuclear antibody**

- Useful Laboratory Tests in Evaluation of SLE

Complete Blood Count	Anemia, leukopenia, thrombocytopenia
Differential	Check for lymphopenia
ESR	Usually elevated (but nonspecific)
Creatinine	± Elevated with renal involvement
Urinalysis	Check for proteinuria, hematuria, casts
RPR/VDRL	False-positive test may occur with SLE
ANA	95% with SLE (use Hep-2 cell line)
dsDNA	Increased risk of renal disease
ssDNA	Sensitive but not specific
Sm	Highest specificity for SLE
nRNP	Decreased risk of renal disease
C3/C4	Decreased with active disease
Antiphospholipid Ab	May occur with SLE
Anti-histone Ab	Drug-induced lupus

Table 99 Features more suggestive of C2 deficiency-associated SLE than classic SLE

1. Childhood onset of photosensitivity
2. Extensive, treatment-resistant skin lesions associated with SCLE, ACLE or DLE
3. Mild or absent renal disease
4. Absent or low-titer ANA and anti-dsDNA antibodies
5. Negative lupus band test
6. Less severe disease overall
7. Pyogenic infections associated with encapsulated bacteria (e.g. *Streptococcus pneumoniae*)
8. Increased risk of atherosclerosis

Stevens–Johnson Syndrome and Toxic Epidermal Necrolysis (TEN)

Etiology and Pathogenesis

- Precise sequence of events is only partially understood. Tissue damage is due to massive keratinocyte cell death via apoptosis, likely by the Fas (CD95)-Fas ligand (CD95L) pathway
- SJS/TEN due to allopurinol – genetic predisposition with HLA-B*5801
- SJS/TEN due to carbamezapine – HLA-B*1502
- SJS/TEN and ocular complications – HLA-DQB1*0601

Clinical Presentation

- Skin lesions tend to appear first on trunk, spreading to the neck, face, and proximal upper extremities
  - **Morphology** – erythematous, dusky red or purpuric macules which are irregular in size and shape. Coalesce together. Nikolsky sign present (dermal–epidermal cleavage occurs). Some patients have targetoid lesions similar to that seen in erythema multiforme. As full-thickness necrosis occurs, lesions become grayish. Fluid fills space between the dermis and epidermis. Tense blisters usually seen only on palmoplantar surfaces where the epidermis is thicker and more resistant to mild trauma
  - Mucosal erosions present in>90% of patients
  - Very painful
- Erythema and erosions of the buccal, ocular, and genital mucosae are present in more than 90% of patients
- Other organs – May involve epithelium of respiratory tract in 25% of TEN patients, GI involvement (esophagitis, diarrhea)
- Definitions
  - SJS<10% of body surface area (BSA)
  - SJS-TEN overlap: 10–30% BSA
  - TEN>30% BSA
- **Factors correlated with poor outcome (see SCORETEN)** – increasing age, extent of epidermal attachment, number of medications, elevation of serum urea and creatinine and glucose, neutropenia, lymphopenia, thrombocytopenia, late withdrawal of drug
- **Complications**
  - Death (occurs 1 in 3 mainly due to *Staph aureus* and *Pseudomonas aeruginosa*)
  - Fluid and electrolyte imbalances
  - Catabolic state
  - Insulin resistance

- o Adult respiratory distress syndrome
- o Multiple organ failure
- o Long-term → scarring of the skin and mucosal surfaces, symblepharon, conjunctival synechiae, entropion, ingrowth of eyelashes, phimosis, vaginal synechiae, nail dystrophy, diffuse hair loss

Labs

- Labs – CBC, CMP, CPK, PT/PTT, amylase, lipase, urea, IgA level
- Blood cultures
- Periodic skin and wound cultures

DDx – erythema multiforme, staph scalded skin syndrome, acute generalized exanthematous pustulosis, generalized fixed drug eruption, paraneoplastic pemphigus, drug-induced linear IgA bullous dermatosis, Kawasaki disease, severe acute GVHD

Histology

- Early → apoptotic keratinocytes observed scattered in the basal and intermediate suprabasal layers of the epidermis
- Later → Subepidermal blister with overlying complete necrosis of the entire epidermis and a sparse perivascular infiltrate composed mostly of lymphocytes

Treatment and Management of TEN

[ ] **Discontinue offending agent! Avoid unnecessary medications. Admit to the burn unit.**
[ ] Punch biopsy – edge of blister for H&E
[ ] Punch biopsy – perilesional for DIF
[ ] Send viral culture and Tzanck Smear of vesicles/bullae
[ ] Intermittent wound cultures
[ ] Blood cultures
[ ] Check IgA level – do not start IVIG without knowing that this is normal first
[ ] Keep wounds moist – polysporin, bactroban, bacitracin. Xeroform gauze ok, but no tape
[ ] Silver-impregnated sheets very helpful to prevent secondary infection
[ ] Gentle handling of patient by staff – to avoid creating new lesions
[ ] No debridement! Only gentle removal of dead skin to prevent further tearing
[ ] Labs – CBC, CMP, CPK, PT/PTT, amylase, lipase, urea, IgA level

[ ] **IVIG** – 1 g/kg/day×3 days (adults) or 0.75 g/kg/day×3 days (children) – follow WBC and BUN QD Make sure IgA level normal before starting.
[ ] Ophthalmology consult
[ ] Hydration critical
[ ] Nutrition critical
[ ] Use a controlled-pressure thermoregulated bed and aluminum survival sheet (if available)
[ ] IVs should be placed in uninvolved skin, if possible
[ ] Pain control – do not use pain patches

Pearls and Pitfalls

– Admit to the burn unit
– No aggressive debridement!

* Side effects of IVIG – injection reaction (≤1 h), headache, flushing, chills, myalgia, wheezing, back pain, nausea, hypotension, anaphylaxis with IgA deficiency, thrombosis, renal failure (sucrose-containing solutions)

Table 100 SCORETEN Severity-of-Illness score

SCORETEN Parameter	Individual Score
Age>40 years	Yes=1, No=0
Malignancy	Yes=1, No=0
Tachycardia>120/min	Yes=1, No=0
Initial surface of epidermal detachment	Yes=1, No=0
Serum urea>10 mmol/l or>58 mg/dl	Yes=1, No=0
Serum glucose>14 mmol/l or>255 mg/dl	Yes=1, No=0
Bicarbonate<20 mmol/l or<20 mEq/l	Yes=1, No=0
SCORETEN (sum of individuals scores) and Associated Mortality – only useful in first 24 h	
0–1 → 3.2%	
2 → 12.1%	
3 → 35.3%	
4 → 58.3%	
> or=5 → 90%	

Trent JT et al. Analysis of intravenous immunoglobulin for the treatment of toxic epidermal necrolysis using SCORTEN. *Arch Dermatol* 2003; 139: 39–43
Bastuji-Garin, Fouchard N, Mertocchi M, Roujeau JC, Revuz J, Wolkenstein P. SCORTEN: A severity-of-illness score for toxic epidermal necrolysis. *J Invest Dermatol* 2000; 115: 149–153

Tinea

Common Fungal Isolates and Their Significance

Courtesy of Judy Warner

At the UAB Fungal Reference Laboratory, protocols dictate that for a nail specimen only the dermatophytes and the non-dermatophyte causes of Onychomycosis will be reported. For skin specimens, all organisms will be reported since the laboratory has no knowledge of the patient's immunocompetency. If you ever question if the organism is the "real" cause, repeat the culture and see if the same organism is isolated.

Here are some of the most common isolates and pathogens. This list includes the most common isolates that might be reported to you that may or may not be the pathogen in the case. The true pathogens such as all the dermatophytes and dimorphic molds have not been included.

Table 101 Common fungal isolates and their significance

Organism	Clinical Significance
Acremonium sp.	Is a non-dermatophyte cause of onychomycosis but is a common contaminant
Aspergillus sp.	There are several species all important in the immunocompromised patient but only Aspergillus flavus, Aspergillus terreus, and Aspergillus versicolor are considered causes of onychomycosis
Aureobasidium pullulans	Will occasionally cause a cutaneous infection but is a common contaminate
Bipolaris sp.	A common contaminate but may be important in the immunocompromised patient
Candida albicans	Most common cause of candidiasis but can be found as normal flora of the skin and mouth and vaginal mucosa
Candida krusei	Causes infections in immunocompromised patients and is resistant to fluconazole
Candida parapsilosis	Common cause of paronychia. But is normal flora on the skin
Candida tropicalis	Can cause disease in immunocompromised patients but is normal skin flora
Chaetomium sp.	Occasionally a cause of onychomycosis; isolated from dirt
Cladophialophora sp.	Nonpathogenic sp are called Cladosporium sp. Can cause chromoblastomycosis. But are a common contaminant
Curvularia sp.	Rarely a cause of infection. But a very common contaminant
Epicoccum sp.	Contaminant
Exophiala sp.	Can cause phaeohyphomycoses and tinea nigra, but can be contaminant
Fonsecaea sp.	Agent of chromoblastomycosis – will make sclerotic cells. But is also a common contaminant from soil and plants
Fusarium sp.	A non-dermatophyte cause of onychomycosis – it can be a common contaminant
Malassezia furfur	Causes tinea versicolor and Seb derm. This organism is seen on KOH/Calcofluor but will only grow in culture with an oil overlay
Nigrospora sp.	Common contaminant

(continued)

Organism	Clinical Significance
Paecilomyces lilacinus	A common contaminant now thought to be a non-dermatophyte cause of onychomycosis
Penicillium sp.	Usually nonpathogenic
Phialophora sp.	A cause of chromoblastomycosis, and yet can be a contaminant
Phoma sp.	A common plant pathogen that makes large pycnidia. Rare cases of subcutaneous phaeohyphomycosis have been seen
Pithomyces sp.	No infections reported. A common saprophytic mold
Rhodotorula sp.	Is a common contaminant but can colonize immunocompromised patients
Scedosporium apiospermum	**Scedosporium apiospermum** is the asexual stage of **Pseudallescheria boydii.** Systemic infections are most common maybe subcutaneous of cutaneous
Scopulariopsis sp.	A non-dermatophyte cause of onychomycosis
Scytalidium sp.	A non-dermatophyte cause of onychomycosis and skin infections
Trichosporon sp.	Causes white peidra and can be invasion and cause superficial and subcutaneous infections. Can also be a contaminant
Wangiella dermatitidis	Causes phaeohyphomycoses and can be disseminated in some patients. Is also isolated from soil and plant material
Zygomycetes: Mucor sp. Rhizopus sp. Rhizomucor sp.	Are all causes of zygomycosis but are very common contaminants

Tinea Pedis

Etiology and Pathogenesis

- Term used for a dermatophyte infection of the soles of the feet and the interdigital spaces
- **Etiology**
  - **Dermatophytes** – *Trichophyton rubrum*(*most common worldwide*), *T. mentagrophytes,* and *Epidermophyton floccosm, Trichophyton tonsurans* (reported in children)
  - **Non-dermatophytes** – *Scytalidium dimidiatum, Scytalidium hyalinum,* and, rarely, *Candida* species
- **Pathogenesis**
  - Dermatophyte fungi invade the superficial keratin of the skin via keratinases
  - Dermatophyte cell walls contain mannans, which can inhibit body's immune response
  - *T. rubrum* contains mannans that may reduce keratinocyte proliferation, resulting in a decreased rate of sloughing and a chronic state of infection
  - Temperature and serum factors, such as beta globulins and ferritin, appear to have a growth-inhibitory effect on dermatophytes – not completely understood
  - Sebum also is inhibitory, thus partly explaining the propensity for dermatophyte infection of the feet, which have no sebaceous glands

Clinical Presentation and Types

- **Interdigital** – erythema, maceration, fissuring, and scaling, most often seen between the fourth and fifth toes. Pruritus common. Dorsal foot usually clear, but can have extension onto plantar surface. Can be associated with *dermatophytosis complex*, which is infection with fungi followed by an infection with bacteria
- **Chronic hyperkeratotic** – characterized by chronic plantar erythema with slight scaling to diffuse hyperkeratosis. This type can be asymptomatic or pruritic. Also called moccasin tinea pedis, after its moccasin-like distribution. Both feet are usually affected. Dorsal surface of the foot is clear, but, in severe cases, the condition may extend onto the sides of the foot
- **Inflammatory/vesicular** – Painful, pruritic vesicles or bullae, most often on instep of plantar surface. Lesions contain either clear or purulent fluid; after they rupture, scaling with erythema persists. Cellulitis, lymphangitis, and adenopathy can complicate this type. Can be associated with eruption called the dermatophytid reaction, which develops on the palmar surface of one or both hands and/or the sides of the fingers (can mimic dyshidrosis). Close inspection of feet is necessary in patients with vesicular hand dermatoses. Dermatophytid reaction resolves when tinea pedis infection is treated, and tx of hands with topical steroids can hasten resolution

- **Ulcerative** – Rapidly spreading vesiculopustular lesions, ulcers, and erosions, typically in the web spaces. Often accompanied by a secondary bacterial infection. May be accompanied by cellulitis, lymphangitis, pyrexia, and malaise. Occasionally, large areas, even the entire sole, can be sloughed. Seen in immunocompromised, diabetics

Labs

- KOH; when blisters present – scrape roof of vesicle for highest fungal yield
- Fungal culture; use media without cycloheximide, which inhibits non-dermatophytes

DDx – candida, ACD, dyshidrosis, erythema multiforme, erythrasma, friction blisters, PRP, psoriasis, syphilis, autoimmune blistering disease, bacterial infection, xerosis, eczematous dermatitis, irritant contact dermatitis

Histology – parakeratosis with "sandwich sign" (basket weave stratum corneum) or compact hyperkeratosis. See hyphal structures on PAS. Sparse lymphocytic infiltrate.

Treatment

- Topical
  - Clotrimazole 1% cream BID – for 2–6 weeks
  - Spectazole 1% cream BID – 4 weeks
  - Ketoconazole 1% cream BID – 4 weeks
  - Miconazole cream and lotion BID – 2–6 weeks
  - Oxiconazole 1% cream BID – 4 weeks
  - Sertaconazole cream BID – 4 weeks
  - Ciclopirox 1% cream (Loprox) BID – 4 weeks
  - Naftifine 1% cream and gel (Naftin) → cream QD×4 weeks; gel BID×4 weeks
  - Terbinafine (Lamisil) cream BID – 1–4 weeks
  - Butenafine 1% cream (Mentax) – Apply BID for 1 week or QD for 4 weeks
  - Special conditions
    - Moccasin-type tinea pedis is often recalcitrant to topical antifungals alone, owing to the thickness of the scale on the plantar surface. The concomitant use of topical urea or other keratolytics with topical antifungals should help
    - Moccasin tinea pedis caused by *Scytalidium* species – Whitfield solution (contains benzoic and salicylic acids), can be beneficial

- **Oral** – consider if concomitant onychomycosis, extensive disease, diabetics, peripheral vascular disease, or immunocompromised
  - Itraconazole (Sporanox) – 200 mg PO qd for 1 week; not to exceed 400 mg/day; increase in 100-mg increments if no improvement (administer >200 mg/day in divided doses)
  - Terbinafine (Lamisil) – 250 mg PO qd for 1–2 week
  - Fluconazole (Diflucan) – 150 mg PO q week for up to 4 week

Pearls and Pitfalls

– **Prevention**
  - Wear protective footwear in communal areas – may decrease the likelihood of infection
  - Because infected scales can be present on clothing, frequent laundering is a good idea
  - Minimize foot moisture by limiting the use of occlusive footwear and should discard shoes that may be contributing to recurrence of the infection
  - Treat hyperhidrosis, if present
  - Weekly antifungal spray or antifungal powder to shoes

Tinea Pedis Handout (*Courtesy of Dr. Elewski*)

To prevent further infections with tinea pedis, "athlete's foot", we suggest you follow the following instructions:

1. Avoid going barefoot in public facilities especially gymnasiums, locker rooms, and other athletic facilities
2. Never wear someone else's shoes
3. When staying in hotels, never go without footwear in rooms as fungal particles may be living in the carpeting and on the bathroom floors
4. Use an antifungal powder or spray such as Tinactin powder, Micatin powder, or Zeasorb AF in your shoes at least once a week
5. Older tennis shoes and well-worn shoes should be thrown away as they may be heavily contaminated with fungal particles
6. Wear shoes that are not too narrow and made of materials that allow one's feet to "breathe", such as leather
7. Wear socks made of natural materials such as cotton and wool as opposed to synthetic materials such as rayon and polyester
8. If you see any signs of athlete's foot recurring, restart the prescription product we gave you as soon as possible. You might also consider an over-the-counter product such as Micatin or Lotrimin
9. Be sure other family members who may be infected are adequately treated
10. If you have any questions, please do not hesitate to call our office

Tinea Versicolor

Etiology and Pathogenesis

- Eleven species of *M furfur* have been described, with **Malassezia globosa** being the usual form isolated in persons with tinea versicolor
- Risk factors that lead to the conversion of the saprophytic yeast to the parasitic, mycelial morphologic form include a genetic predisposition; warm, humid environments; immunosuppression; malnutrition; and Cushing disease
  - Not considered contagious b/c the organism is a normal inhabitant of skin

Clinical Presentation

- A common, benign, superficial cutaneous fungal infection usually characterized by hypopigmented or hyperpigmented macules and patches on the chest and the back. In patients with a predisposition, the condition may chronically recur. The fungal infection is localized to the stratum corneum
- Affected skin may be either hypopigmented or hyperpigmented or red-brown
  - In the case of hypopigmentation, tyrosinase inhibitors (resulting from the inhibitory action of tyrosinase of dicarboxylic acids formed through the oxidation of some unsaturated fatty acids of skin surface lipids) competitively inhibit a necessary enzyme of melanocyte pigment formation
  - In hyperpigmented macules in tinea versicolor, the organism induces an enlargement of melanosomes made by melanocytes at the basal layer of the epidermis

Labs

- Wood's light – can be used to demonstrate the coppery-orange fluorescence of tinea versicolor. However, in some cases, the lesions appear darker than the unaffected skin under the Wood light, but they do not fluoresce
- KOH examination – demonstrates the characteristic short, cigar-butt hyphae that are present in the diseased state
  - KOH finding → Spaghetti and meatballs or Ziti and meatballs
  - For better visualization, ink blue stain, Parker ink, methylene blue stain, or Swartz-Medrik stain can be added to the KOH preparation

DDx – erythrasma, pityriasis alba, guttate psoriasis, seb derm, tinea corporis, vitiligo, CARP

Histology – See hyphae and budding yeast in the stratum corneum (best seen with PAS or GMS stains), but skin otherwise looks normal. May see slight perivascular inflammation, but not always.

Treatment

- Patients should be informed that tinea versicolor is caused by a fungus that is normally present on the skin surface and is therefore not considered contagious
- The condition does not leave any permanent scar or pigmentary changes, and any skin color alterations resolve within 1–2 months after treatment has been initiated
- Recurrence is common, and prophylactic tx may help reduce high rate of recurrence
- **Selenium sulfide** – lotion is liberally applied to affected areas of the skin daily for 2 weeks; each application is allowed to remain on the skin for at least 10 min prior to being washed off. In resistant cases, overnight application can be helpful
  - **Selsun Blue Shampoo**
- **Sodium sulfacetamide**
- **Topical antifungals** – can be applied every night for 2 weeks. Weekly application of any of the topical agents for the following few months may help prevent recurrence. Can be expensive in patients with widespread disease
  - **Clotrimazole cream** – Gently massage into affected area and surrounding skin areas BID for 2–6 weeks
  - **Terbinafine cream** – apply BID for 2–4 weeks
  - **Ketoconazole cream** – Rub gently into affected area BID for 2–4 weeks
  - **Naftin cream/gel** – apply QD for 2–4 weeks
  - **Econazole (Spectazole)** – apply QD-BID
  - **Oxiconazole (Oxistat)** – apply QID
  - **Ciclopirox olamine (Loprox)** – apply BID for 1–4 weeks
- **Ketoconazole** – a single-dose 400-mg treatment on Day 1; repeat in 7 days
- Fluconazole has been offered as a single 150–300-mg weekly dose for 2–4 weeks
- Itraconazole is usually given at 200 mg/day for 7 days

Pearls and Pitfalls

- Instruct patient taking ketoconazole to take with an acidic beverage such as orange juice or soda, which will help with absorption. Additionally, take the medication 1 h prior to exercising and sweating. Medication excreted in the sweat and is most effective this way
- Oral therapy does not prevent the risk of recurrence; patient will still need to take prophylactic measures in many cases
- Oral terbinafine does not work for tinea versicolor, although *in vitro* studies suggest fungistatic activity. Topical terbinafine does seem to help, however

Tuberculosis of the Skin

Table 102 Tuberculosis of the skin

	Tuberculous Chancre	Tuberculosis Verrucosa Cutis	Lupus Vulgaris	Scrofuloderma	Tuberculous Gumma	Tuberculosis Cutis Orificialis
	Primary (exogenous) inoculation	Exogenous reinfection	Hematogenous, lymphatic or contiguous spread from distant site of TB infection	Contiguous spread onto skin from underlying TB infection	Hematogenous spread	Autoinoculation from underlying advanced visceral tuberculosis
	Non-sensitized host	Sensitized host with strong immunity	Sensitized host with moderate to high immunity	Sensitized host with low immunity	Immunosuppressed host	Sensitized host with diminishing immunity
	Pauci- or multi-bacillary, depending on stage of infection and strength of immune response	Paucibacillary	Paucibacillary	Multi- or paucibacillary	Multi-bacillary	Multi-bacillary
	• Painless red-brown papule that ulcerates • Tuberculosis primary complex: regional LN, 3–8 weeks post infection	• Slowly growing verrucous plaques with irregular borders • Typically on hand • Most common form • TB skin test +	• Brownish-red plaque • "Apple-jelly" color on diascopy • Head/neck involvement in 90% of cases	• Subcutaneous nodules with purulent or caseous drainage • May develop sinuses and ulcers with granulating bases • Occurs most commonly over cervical lymph nodes	• Subcutaneous abscesses • May form fistulas and ulcers • Typically on trunk, head, or extremities	• Punched-out ulcers with undermined edges • On mucocutaneous junctions of mouth, genitalia

Tzanck Smear

Courtesy of Dr. Matthew Wood

-Suitable for HSV, VZV, CMV, or even tumors, if a rapid diagnosis is needed.

Choose a fresh vesicle (less than 3 days old, and **not crusted**).

Deroof the vesicle carefully with a #15 blade and scrape the base with moderate pressure. Remember you are trying to scrape away the acantholytic cells.

Gently smear onto the slide.

Repeat. The more cells you get on the slide, the more likely you are to get the diagnosis, but be careful to smear it into a thin coat, because if cells are sitting on top of one another, it makes it difficult to interpret.

Allow to air dry.

Apply a few drops of mineral oil, then coverslip. The large coverslips are best, as they allow you more room for the smear. If not available, two of the smaller coverslips side by side will do.

Scan on low power (high power is for wimps), looking for multinucleate keratinocytes, acantholytic keratinocytes, and enlarged nuclei with peripheral margination of chromatin. Any of these are diagnostic of *herpesviridae* infection.

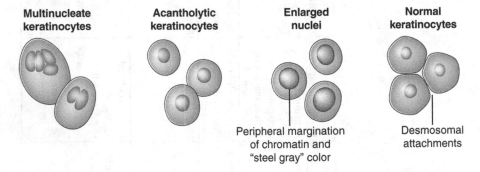

| Multinucleate keratinocytes | Acantholytic keratinocytes | Enlarged nuclei | Normal keratinocytes |

Peripheral margination of chromatin and "steel gray" color

Desmosomal attachments

Tip for beginners: use a tongue depressor to scrape your buccal mucosa and smear it, just the same as above. Stain it up and compare the cytology of these normal keratinocytes to those you see in the Tzanck.

Fig. 21 Microscopic features of a herpetic infection: (**a**) Multinucleated keratinocytes (**b**) Acantholytic keratinocytes (**c**) Enlarged nuclei with peripheral margination of chromatin and "steel gray" color

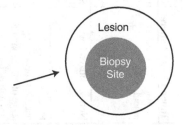

Lesion

Biopsy Site

Fig. 22 Where to biopsy a herpetic lesion for H&E

Ulcers

Table 103 Comparison of clinical findings in the three major types of leg ulcers

	Venous	Arterial	Neuropathic
Location	Medial malleolar region	Pressure sites Distal points (toes)	Pressure sites
Morphology	Irregular borders	Dry, necrotic base "Punched out"	"Punched out"
Surrounding Skin	Pigmentation secondary to hemosiderin	Shiny atrophic skin with hair loss	Thick callus
Other physical exam findings	Varicosities Leg/ankle edema +/– stasis dermatitis +/– lymphedema	– Weak/absent peripheral pulses – Prolonged capillary refill time (> 3–4 s) – Pallor on leg elevation (45° for 1 min) – Dependent rubor	–Peripheral neuropathy with ↓ sensation +/– foot deformities

- **Treatment of Venous Ulcers**
  - Important to measure ABI to rule out arterial disease
    - ABI < 0.8 indicates arterial disease; compression only with caution
    - ABI < 0.5 – compression is contraindicated
  - Compression
    - Compression is better than no compression
    - High compression is better than low compression; contraindicated in arterial dz
    - Stockings need to be replaced at least every 6 months
  - Moist wound environment accelerates healing; occlusion decreases infection rates
  - Debridement can be helpful
  - Antiseptics
    - Avoid – chlorhexidine, betadine, hydrogen peroxide, astringents, and bleach for open wounds → cytotoxic and likely impair epithelialization and delay healing
  - Pentoxifylline (decrease TNF-α) – 800 mg TID; SE – GI upset, dizziness
  - Treatment pearls (*courtesy of Dr. Aton Holzer*) –
    - Pentoxifylline (Trental) – 400 mg PO TID **plus**
    - Folate 1 mg PO QD **plus**
    - Doxycycline 100 mg PO BID (inhibits MMPs) **plus**
    - Silvadene (if no allergy to sulfa)
  - Apligraf® – FDA approved for tx of venous and diabetic foot ulcers that fail to heal despite adequate clinical tx
- **Treatment of Arterial Ulcers**
  - Goal is to reestablish adequate arterial supply; patients should be referred to a vascular surgeon for assessment and treatment

○ Encourage lifestyle changes → lose weight, stop smoking, control HTN and diabetes, lower lipids, exercise under direction of MD. Aspirin/Plavix may be indicated.

○ Debridement can be detrimental and should be avoided

- **Treatment of Neuropathic and Diabetic Ulcers**
  ○ Management → Aggressive debridement, tx of associated arterial dz, offloading of pressure, restoring circulating to lower extremity when necessary, tx infection if present
  ○ Education and preventative measures must be stressed
    - Inspect feet daily. Applying a lotion to the feet daily may help them do this. If vision impaired, have someone help them
    - Wash feet daily in warm water; dry between the toes
    - Always test water temperature before bathing
    - Inspect insides of the shoes before putting them on
    - Do not remove corns or apply strong chemicals to the feet
    - Cut nails straight across
    - Wear properly fitting shoes; new shoes should be worn for 1–2 h daily only. Check feet for red spots afterwards
    - Avoid open-toed shoes and pointed shoes
    - Never walk barefoot
  ○ Debridement can be helpful
  ○ Apligraf® – FDA approved for tx of venous and diabetic foot ulcers that fail to heal despite adequate clinical tx
  ○ Hyperbaric oxygen therapy may be helpful
  ○ Short-contact topical tretinoin solution (0.05%) – apply for 10 min daily, then wash off
  ○ Becaplermin (human platelet-derived growth factor) – FDA-approved for adjunctive tx for diabetic neuropathic ulcers

References:

(1) Fonder MA, Lazarus GS, Cowan DA, et al. Treating the chronic wound: A practical approach to the care of nonhealing wounds and wound care dressings. J Am Acad Dermatol 2008; 58(2): 185–206.
(2) Tom WL, Peng DH, Allaei A, et al. The effect of short-contact topical tretinoin therapy for foot ulcers in patients with diabetes. Arch Dermatol 2005; 141(11): 1373–7.
(3) Phillips TJ, Dover JS. Leg Ulcers. J Am Acad Dermatol 1991; 25: 965–87.

Urticaria

Etiology and Pathogenesis

Table 104   Some causes of urticaria

Causes of Urticaria		
Infections	Bacterial	Cholecystitis Cystitis Dental abscess *Helicobacter pylori* Hepatitis Otitis Pneumonitis Sinusitis Vaginitis
	Fungal	Tinea Candida
	Other	Scabies Helminth Protozoa *Trichomonas* Syphilis
Drugs & Chemicals	Salicylates NSAIDs Opiates Radiocontrast material Penicillin (medication, milk, blue cheese) Sulfonamides Sodium benzoate Douches Ear drops or eyedrops Insulin Menthol (cigarettes, toothpaste, iced tea, lotions, lozenges, candy) Tartrazine (vitamins, birth control pills, antibiotics, yellow #5)	
Foods	Nuts Berries Fish Seafood Bananas Grapes Tomatoes Eggs Cheese	
Inhalants	Animal dander Pollen	

Causes of Urticaria	
Systemic Disease	Rheumatic fever Juvenile rheumatoid arthritis Leukemia Lymphoma Connective tissue disease (lupus, RA, Sjögren's) HIV/AIDS
Endocrinopathies	Thyroid disease Diabetes mellitus Pregnancy Menstruation Menopause
Physical Stimuli	Light Pressure Heat Cold Water Vibration

Contactants	Wool
	Silk
	Occupational exposures
	Potatoes
	Antibiotics
	Cosmetics
	   Dyes
	   Hairspray
	   Nail polish
	   Mouthwash
	   Toothpaste
	   Perfumes
	   Hand cream
	   Soap
	Insect repellant

Familial Disorders	Hereditary angioedema Muckle-Wells syndrome

Reference: Lee AD and Jorizzo JL. Urticaria. In: Callen JP, Jorizzo JL (eds). Dermatological Signs of Internal Disease , 4th edn. Saunders Elsevier, 2009: 53–62

- Urticaria may be immunologic or non-immunologic
  - **Immunologic** – autoantibodies against FcεRI or IgE, IgE-dependent (allergic), immune complex (vasculitic), complement- and kinin-dependent (C1 esterase inhibitor deficiency)
  - **Non-Immunologic** – direct mas cell-releasing agents (e.g., opiates), vasoactive stimuli (e.g., nettle stings), aspirin and other NSAIDs, angiotensin-converting enzyme (ACE) inhibitors

Clinical Presentation and Types

- Pink to erythematous urticarial wheals that come and go within 24 h. Angioedema involves deeper dermis and subcutaneous tissues and may lead to anaphylaxis
- **Physical Urticarias**
    - o **Due to mechanical stimuli** – sites of friction (collars, cuffs of clothes), after scratching
    - o **Delayed pressure urticaria** – deep erythematous swellings at sites of sustained pressure to the skin (elastic of socks, under bra, in genital area after intercourse), after a delay of 30 min to 12 h. Usually painful, pruritic, or both. May get systemic features
    - o **Vibratory urticaria** – jogging, lawnmowers, motorcycles, jack hammers. May be acquired or familial (AD)
- **Urticaria due to Temperature Changes**
    - o **Heat and stress exposure** – occur within 15 min of sweat-induced stimuli such as moving from hot to cold room, drinking alcohol, eating spicy foods, in hot weather
    - o **Exercise-induced urticaria or anaphylaxis** – produced by exercise
    - o **Adrenergic urticaria** – presence of blanched vasoconstricted skin surrounding pink wheals induced by sudden stress. Can be reproduced by intradermal injections of norepinephrine
    - o **Localized heat contact urticaria** – very rare. Lesions develop within minutes of coming into contact with any heat source. Systemic symptoms may occur
    - o **Primary cold contact urticaria** – usually idiopathic. May follow respiratory infections, bites/stings, HIV. Seen commonly in young adults. Itching, burning, and whealing occur in cold-exposed areas minutes after rewarming the skin. May occur after contact with cold objects such as ice cubes. Mean duration is 6–9 years
    - o **Secondary cold contact urticaria** – extremely rare. Due to serum abnormalities such as cryoglobulins or cryofibrinogenemia, hepatitis B or C, mononucleosis or lymphoproliferative disease. See other manifestations such as Raynaud's or purpura. Lesions may last longer than 24 h
    - o **Reflex cold urticaria** – generalized cooling induces widespread whealing. Can experience life-threatening reactions by diving into a cold lake. Ice cube test is negative
    - o **Familial cold urticaria** – this condition allelic with Muckle–Wells (see *periodic fevers*). Mutation in CIAS1 (cryopyrin). Burning, itching plaques that can last 48 h. Anakinra may help
- **Urticaria due to Other Exposures**
    - o **Solar urticaria** – itching and whealing with UV exposure. Wheals last for < 1 h, but can get headache, syncope. Primary form seen with type I hypersensitivity and secondary form may be seen with porphyria
    - o **Aquagenic urticaria** – contact with water of any temperature induces lesions. Physical urticarias must be differentiated

- **Urticarial Vasculitis** – vaculitis that mimics urticaria clinically, but LCV on pathology. Lesions may leave behind bruising (because of vessel damage) and may last longer than 24 h. Lesions painful and pruritic. Angioedema occurs in 40%. See arthralgias. May see GI, renal dz. Rarely see Raynaud's, lymphadenopathy, splenomegaly, eye problems, pseudotumor cerebri, muscle and heart involvement. Patients with hypocomplementemia tend to have more frequent and more severe systemic involvement and course less favorable. May have – SLE, hep B/C, Lyme, mononucleosis, drug (cimetidine, diltiazem), hypergammaglobulinemia, hematologic disorders
- **Distinctive Urticarial Syndromes**
  - **Muckle–Wells syndrome** –*see periodic fevers*
  - **Familial Mediterranean fever** –*see periodic fevers*
  - **Systemic capillary leak syndrome (Clarkson syndrome)** – rare, acquired disorder characterized by episodic massive plasma exudation from vessels, potentially leading to life-threatening hypotension (analogous to anaphylaxis). Associated with IgG paraproteinemia. Medications such as IL-2 can produce this

Labs and Imaging to Consider – CBC, renal function tests, LFTs, thyroid function tests, iron, B12, folate, ANA, dsDNA, rheumatoid factor, ESR, C3, C4, cryoglobulins, cryofibrinogen, urinalysis, syphilis serologies, anti-DNase B or streptococcal serologies, hepatitis B and C, mononucleosis serologies, *Helicobacter pylori* (IgM and IgG titers), stool specimen for ova and parasites (three samples), sinus x-rays, dental x-rays, chest x-ray, skin biopsy to rule out mimickers of urticarial

DDx – (all derm conditions with an urticarial component) – papular urticarial, Sweet's syndrome, urticarial bullous pemphigoid, urticarial vasculitis, acute facial contact dermatitis, urticarial drug eruption, urticarial pigmentosa

Histology

- Perivascular infiltrate of lymphocytes, eosinophils, and some neutrophils with extension of eosinophils into the dermis between collagen bundles. Inflammation very scant
- Some have a neutrophilic predominant pattern (a minority of patients), but no diagnostic significance
- Dermal edema (highly subjective)

Treatment

- Antihistamines
  - Hydroxyzine, doxepin, cetirizine, loratadine, desloratadine, fexofenadine, levocitirizine, diphenhydramine
- Leukotriene receptor antagonists
  - Montelukast 10 mg QD, Zafirlukast 20 mg BID
- Nifedipine (blood pressure medication) has mast cell stabilizing properties → 5–20 mg TID
- Other – Corticosteroids, cyclosporine, colchicine, dapsone, hydroxychloroquine, sulfasalazine (delayed pressure urticarial), methotrexate, mycophenolate mofetil, PO tacrolimus, plasmapheresis, PUVA, IVIG, omalizumab
- Non-drug therapies
  - Exclusion of food additives and natural salicylates from the diet has been advocated in a number of reports
  - Rice/Lamb diet – can only eat water, green tea, white rice, lamb, and white sugar. If symptoms have improved after 2 weeks, can slowly add back foods, one at a time. If no improvement at all, diet unlikely to be source of urticaria

Pearls and Pitfalls

- Check G6PD level prior to start dapsone or sulfasalazine
- Patients with a neutrophilic predominant pattern on path may do better with dapsone or colchicine if antihistamines alone are ineffective
- NSAIDs have been used to treat delayed pressure urticarial but may exacerbate chronic urticarial
- Check for porphyria if solar urticaria is present
- Give EpiPen or EpiPen Jr. if any signs/symptoms of anaphylaxis and refer to allergist
- Let history and clinical exam dictate what labs are ordered
- Lesions lasting longer than 24 h – urticarial vasculitis, secondary cold contact urticaria (croglobulins, cryofibrinogenemia, hep B/C, mono, lymphoproliferative disease), familial cold urticaria
- In SLE with urticaria, think about autoantibodies to C1q
- Consider ice cube test (wrap ice cube in bag to ensure that it is cold, not water, that is causing the urticaria)
- Over 75% of cases are idiopathic

Vasculitis

Etiology and Pathogenesis

Causes of Leukocytoclastic Vasculitis	
Drug Reaction *(10–15%)*	**Most common: NSAIDs** (including COX-2 inhibitors), **beta lactam ABX** (including PCN), **diuretics**, Anti-TNF agents, G-CSF, hydralazine, leukotriene inhibitors, minocycline, quinolones, streptokinase, propylthiouracil/other thyroid agents
	Occasionally: ACE inhibitors, allopurinol, beta-blockers, coumarins, furosemide, interferons, macrolides ABX, phenytoin, quinine, retinoids, sirolimus, sulfonylureas, thiazides, TMP-SMX, vancomycin
	Rare: amiodarone, aspirin, atypical antispscyhotics, bortezomib, cocaine, gabapentin, insulin, leflunomide, levamisole, mefloquine, metformin, methamphetamine, phenothiazines, quinidine, radiographic contrast media, rituximab, SSRIs, vitamins, food/drug additives, foods (e.g. gluten)
Connective Tissue Disease	**SLE, rheumatoid arthritis, Sjögren's syndrome**, mixed connective tissue disease, polyartertitis nodosa, dermatomyositis, seronegative spondyloarthropathies, sarcoidosis
Allergic Vasculitis	Henoch-Schönlein purpura, hypersensitivity vasculitis, urticarial vasculitis, Churg-Strauss syndrome, Polyartetitis nodosa, Wegener's
Cutaneous Diseases	Erythema multiforme, erythema elevatum diutinum, PLEVA, Behçet's syndrome, Finkelstein's acute hemorrhagic edema of infancy
Bacterial and Atypical Mycobacterial Infections	**Beta-hemolytic Streptococcus**, *Neisseria meningitides*, Staphylococcus, meningococcemia, gonococcemia, tuberculosis, leprosy
Viral Infections	Hepatitis B, **hepatitis C** (probably through cryoglobulins), EBV, HIV, coxsackie, echovirus, parvovirus B19, CMV(rare), varicella zoster virus (rare), influenza – including vaccine (rare)
Rickettsial Infections	Rocky Mountain Spotted Fever
Fungal Infections & Spirochete Infections	Syphilis
Inflammatory Bowel Disease	**Crohn's disease, Ulcerative colitis**
Proteins	Serum sickness, hyposensitization, cryoglobulinemia, dysproteinemia
Malignancy *(2–5%)*	Lymphoproliferative d/o – esp. **Hairy Cell Leukemia**, Hodgkin's lymphoma, myeloma, leukemia, lymphoma, lung CA, colon CA
Genetic *(rare)*	Immunodeficiency syndromes Familial Mediterranean fever and other periodic fever syndromes

Clinical Presentation

Table 105 Clinical manifestations of vasculitis based on vessel size affected

Large[1] Arteries	Medium Arteries	Medium Arteries and Small Vessels	Small Vessels (leukocytoclastic)
Primary • Giant cell arteritis • Takayasu's arteritis **Secondary** • Aortitis assoc with RA • Infection (syphilis, TB)	**Primary** • Classical PAN • Kawasaki disease **Secondary** • Hepatitis B associated PAN	**Primary** • Wegener's granulomatosis[2] • Churg-Strauss syndrome[2] • Microscopic polyangiitis[2] **Secondary** • Vasculitis secondary to RA, SLE, Sjögren's syndrome • Drugs • Infection (e.g. HIV)	**Primary** • Henoch-Schönlein purpura • Cryoglobulinemia • Cutaneous leukocytoclastic angiitis **Secondary** • Drugs (sulfonamides, PCNs, thiazide diuretics, etc.) • Hepatitis C associated • Infection
Limb claudication Asymmetric blood pressure Absence of pulses Aortic dilation Bruits Constitutional symptoms[3]	Subcutaneous nodules Ulcers (deep) Livedo reticularis Pitted palmar/digital scars Digital gangrene Mononeuritis Aneurysms Infarct Erythematous nodules Hypertension (renal artery) Constitutional symptoms[3]	(see medium-sized and small vessels)	Purpura Infiltrated erythema Urticaria Vesiculobullous lesions Ulcers (superficial) Splinter hemorrhages Scleritis, episcleritis, uveitis Palisaded neutrophilic granulomatous dermatitis Glomerulonephritis Gastric colic Pulmonary hemorrhage Constitutional symptoms[3]

[1] Large vessels (aorta and its branches) are not found in the skin. However, large-vessel vasculitic syndromes, giant cell arteritis, and Takayasu arteritis can rarely involve muscular arteries and small vessels of the skin.

[2] Diseases most commonly associated with ANCA (antimyeloperoxidase and antiproteinase 3 antibodies), with significant risk of renal involvement and which are most responsive to immunosuppression with cyclophosphamide.

[3] Fever, weight loss, malaise, arthralgia, and arthritis are common to vasculitic syndromes of all vessel sizes.

References:

1. Chen KR, Carlson JA. Clinical approach to cutaneous vasculitis. Am J Clin Dermatol. 2008; 9(2): 71–92.
2. Watts RA and Scott DGI. Epidemiology of vasculitis. In: Ball GV, Bridges SL (eds). Vasculitis, 2nd edn. New York: Oxford Univ Press, 2008: 7–21.

Labs

- **Basic Laboratory Studies for Patients with Confirmed Cutaneous Vasculitis**
  - Necessary
    - Complete blood count with differential
    - Basic Metabolic profile (including BUN, Creatinine, glomerular filtration rate)
    - Liver function tests
    - Erythrocyte sedimentation rate (ESR)
    - C-Reactive Protein (CRP)
    - Urinalysis
    - Cryoglobulins, serum/urine protein and immunofixation electrophoresis
    - Hepatitis C antibody, Hepatitis B surface Ag, HIV antibody
    - ANCAs (myeloperoxidase and proteinase-3) – should be done by indirect immunofluorescence for screening and ELISA to confirm (some labs use ELISA as the screening. UAB uses IIF.)
    - ANA, anti-SSA (Ro), anti-SSB (La)
    - Stool guiac
  - Optional
    - C3, C4, CH50
    - Rheumatoid factor (Usually IgM, but can also check IgA, IgG Rheumatoid factor)
    - Antistreptolysin O
    - Blood cultures
- Radiographic Examination
  - Chest X-ray

Histology – depends on type of vasculitis

- H&E
- Direct immunofluorescence (< 24 hrs optimal)

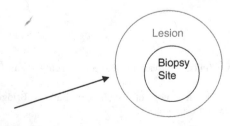

Fig. 23 Where to biopsy vasculitis lesion for DIF

DDx

Table 106 Mimickers of vasculitis

Relative Frequency	Mimicker	Mechanism
Common	Antiphospholipid antibody syndrome	Thrombosis
	Cholesterol embolization	Embolus
	Septic vasculitis[a]	Infection and embolus
	Infective endocarditis[a]	Infection and embolus
	Pigmented purpuric dermatitis	Hemorrhage
	Solar purpura	Hemorrhage
	Purpura fulminans	Thrombosis
	Warfarin necrosis	Thrombosis
	Livedo vasculopathy	Thrombosis
Less frequent than vasculitis	Hypothenar hammer syndrome	Vascular trauma
	(fibromuscular dysplasia)	Hemorrhage
	Scurvy	Thrombosis
	Thrombotic thrombocytopenic purpura	
Rare	Amyloidosis	Vessel-wall pathology
	Calciphylaxis	Vessel-wall pathology
	Cardiac myxoma	Embolus
	Ergotamine and cocaine abuse	Vasospasm
	Angiotropic B-cell lymphoma	Intravascular proliferation/embolus

[a] *Can also present as an authentic vasculitis with immune complex deposition*
Reference: Used with permission from Elsevier. Chen KR, Carlson JA. Clinical approach to cutaneous vasculitis. Am J Clin Dermatol. 2008; 9(2): 71–92

Treatment and Management

- **Management and Treatment (See Therapeutic Ladder)**
  - Determine whether the cutaneous vasculitis is primary or secondary to an underlying condition
    - Assess for history of – infections, drugs, inflammatory disease, previous history of associated disorders, neoplasm
  - Evaluate the patient for systemic involvement (labs help with this)
  - Elevation of the legs or compression stockings may be useful because the disease often affects dependent areas

Table 107 Therapeutic ladder for patients with vasculitis

Disorder	1st Line	2nd Line	3rd Line
Cutaneous Small vessel vasculitis	• d/c incriminated drugs • Supportive care • Treat underlying infections, neoplasm • NSAIDs • Antihistamines	• Colchicine (0.6 mg BID-TID) • Dapsone (50–200 mg/day) • Corticosteroids	• Azathioprine (2mg/kg/d) • Methotrexate
Henoch-Schönlein purpura	• Supportive Care	• Dapsone • Colchicine • Corticosteroids • Corticosteroids + Azathioprine • Corticosteroids + cyclophosphamide	• IVig • Aminocaproic acid • Plasmapheresis • Factor XIII
Acute hemorrhagic edema of infancy	• Supportive Care	• Antihistamines	• Corticosteroids
Urticarial vasculitis	• Antihistamines • Indomethacin • Dapsone (100–200mg/d) • Hydroxychloroquine (200–400 mg/d) • Corticosteroids	• Azathioprine • Colchicine (0.6 mg BID-TID)	• Mycophenolate mofetil • Rituximab
Erythema elevatum diutinum	• NSAIDs • Intralesional corticosteroids	• Dapsone • Colchicine • Hydroxychloroquine • Tetracyclines	• Niacinamide • Plasmapheresis
Cryoglobulinemic vasculitis (+HCV)	• Low antigen diet • Interferon + Ribavirin • Corticosteroids	• Corticosteroids + Cyclophosphamide	• IVig • Rituximab • Plasmapheresis
Cutaneous polyarteritis nodosa	• Treat underlying infections • d/c incriminated drugs • NSAIDs • Corticosteroids (topical, Intralesional or oral)	• Methotrexate (7.5–15 mg/wk) • Dapsone or sulfapyridine • IVig	• Pentoxifylline • Colchicine • Azathioprine or mycophenolate mofetil • Anti-TNF agents
Classic PAN (+HBV)	• Corticosteroids • Corticosteroids + Plasmapheresis + interferon/lamivudine	• Corticosteroids + Cyclophosphamide	• IVig
Microscopic polyangiitis	• Corticosteroids	• Corticosteroids + cyclophosphamide	• Azathioprine • Mycophenolate mofetil • IVig

(continued)

Table 107   (continued)
Table 107   Therapeutic ladder for patients with vasculitis

Disorder	1st Line	2nd Line	3rd Line
Wegener's granulomatosis (induction)	• Corticosteroids + Cyclophosphamide • Corticosteroids + Methotrexate	• TMP-SMX	• Mycophenolate mofetil • IVig • Corticosteroids + Rituximab • Plasmapheresis
Wegener's granulomatosis (relapse)	• Corticosteroids + Cyclophosphamide	• IVig	• Mycophenolate mofetil • Rituximab
Churg-Strauss syndrome	• Corticosteroids	• Corticosteroids + Cyclophosphamide	• IVig +/− plasmapheresis
Autoimmune connective tissue disease-associated vasculitis	• Corticosteroids • Corticosteroids + Cyclophosphamide (for severe systemic vasculitis)	• Corticosteroids + Azathioprine • Corticosteroids + Methotrexate	• Corticosteroids + Methotrexate • Corticosteroids + plasmapheresis

Reference: Used with permission from Elsevier. Chung L, Kea B and Fiorentino DF. Cutaneous vasculitis. In: Bolognia JL, Jorizzo JL, Rapini RP(eds). Dermatology, 2 nd edn. London: Mosby, 2009: 347–367

Vitiligo

Etiology and Pathogenesis

- Multifactorial disorder related to genetic and nongenetic factors
- Familial predisposition – susceptibility genes include *SLEV1* and *NALP1*
- Theories to etiology – autoimmune destruction, intrinsic defect of melanocytes, defective free radical defense(s), reduced melanocyte survival, viral infection, membrane lipid alterations in melanocytes, deficiency of unidentified melanocyte growth factor(s)

Clinical Presentation

- The widely used classification of vitiligo as localized, generalized, and universal types is based on the distribution, as follows:
  - **Localized**
    - Focal – One or more macules in one area but not clearly in a segmental or zosteriform distribution
    - Segmental – One or more macules in a quasidermatomal pattern
    - Mucosal – Mucus membrane alone
  - **Generalized**
    - Acrofacial – Distal extremities and face
    - Vulgaris – Scattered macules
    - Mixed – Acrofacial and vulgaris involvement, or segmental and acrofacial and/or vulgaris involvement
    - Universal – Complete or nearly complete depigmentation
  - When progression, prognosis, and treatment are considered, vitiligo can be classified into two major clinical types: segmental and nonsegmental
    - Segmental vitiligo usually has an onset early in life and rapidly spreads in the affected area
    - The course of segmental vitiligo can arrest and depigmented patches can persist unchanged for the life of the patient
    - The nonsegmental type includes all types of vitiligo except segmental vitiligo
- Common distribution = around eyes, mouth, genitals, and hands
- **Trichrome vitiligo** – lesions show a tan zone between the normal skin and completely depigmented skin
- **Quadrichrome vitiligo** – lesions show tan and dark brown between normal skin and depigmented skin
- **Isomorphic Koebner phenomenon** – vitiligo develops in sites of specific trauma
- Vitiligo may be associated with halo nevi, other autoimmune diseases, especially thyroid disease (Graves' disease, Hashimoto's thyroiditis), and diabetes mellitus.

Other associated autoimmune diseases include pernicious anemia, Addison disease, and alopecia areata

- Syndromes
  - **Vogt–Koyanagi–Harada (VKH) syndrome** – multisystem disorder characterized by uveitis, aseptic meningitis, otic involvement, poliosis and vitiligo, especially of the head and neck
  - **Alezzandrini syndrome** – whitening of scalp hair, eyebrows, eyelashes, as well as depigmentation of the skin of the forehead, nose, cheek, upper lip, and chin. Occur on same side as unilateral visual changes. Believed to be closely related to VKH
  - **APECED (autoimmune polyendocrinopathy-candidiasis-ectodermal dysplasia)** also have vitiligo. *AIRE* gene defect

Labs – TSH, fasting glucose or glycosylated hemoglobin, CBC+diff, B12, folate, ferritin, ANA, rheumatoid factor

DDx – leprosy, piebaldism, idiopathic guttate hypomelanosis, nevus anemicus, Bier spots, tinea versicolor, tuberous sclerosis, nevus depigmentosus, GVHD

Histology – decreased or absent melanin and melanocytes in basal layer, which may be difficult to see on H&E. Special stains for melanin may be needed. Perivascular lymphocytic infiltrate only in early lesions.

Treatment

- PUVA (PO or topical)
  - Two or three treatments per week for many months are required before repigmentation from perifollicular openings merges to produce confluent repigmentation
  - The best results can be obtained on the face and on the proximal parts of extremities
  - Vitiligo on the back of hands and feet is very resistant to therapy
- Narrowband UVB – three times a week
- Excimer laser (produces monochromatic rays at 308-nm)two to three times a week to treat limited, stable patches of vitiligo
- Topical corticosteroids BID
- Protopic ointment 0.1% BID
  - Combination treatment with Protopic 0.1% plus the 308-nm excimer laser is superior to monotherapy with the excimer laser alone for UV-resistant vitiliginous lesions
  - Don't use protopic ointment 0.1% in conjunction with light therapies such as PUVA or NbUVB (may increase risk of malignancy)

- Calcipotriene (Dovonex)
  - Topical calcipotriene and narrowband UV-B or PUVA results in improvement appreciably better than achieve with monotherapy
- Punch grafts
  - Punch biopsy specimens from pigmented donor site transplanted into depigmented sites
  - Repigmentation and spread of color begin about 4–6 weeks after grafting
  - The major problem is a residual, pebbled, pigmentary pattern
- Minigrafts
  - Small donor grafts are inserted into the incision of recipient sites and held in place by a pressure dressing
  - The graft heals readily and begins to show repigmentation within 4–6 weeks
  - Some pebbling persists but is minimal, and the cosmetic result is excellent
- Suction blister
  - Epidermal grafts can be obtained by vacuum suction usually with 150 mmHg
  - The recipient site can be prepared by suction, freezing, or dermabrasion of the sites, 24 h before grafting
  - The depigmented blister roof is discarded, and the epidermal donor graft is placed on the vitiliginous areas
- Micropigmentation
  - Tattooing can be used to repigment depigmented skin in dark-skinned individuals
  - Color matching is difficult, and the color tends to fade. Skin can be dyed with dihydroxyacetone preparations, though the color match is often poor
- **Depigmentation**
  - If patient does not respond to repigmentation therapies, could consider depigmentating all areas of the body to make skin color uniform. Use only in select patients – could have long-term social and emotional consequences. Consider pysch evaluation prior to this
  - 20% cream of monobenzylether of hydroquinone is applied BID for 3–12 months
  - Burning or itching may occur
  - Allergic contact dermatitis may be seen

Pearls and Pitfalls

– Recommend taking photographs at each visit to visually monitor progress. Patients find this very encouraging and can help you assess whether the treatment is working or not
– Uveitis is the most significant ocular abnormality seen in vitiligo, but rare. Send to ophthalmology if eye symptoms present

- Some clinicians, if using topicals, will:
  - Prime the skin with clobetasol QHS × 2 weeks then switch to protopic × 2 weeks and continue alternating for 3 months
- Vitamins may be helpful
  - Folic acid 5 mg/day (write for 1 mg tabs – 2 tabs in AM, 2 in PM, 1 at lunch)
  - Multivitamin daily
  - Ascorbic acid – 1,000 mg QD
  - Vitamin B12 – 1,000 mcg QD
  - Vitamin E
  - Alpha lipoic acid

References:

(1) Juhlin L, Olsson MJ. Improvement of vitiligo after oral treatment with vitamin B12 and folic acid and the importance of sun exposure. Acta Derm Venereol. 1997; 77(6): 460–2.
(2) Dell'Anna ML et al. Antioxidants and narrow band-UVB in the treatment of vitiligo: a double-blind placebo controlled trial. Clin Exp Dermatol. 2007; 32(6): 631–6.

Vulvodynia

Etiology and Pathogenesis

- Unknown. Theories – chronic subclinical yeast infection, treatments for yeast sensitizing skin, genetics (many homozygous for allele 2 in interleukin-1β receptor antagonist which is assoc with prolonged inflammatory response), hormones, from pelvic floor disorders, a neuropathic disorder
- Risk for vulvodynia increases with multiple assaults – yeast infection, urogenital infections, trichomonas, HPV

Clinical Presentation

- Vulvar discomfort most often described as burning pain without relevant visible findings or a specific, clinically identifiable, neurologic disorder
  - Patients describe chronic vulvar burning, stinging, irritation, rawnesss, and rarely, pruritus
  - May be triggered by sexual intercourse or nonsexual activities such as walking
- Exam – complete genitourinary exam recommended and should include speculum
  - Wet mount often helpful – evaluate pH, white blood cells, yeast
- Conditions such as interstitial cystitis, headaches, fibromyalgia, irritable bowel syndrome, depression are overrepresented in women with vulvodynia

Labs

- Fungal culture – rule out yeast/fungal etiology
- Routine vaginal culture – some will have heavy growth of group B *Streptococcus*. Some feel this occasionally produces vulvar burning or irritation, although it can be an asymptomatic colonizer

DDx – candida, irritant dermatitis, allergic contact dermatitis, lichen planus (especially erosive type), lichen sclerosus et atrophicus, bullous disorder (cicatricial pemphigoid, pemphigus vulgaris, bullous pemphigoid), erythema multiforme, fixed drug eruption, atrophic vaginitis (premenopausal women), malignant and premalignant conditions

Histology

- No specific findings, but biopsy of a specific skin lesion may be useful to rule out other conditions

Treatment

Treatment involves both approaches
- **Non-medication approach**
  - Validate symptoms in a supportive manner
  - Discontinue irritants such as excessive washing, irritating lubricants, douching, tight clothing, sanitary pads, hair dryer, nonessential meds
  - Apply lubrication during sexual activity (astroglide, vegetable oil)
  - Cold compresses prn
  - Refer to specialist to address underlying depression, if present
  - Education and handouts to patient and her partner
  - Refer patient and partner for sexual counseling and cognitive-behavioral therapy
  - Pelvic floor training (some physical therapists perform this) – surface electromyography and biofeedback
- **Medical approach**
  - Treat any objective abnormalities
  - **Topical medications**
    - Topical estrogens (estradiol vaginal cream) may be used
    - Apply topical anesthetic (lidocaine 5% jelly or xylocaine 2% jelly or 5% ointment) for pain 20 min prior to sexual activity. Condom may help decrease penile numbness and rare risk of toxicity.
    - Amitriptyline 2%, baclofen 2%
    - Capsaicin cream 0.025%
    - Nitroglycerin – headache is a significant side effect
  - **Oral medications**
    - Tricyclic medications (TCA) – such as amitriptyline or desipramine (≤150 mg). Start amitriptyline at half of a 10 mg tablet
    - Venlafaxine extended release (150 mg/day)
    - Duloxetine (60 mg BID)
    - Gabapentin (≤ 3,600 mg/day)
    - Pregabalin (≤ 300 mg BID)
  - **Injectable medications**
    - Triamcinolone 10 mg/mL, 0.2–0.4 mL into trigger point
    - Botulinum toxin A injections
  - Surgery (for vestibulodynia only)

Pearls and Pitfalls

- Vulvodynia is a diagnosis of exclusion
- Take a thorough history of how patients are treating this area – unusual or harsh chemicals often being used to relieve symptoms, although these typically compound the problem
- Refer patient for membership in National Vulvodynia Association (www.nva.org)
- Topical and oral corticosteroids not helpful for vulvar pain unless there is an accompanying inflammatory skin disease
  - However, intralesional steroids may be helpful if trigger point is identified
- Tricyclic antidepressants (TCA)
  - Do not use TCA if patient already on an SSRI
  - If using TCA, tell patient that this is being used for its benefit in neuropathic pain
  - Side effects can include – constipation, weight gain, urinary retention, tachycardia, blurred vision, confusion, drowsiness
  - Desipramine less sedating but more likely to cause anxiety and tremulousness

Reference:

Groysman V. Vulvodynia: New concepts and review of the literature. Dermatol Clin. 2010; 28: 681–96.

Wegener's Granulomatosis

Etiology and Pathogenesis

- Multisystem disease characterized by necrotizing granuloma of the upper and lower respiratory tracts, disseminated necrotizing vasculitis (affecting small- and medium-sized vessels), and glomerulonephritis
- Etiology from genetic and environmental factors – polymorphism in the PR3 promoter has been associated. *Staphylococcus aureus* may also play a role as nasal carriage is associated with relapse

Clinical Presentation and Types

- General: Patients may be febrile and appear ill
- Patients typically present at age 35–55 years. Less than 15% of cases occur in children
- **Neurologic**: Patients may have mononeuritis multiplex, neuropathy, stroke, seizure, cerebritis, or meningitis
- **Head, ears, eyes, nose, and throat**
  - Ocular findings include conjunctivitis, keratitis, and scleritis
  - Proptosis may signal retrobulbar granuloma
  - Xanthelasma has been reported
  - Nearly 75% of patients present with ear, nose, and throat findings
  - Subglottic stenosis and tracheal stenosis may prove fatal if not treated
  - Sinusitis and disease in the nasal mucosa are the most common findings
  - Purulent or sanguinous nasal discharge may be seen
  - Otitis media may be present; deformation or destruction of the pinnae or nose (saddle nose) is rare
  - Oral involvement is rare; however, a classic presentation includes "strawberry gingival hyperplasia"
- **Cutaneous**
  - Cutaneous findings are variable and usually nonspecific
  - Palpable purpura, papules, subcutaneous nodules, and ulcerations are the most common findings. Papulonecrotic lesions common and usually occur on extremities (especially around elbows)
  - Gingiva – often red, friable, hyperplastic
  - Ulcerations may resemble pyoderma gangrenosum
  - Petechiae, vesicles, pustules, hemorrhagic bullae, livedo reticularis, digital necrosis, subungual splinter hemorrhages, and genital ulcers resembling SCC have been reported
  - The lower extremities are most commonly affected
  - Cutaneous manifestations occur in 35–50% of patients, and they may be the presenting sign of disease in 13% of patients

- **Morbidity and Mortality**: The most common causes of death for persons with WG include renal and respiratory failure, infection, malignancy, and, less often, heart failure and myocardial infarction. The 1-year survival rate in persons with untreated disease is estimated at 18%
- The **lungs** are affected in 85% of patients. Disease severity is usually related to renal involvement, which occurs in 75% of patients

Labs and Imaging to Consider

- Antineutrophil cytoplasmic autoantibodies
  - c-ANCA with PR3 specificity is most specific for WG
  - c-ANCA is found in 80–95% of active cases
  - Titers may be used to monitor disease activity
  - As many as 25% of active cases of WG express perinuclear antibodies (p-ANCA) specific to myeloperoxidase
- CBC count+diff: Mild anemia and leukocytosis are common. Eosinophilia is more common in persons with Churg–Strauss syndrome than in those with WG
- Urinalysis: RBCs, casts, and albumin may be found with renal involvement
- Rheumatoid factor: levels may be slightly elevated
- Electrolytes: Elevated BUN and creatinine levels may signify renal involvement. Calculated creatinine clearance may be elevated
- ESR may be elevated
- CXR – Pulmonary infiltrates and granulomas seen with lower resp tract involvement
- Sinus radiography – Bony destruction, thickening, and sclerosing osteitis of the nasal cavity, mastoid air cells, and maxillary sinuses is reported

DDx – Sweet syndrome, Churg–Strauss syndrome, Henoch–Schönlein purpura, Leishmaniasis, pyoderma gangrenosum, relapsing polychondritis, rhinoscleroma, syphilis, temporal (Giant Cell) arteritis, Yaws, polyarteritis nodosa, microscopic arteritis, cryoglobulinemic vasculitis, lethal midline granuloma, lymphamatoid granulomatosis

Histology

- Histopathologic findings may be as variable as cutaneous manifestations
- Vasculitis, granulomatous vasculitis, extravascular palisading granulomas, and leukocytoclastic vasculitis are reported most commonly, although more than half of all skin biopsy specimens return nonspecific findings
  - Necrotizing vasculitis is usually correlated with petechiae, purpura, and ecchymoses (especially on the lower extremities)
  - Palisading granulomas are most commonly observed with indurated nodules on the upper extremities
  - Granulomatous vasculitis is associated with erythematous papules, nodules, and ulcerations

Treatment

- Aggressive medical tx usually necessary to control pulmonary and renal involvement
- Tx with **cyclophosphamide** (CYC) at 2 mg/kg/day up to 200 mg/day and **corticosteroids** at 0.5–1 mg/kg/day up to 80 mg/day is the tx of choice for remission induction
- Glucocorticoids are tapered after 1 month of therapy and discontinued within 6–9 months. CYC is discontinued one full year after remission
- After 3–6 months beyond induction of remission… these may be useful adjuncts for transition to remission–maintenance therapy
  - **Azathioprine** 2 mg/kg/day with corticosteroid therapy
  - **Methotrexate** 0.3 mg/kg/week PO/IM; not to exceed 20 mg
  - **Leflunomide**
- Reported to be useful in a small number of patients
  - **Bactrim** 160 mg TMP/800 mg SMZ PO q 12 h for 10–14 days
  - **Potassium iodide (SSKI)** – 300–500 mg PO (6–10 gtt) tid
- **Infliximab** may be used at dosages of 3–5 mg/kg for adjunctive treatment of WG, with infusions every 4 weeks following induction. Anecdotal evidence indicates a dose–response phenomenon, with higher doses leading to more remissions
  - 3–5 mg/kg IV at weeks 0, 2, and 6, with maintenance infusions given q 4–6 week after induction; may be increased up to 10 mg/kg
- Remission with **rituximab** therapy has been shown in a small number of patients with disease refractory to other medications
  - **Rituximab** 375 mg/m^2 q week for 4 week

Pearls and Pitfalls

- Predictors of treatment resistance include female sex, black race, and presentation with severe renal disease
- Predictors of relapse following remission include anti-PR3 seropositivity, upper respiratory tract involvement, and lung involvement

Wet Wraps

* Useful for severe eczematous eruptions, erythroderma

Instructions:

(1) Shower or bathe first
(2) Pat skin dry – do not rub dry
(3) Immediately apply triamcinolone 0.1% **ointment** (some clinicians prefer creams, although these can be more irritating)
(4) Submerge clean towels (that haven't been washed in detergent with fragrances or dryer sheets) in warm water and wring out excess water
(5) Wrap the patient in warm towels and leave on for 1.5 h. Make sure towels are not burning hot
(6) Remove the towels after 1.5 hours. Leave the ointment on
(7) Repeat daily to twice daily based on doctor's instructions
(8) May apply a moisturizing ointment such as Vaseline throughout the day

* May have the patient apply tight-fitting pajamas or long-johns, instead of towels, that have been moistened in warm water.

NOTES

Index

A

Acanthosis nigricans (AN)
  acral, 206
  classification, 205
  diagnostic pitfalls, 207
  differential diagnosis, 207
  drug-induced, 206
  etiology, 205
  familial, 206
  labs, 206
  mixed-type, 206
  obesity associated, 205
  paraneoplastic syndromes, 399–400
  prevention, 207
  syndromic, 206
  treatment, 207
  unilateral and aka nevoid, 206
ACC. *See* Aplasia cutis congenita (ACC)
Ackerman tumor. *See* Oral florid papillomatosis
Acneiform, drug reactions, 185
Acne keloidalis nuchae (AKN)
  AK's, 218–220
  clinical presentation, 215
  diagnostic pitfalls, 220
  differential diagnosis, 215
  etiology and pathogenesis, 215
  medical treatment and management, 215
  prevention, 217
  surgical treatment, 216–217
Acne vulgaris
  benzoyl peroxide and topical antibiotics,
      210–211
  clinical presentation and types, 208–209
  diagnostic pitfalls, 214
  differential diagnosis, 209
  etiology and pathogenesis, 208

  labs, 209
  oral antibiotics, 212–213
  oral contraceptives, 213
  procedures, 214
  systemic retinoids, 213
  topical retinoids, 210
  treatment, 210
Acquired angioedema, 399
Acquired digital fibrokeratoma, 73
Acquired ichthyosis, 400
Acquired perforating dermatosis, 417
Acral erythema, drug reactions, 185
Acral lentiginous melanoma, 370
Acremonium sp., 80, 514
Acrodermatitis continua
      of Hallopeau, 453
Acrodermatitis enteropathica
  clinical presentation, 83–84
  diagnostic pitfalls, 85
  differential diagnosis, 84
  etiology and pathogenesis, 83
  histology, 84
  labs, 84
  treatment, 84
  zinc deficiency, 94
Acrokeratoelastoidosis, 118
Acromegaly + hypertrichosis, 56
Actinic folliculitis, 310
Actinic keratoses (AK)
  clinical presentation, 218
  diagnostic pitfalls, 220
  differential diagnosis, 218
  etiology and pathogenesis, 218
  histology, 218
  treatment, 218–220
Actinic LP, 350

J.A. Cafardi, *The Manual of Dermatology*,
DOI 10.1007/978-1-4614-0938-0, © Springer Science+Business Media LLC, 2012

Basal cell carcinoma (BCC) (*cont.*)
   treatment, 236–237
Bazex–Dupré–Christol syndrome, 97
      See also Bazex syndrome
Bazex syndrome, 236
BCC. *See* Basal cell carcinoma (BCC)
Beau's lines, 70
Beckwith–Wiedemann syndrome, 97, 99, 100
Bednar tumor, 277
Behçet's syndrome
   clinical presentation, 238
   diagnostic pitfalls, 239
   differential diagnosis, 239
   etiology and pathogenesis, 238
   histology, 239
   labs, 238–239
   treatment and management, 239
Beighton's sign, 486
Benzalkonium chloride, 404
Benzocaine, 404
Beradinelli-Seip syndrome, 56
Berliner's sign, 486
Beta-hydroxy acid, salicylic acid, 157
Bexarotene, 269
Biette's collarette, 506, 507
Bilateral bursitis, Verneuil, 506
Bilobed nails, 70
Biotin deficiency/multiple carboxylase
      deficiency, 95
Bipolaris sp., 80, 514
Bisphosphonates, 178
Björnstad syndrome, 48
Blastomycosis, 386
Blau syndrome, 420, 476
Bloch–Sulzberger syndrome, 112
Bloom's syndrome, 97
Blue nails, 70
Bocquet's criteria, 287
Botox cosmetic, 159–160
Bowenoid papulosis, 256
Brachyonychia, 70
Brauer lines, 87
Brocq's alopeica
   clinical presentation, 23
   etiology and pathogenesis, 23
   histology, 23
   labs, 23
   treatment, 24
Brunauer–Fuhs–Siemens syndrome
      (Striate PPK), 118
Bubble hair, 51
Bullous
   impetigo, 95
   LP, 350

lupus
   clinical presentation, 240
   diagnostic pitfalls, 241
   differential diagnosis, 240
   etiology and pathogenesis, 240
   histology, 241
   labs, 240
   treatment, 241
morphea, 382
pemphigoid
   clinical presentation, 242
   diagnostic pitfalls, 244
   differential diagnosis, 242
   drug reactions, 185
   etiology and pathogenesis, 241–242
   labs and histology, 242
   treatment and management, 243–244
   variants, 242
Buschke–Löwenstein tumor, 257
Buschke–Ollendorff syndrome, 99

C

CAHMR syndrome, 56
Calciphylaxis
   clinical presentation, 246
   diagnostic pitfalls, 247
   differential diagnosis, 246
   etiology and pathogenesis, 245
   histology, 246
   labs, 246
   treatment and management, 246–247
Canakinumab (Ilaris), 418
Candida
   C. albicans, 80, 514
   C. dermatitis, 94
   C. krusei, 80, 514
   C. parapsilosis, 80, 514
   C. tropicalis, 80, 514
Cantu syndrome, 56
Capillaritis, 425
Carcinoid syndrome, 400
Carney complex, 100
CARP. *See* Confluent and reticulated
      papillomatosis (CARP)
Carvajal syndrome, 50, 100, 119
Castleman's disease, 343
CCCA. *See* Central centrifugal cicatricial
      alopecia (CCCA)
Central centrifugal cicatricial alopecia (CCCA)
   clinical presentation, 25–26
   etiology and pathogenesis, 25
   histology, 26
   treatment, 26